OXFORD MEDICAL PU

Clinical Medicine

Key questions answered

Clinical Medicine

Key questions answered

Wai-Ching Leung
Senior Registrar in Public Health Medicine,
Sunderland Health Authority,
Sunderland, UK

OXFORD NEW YORK TOKYO
OXFORD UNIVERSITY PRESS
1998

Oxford University Press, Great Clarendon Street, Oxford OX2 6DP

Oxford New York
Athens Auckland Bangkok Bogota Buenos Aires
Calcutta Cape Town Chennai Dar es Salaam Delhi
Florence Hong Kong Istanbul Karachi Kuala Lumpur
Madrid Melbourne Mexico City Mumbai Nairobi Paris
Singapore Taipei Tokyo Toronto Warsaw

and associated companies in
Berlin Ibadan

Oxford is a trade mark of Oxford University Press

Published in the United States
by Oxford University Press, Inc., New York

A catalogue record for this book is available from the British Library

Library of Congress Cataloging in Publication Data
Leung, Wai-Ching.
Clinical medicine: key questions answered / Wai-Ching Leung.
(Oxford medical publications)
1. Clinical medicine–Examinations, questions, etc. I. Title. II. Series
{DNLM: 1. Clinical Medicine examination questions.
WB 18.2 L653c 1998 / Not Acquired}
RC58.L39 1998 616'.0076–DC21 98–15855
ISBN 0 19 262891 7 (Pbk)

Typeset by Jayvee, Trivandrum, India
Printed in Great Britain by
Biddles Ltd, Guildford & King's Lynn

Preface

Revision for the Final MB is often a daunting experience for students. They are required to take written, oral and clinical examinations in a wide range of subjects and specialties, in some of which they last received tuition more than a year previously. In addition, on the General Medical Council's recommendation a number of subjects have recently been given prominence in the undergraduate curriculum, such as Law and Ethics, Health Service organization, Public Health and General Practice, for which there are currently few appropriate undergraduate textbooks and revision books. The General Medical Council has recommended both horizontal and vertical integration of the medical curriculum, but many medical schools have achieved horizontal integration only for the first 2–3 years of the curriculum. Most fourth and fifth year curricula are not horizontally integrated, and are unlikely to be so for the near future.

Candidates taking the Final MB examination or continuous assessments therefore face several problems in their revision.

They may be unaware of their relative strengths and weaknesses in the different subjects and specialties. As a result, they may allocate their revision time unwisely and may even inadvertently totally neglect some important subjects.

To revise the whole curriculum students would need to buy revision books in each subject and specialty. This would be extremely expensive, and there is also a risk that the students may also be tempted to spend more time than is appropriate on one subject.

Students may be tempted to ignore the relative 'new' undergraduate subjects, on which there are currently few revision books, to their detriment in the examinations or assessments.

Multiple choice questions are still widely used in the Final MB and continuous assessments, in conjunction with short answer questions and structured answer questions. As they are reliable and can be objectively scored, multiple choice questions are also uniquely suited for self-assessment during revision.

This book has been written to assist medical students to overcome the problems outlined above. It is also useful for students to consolidate their knowledge at the end of each specialty attachment. It consists of over 700 questions in total. Each of the first 10 chapters covers an important subject or specialty in the Final MB curriculum. The number of questions in each section varies to reflect the subject's relative importance in the examination. For example, there are 150 questions in General Medicine, but only 60 questions in most other specialties. It is hoped that students will devote an appropriate proprortion of their revision time to each subject and specialty. The final chapter consists of 60 multiple choice questions using a problem-based approach, and covers all specialties. Answers with explanations are provided for all questions. It is hoped that students will find this helpful in integrating the knowledge and skills obtained throughout their medical training.

W.-C.L.

Sunderland
May 1998

Advice on answering multiple choice questions

Multiple choice questions are commonly used both in the Final MB and in most post-graduate examinations. They are also valuable self-assessment tools.

Each question has a stem followed by five items numbered a–e. You are required to answer whether each of the items a–e is true or false.

Techniques for answering multiple choice questions

Organize your time

You must find out the time allowed in the examination, and the number of questions to be answered. Work out when you should have completed a quarter, half and three-quarters of the questions, and monitor your progress throughout.

Answer the questions reasonably quickly. Mark those you are not sure of with a pencil on the question paper. You can return to them afterwards. Allow plenty of time to transfer your answers to the computer question paper.

Read the questions carefully

It is especially important to read the questions carefully in multiple choice examinations. The difference in one word can change the answer from true to false and vice versa.

The items in each question are independent of each other. For example, if you are answering item e, you should ignore the text given in items a–d.

It is also vital to interpret important words correctly. For example,

'. . . recognized feature of . . .' means '. . . it may be a feature of the disease, even though it may be only 1% of the patients with this disease'.

'. . . characteristic feature of . . .' means '. . . the presence of the feature makes the diagnosis very likely . . .'

'. . . is diagnostic of . . .' means '. . . one can be certain of the diagnosis if the feature is present . . .'

What to do about questions you are not sure of

Before you attend the examination, you should find out in advance:-
whether you have an option of stating 'don't know';
whether you would score a negative mark for giving the wrong answer.

Negative marking

The 'negative marking' system operates for most examinations. You score +1 for each correct answer and -1 for each wrong answer. In some examinations, you score 0 if you do not put down any answers. In others, you are required to put 'don't know' to score 0. Otherwise you score -1 mark. It is important to find out in advance about the system to be used in your examination.

It is debatable what the best strategy is if you do not know the answer. Statistically, total random guesses to some questions should not affect your score, and that you should improve your score if you attempt the questions you are not sure of by educated guessing.

However, random guessing is risky. Although it has an equal chance of increasing or decreasing your score, you might not want to take that risk if you are on the borderline. Also some students are better than others at guessing. You may wish to use the following tests to estimate how good you are at this. Mark the items you are not sure of as you answer, and simply add up the scores to these questions. If your total score for these questions is positive, you would on the whole benefit by guessing.

No negative marking

In some medical schools, you are awarded +1 for a correct answer, but 0 mark if you either give a wrong answer or give no answer. In this case, it is obvious that you should answer all parts of each question, giving educated guesses for the items you are unsure of.

Do not calculate your score

You can never be sure of the pass mark or the number of questions you have got right. Hence, it is very dangerous to calculate your score and stop answering once you think you have scored enough to pass.

Contents

Abbreviations

ACE	angiotensin converting enzyme
ACTH	adrenocorticotrophic hormone
ADH	antidiuretic hormone
AFP	alphafetoprotein
AIDS	acquired immunodeficiency syndrome
ALT	alanine aminotransferase
ANA	antinuclear antibodies
APTT	activated partial thromboplastin time
APUD	amine precursor uptake and decarboxylation (cells)
AST	aspartate aminotransferase
AV	atrioventricular
CABG	coronary artery bypass graft
CEA	carcinoembryonic antigen
CMV	cytomegalovirus
CNS	central nervous system
CSF	cerebrospinal fluid
CT	computed tomography
CTG	cardiotocography
DDAVP	desmopressin
DIP	distal interphalangeal joints
ECG	electrocardiogram
ECT	electroconvulsive therapy
EEG	electroencephalogram
ELISA	enzyme-linked immunoadsorbent assay
EMG	electromyelography
ER	oestrogen receptor
ERCP	endoscopic retrograde cholangiopancreatography
ESR	erythrocyte sedimentation rate
FEV_1	forced expiratory volume in 1s
FH	family history
FSH	follicle stimulating hormone
GABA	γ-aminobutyric acid
GH	growth hormone
GnRH	gonadotropin releasing hormone
β-hCG	human chorionic gonadotropin
5-HIAA	5-hydroxyindole acetic acid

HIV	human immunodeficiency virus
HLA	histocompatibility leucocyte antigen
HMG CoA	3-hydroxy-3-methylglutaryl coenzyme A
IDDM	insulin dependent diabetes mellitus
INR	International normalized ratio (prothrombin ratio)
IVU	intravenous urography
JVP	jugular vein pulse
LATS	long-acting thyroid stimulator
LDH	low-density lipoprotein
LH	luteinizing hormone
MAO	monoamine oxidase
MAOI	monoamine oxidase inhibitors
MCHC	mean corpuscular haemoglobin concentration
MCP	metacarpophalangeal joints
MCV	mean corpuscular (red cell) volume
MMR	measles, mumps, rubella (vaccination)
MRI	magnetic resonance imaging
NIDDM	non-insulin dependent diabetes mellitus
PCR	polymerase chain reaction
PEFR	peak expiratory flow rate
PIP	proximal interphalangeal joints
PSA	prostatic specific antigen
PTH	parathyroid hormone
PUVA	psoralens with UVA therapy
QALY	quality adjusted life year
SA	sinoatrial
SIADH	syndrome of inappropriate antidiuretic hormone secretion
SLE	systematic lupus erythematosus
SSRI	selective serotonin reuptake inhibitors
T_3	triiodothyronine
TENS	transcutaneous electrical nerve stimulation
TIBC	total iron binding capacity
TNM	tumour, lymph node, metastasis (tumour staging)
TORCHS	Toxoplasmosis, rubella, cytomegalovirus, hepatitis, syphilis infection
TRAb	TSH-receptor antibodies
TRH	thyrotropin releasing hormone
TSH	thyroid stimulating hormone
VC	vital capacity
VMA	vanillylmandelic acid
VZIG	varicella zoster immunoglobulin

1 *General medicine*

Questions

1.1 *Which of the following statements about hypothermia is/are true?*

a it is defined as fall of oral temperature to below 35°C
b it may be caused by hypothyroidism
c the J wave on the ECG is characteristic
d it is often associated with a low blood pressure
e death may be diagnosed in hypothermic patients with absent pupillary reflex

1.2 *Symptoms and signs of symptomatic HIV infection include*

a weight gain
b oral candida
c fever
d constipation
e splenomegaly

1.3 *Which of the following statements about typhoid fever is/are true?*

a it is caused by cocci
b it has an incubation period of about 3–4 weeks
c headache and muscle ache as common symptoms in the first week
d it may be associated with rose spots
e about 50% of the patients become chronic carrier of the organism

1.4 *The first heart sound*

a results from closure of the pulmonary valve
b is best heard at the apex
c is loud in mitral regurgitation
d is accentuated in pulmonary hypertension
e is usually soft in mitral stenosis

1.5 *An exercise ECG*

a may detect evidence of ischaemia not apparent in a resting ECG
b may detect stress-induced arrhythmia not apparent in a resting ECG

c is useful in the assessment of severe aortic stenosis
d is useful in the assessment of unstable angina
e should be performed with regular monitoring of symptoms and blood pressure

1.6 *Features of pulmonary oedema on a chest radiograph may include*

a pulmonary oligaemia
b Kerley 'B' lines
c enlarged hilar vessels
d pleural effusion
e reduced cardiothoracic ratio

1.7 *Which of the following are appropriate measures in acute pulmonary oedema?*

a lie the patient flat
b administer 100% oxygen
c administer intravenous morphine
d administer intravenous frusemide
e administer intravenous isosorbide dinitrate

1.8 *Sinus bradycardia*

a may occur physiologically in athletes
b may be associated with absent P waves
c may follow myocardial infarction
d can be treated with intravenous atropine if symptoms occur
e may be caused by fever

1.9 *Atrial fibrillation*

a is associated with a slow atrial rate
b is associated with an irregular irregular pulse
c is almost always symptomatic
d is a predisposing factor for stroke
e may be restored to sinus rhythm by elective DC cardioversion

1.10 *Ventricular tachycardia*

a may respond to carotid sinus massage
b is characteristically associated with a narrow QRS complex on the ECG
c may cause syncope
d may be treated by intravenous lignocaine
e may not require treatment

1.11 *Which of the following are recognized treatments for supraventricular tachycardia?*

a Valsalva manoeuvre

b intravenous adenosine
c intravenous verapamil and propranolol together
d intravenous lignocaine
e oral amiodarone

1.12 *In third degree heart block*

a the pulse is irregularly regular
b the pulse rate is about 90 beats/min
c Wenckebach's phenomenon may be seen on the ECG
d cannon waves may be seen in the neck veins
e the atrial and ventricular rates are identical

1.13 *Angina pectoris*

a can usually be diagnosed by a resting ECG
b may cause breathlessness
c may be exacerbated after a meal
d is often relieved by rest
e can usually be diagnosed by physical examination alone

1.14 *Which of the following are recognized treatments for acute myocardial infarction?*

a 24% oxygen by face mask
b oral aspirin
c intravenous opiates
d intravenous streptokinase
e intravenous beta-blockers such as atenolol

1.15 *Causes of secondary hypertension include*

a polycystic kidney disease
b phaeochromocytoma
c corticosteroid therapy
d mitral stenosis
e Addison's disease

1.16 *Recognized clinical features of a medium-sized pulmonary embolus include*

a haemoptysis
b shortness of breath
c chest pain worse on coughing
d pleural rub
e stridor

1.17 *Physical signs characteristic of mitral regurgitation include*

a a midsystolic murmur

b a murmur best heard at the apex
c a displaced apex beat
d an irregular irregular pulse
e a murmur radiating to the carotids

1.18 *Signs of aortic regurgitation include*

a a collapsing pulse
b reduced pulse pressure
c a murmur best heard on lying the patient on the left
d an early diastolic murmur
e a thrusting apical impulse

1.19 *Which of the following statements about acute pericarditis is/are true?*

a it is often caused by coxsackie B virus in young adults
b the associated pain is often retrosternal
c the associated pain is characteristically worse on movement
d a pericardial friction rub is diagnostic
e opiate is the best analgesia

1.20 *Which of the following statements about chronic type II respiratory failure is/are true?*

a the carbon dioxide level is characteristically reduced
b the serum bicarbonate level is characteristically raised
c it may be caused by asthma
d it may be caused by chronic obstructive airway disease
e it should be treated with high concentration of oxygen

1.21 *Which of the following statements about late-onset asthma is/are true?*

a skin tests are positive in more than 80% of the cases
b the severity of an attack correlates well with the presence of wheezing
c the ratio of FEV_1 (forced expiratory volume in 1 s) to VC (vital capacity) is characteristically reduced
d inhaled sodium cromoglycate is usually highly effective
e there is often a positive history of allergic disorders

1.22 *Pneumococcal pneumonia*

a occurs in the elderly in the majority of the cases
b is associated with a high fever
c characteristically causes consolidation in one affected lobe or segment of the lung
d occurs more frequently in winter
e is usually associated with an increase in neutrophil count

1.23 Tuberculosis may cause

a osteomyelitis
b erythema marginatum
c erythema nodosum
d meningitis
e Cushing's syndrome

1.24 Which of the following statements about bronchial carcinoma is/are true?

a it is the commonest cancer in men
b large cell carcinoma is the commonest type
c risk is directly proportional to the number of cigarettes smoked
d risk is increased by asbestos exposure
e it is commoner in rural than urban dwellers

1.25 Clinical features caused by bronchial carcinoma within the chest include

a cough
b haemoptysis
c Horner's syndrome
d pain in the distribution of a thoracic dermatome
e signs of a pleural effusion

1.26 Extrapulmonary manifestations of bronchial carcinoma not due to metastasis include

a clubbing of the fingers
b sensory neuropathy
c cerebellar ataxia
d ectopic ADH secretion
e hypercalcaemia

1.27 Clinical features of sarcoidosis include

a erythema nodosum
b clubbing of the fingers
c uveitis
d hypercalcaemia
e inappropriate ADH secretion

1.28 Which of the following statements about sarcoidosis is/are true?

a it characteristically causes caseating lesions
b it typically causes a strongly positive Mantoux reaction
c often causes raised plasma level of angiotensin converting enzyme (ACE)

d symptomatic lung lesions may respond to corticosteroid treatment
e pulmonary lesions detected on chest radiograph are almost always symptomatic

1.29 *Causes of a pleural effusion include*

a bacterial pneumonia
b heart failure
c pneumothorax
d pulmonary embolus and infarction
e fibrosing alveolitis

1.30 *Characteristic clinical features of a spontaneous pneumothorax are*

a gradual onset of chest pain
b bilateral chest pain
c displacement of trachea to the affected side
d reduced or absent breath sounds on the affected side
e increased vocal resonance on the affected side

1.31 *Characteristic symptoms of peptic ulcer disease include*

a diffuse abdominal pain
b pain relief by food
c night pain
d persistent symptoms throughout the year
e pain relieved by antacids

1.32 *Which of the following statements about Helicobacter pylori is/are true?*

a it is a gram positive bacterium
b colonization with H. pylori can be demonstrated in over 60% of proven duodenal ulcer
c colonization with H. pylori can be demonstrated in over 60% of proven gastric ulcer
d it can be eradicated by a combination of bismuth and two antibiotics
e it may be diagnosed by the detection of antibodies to serum helicobacter proteins

1.33 *Which of the following class of drugs are recognized treatments for peptic ulcer diseases?*

a antacids
b histamine agonists
c proton pump inhibitors
d non-steroidal anti-inflammatory drugs
e corticosteroids

1.34 *Which of the following clinical features is/are commoner in ulcerative colitis than in Crohn's disease?*

a bloody diarrhoea
b rectal passage of mucus
c ileovesical fistula
d anal fissure
e fat malabsorption

1.35 *Which of the following is/are characteristic clinical features of toxic dilatation of the colon?*

a constipation
b fever
c dehydration
d tachycardia
e abdominal tenderness

1.36 *Which of the following is/are recognized treatments for Crohn's disease?*

a a low protein diet
b oral corticosteroid
c oral sulphasalazine
d oral lactulose
e bowel resection

1.37 *Which of the following statements about pseudomembranous colitis is/are true?*

a Clostridium perfringens is the causative organism
b it is commoner in patients receiving antibiotics
c oral vancomycin is a recognized treatment
d it predisposes to toxic dilatation of the colon
e it is caused by an endotoxin

1.38 *Which of the following statements about irritable bowel syndrome is/are true?*

a it occurs more frequently in women than men
b it occurs more frequently in the elderly
c pellet-like stools are characteristic
d it is sometimes caused by inflammatory bowel disease
e diarrhoea characteristically occurs at night

1.39 *Features of portal hypertension include*

a ascites
b splenomegaly
c raised platelet level

d raised blood pressure
e oesophageal varices

1.40 *Factors which may precipitate hepatic encephalopathy include*

a reduced dietary protein intake
b gastrointestinal bleeding
c infection
d diarrhoea
e surgical portasystemic shunt

1.41 *Causes of acute hepatitis include*

a hepatitis C virus
b hepatitis A virus
c paracetamol
d primary biliary cirrhosis
e gallstones

1.42 *Clinical signs of cirrhosis of the liver include*

a tender liver
b ascites
c clubbing of the fingers
d testicular enlargement
e jaundice

1.43 *Predisposing conditions for hepatocellular carcinoma include*

a hepatitis B infection
b alcohol cirrhosis
c haemochromatosis
d hepatitis A infection
e primary biliary cirrhosis

1.44 *Clinical features of thiamine deficiency include*

a peripheral neuropathy
b night blindness
c heart failure
d memory loss
e rickets

1.45 *Causes of inappropriate ADH secretion include*

a diabetes insipidus
b hyperkalaemia
c head injury
d carcinoma of the bronchus
e compulsory drinking

1.46 *Which of the following are recognized emergency treatments for acute hyperkalaemia?*

a intravenous calcium gluconate 10%
b infusion of dextrose and insulin
c peritoneal dialysis
d haemodialysis
e oral spironolactone

1.47 *Causes of metabolic acidosis include*

a hypokalaemia
b salicylate poisoning
c diabetes ketoacidosis
d chronic renal failure
e persistent vomiting

1.48 *Characteristic features of acute glomerulonephritis include*

a hypertension
b polyuria
c proteinuria
d smoky urine
e nocturia

1.49 *Conditions found more frequently in patients with chronic renal failure include*

a anaemia
b hypertension
c osteomalacia
d metabolic alkalosis
e peripheral neuropathy

1.50 *Which of the following disorders are autosomal dominant in inheritance?*

a Huntington's chorea
b haemophilia A
c congenital spherocytosis
d α1-antitrypsin deficiency
e polyposis coli

1.51 *Which of the following statements about sex-linked recessive disorders is/are true?*

a 50% of the daughters of an affected father are carriers
b 50% of the sons of an affected father have the disorder
c 50% of the daughters of a carrier mother are carriers

d 50% of the sons of a carrier mother have the disorder
e 50% of the daughters of an affected mother are carriers

1.52 *Which of the following hormones are secreted from the anterior pituitary gland?*

a parathyroid hormone
b thyroxine
c growth hormone
d prolactin
e oxytocin

1.53 *Clinical features of a large pituitary gland include*

a neck stiffness
b diplopia
c optic atrophy
d bitemporal hemianopia
e headache

1.54 *Clinical features of acromegaly include*

a lip enlargement
b carpel tunnel syndrome
c large feet
d testicular atrophy
e pretibial myxodema

1.55 *Which of the following features is/are characteristic of cranial diabetes insipidus?*

a oligouria
b polydipsia
c low plasma osmolality
d low urinary osmolality
e no clinical response to desmopressin (DDAVP)

1.56 *Clinical features of hyperthyroidism include*

a weight gain
b palpitations
c tremor
d diminished tendon jerks
e emotional lability

1.57 *Characteristic biochemical results in hyperthyroidism due to Grave's disease include*

a elevated T_3 level
b elevated TSH level
c presence of TSH-receptor antibodies (TRAb)

d elevated thyroxine level
e an exaggerated rise in TSH following an intravenous TRH injection

1.58 *Causes of hypercalcaemia include*

a primary hyperparathyroidism
b secondary hyperparathyroidism
c osteomalacia
d sarcoidosis
e osteoporosis

1.59 *Recognized treatments for hypercalcaemia include*

a oral 1-α-hydroxycholecalciferol
b fluid restriction
c oral phosphate
d intravenous bisphosphonate
e calcitonin injection

1.60 *Causes of Cushing's syndrome include*

a Conn's syndrome
b adrenal adenoma
c small cell carcinoma of the lung
d Cushing's disease
e steroid treatment

1.61 *Causes for secondary hyperaldosteronism include*

a adrenal hyperplasia
b congestive heart failure
c cirrhosis with ascites
d adrenal adenoma
e loss of sodium from the gastrointestinal tract

1.62 *Clinical features of Addison's disease include*

a vomiting
b striae
c hypotension
d pigmentation
e glucose intolerance

1.63 *Non-insulin dependent diabetes mellitus*

a has a HLA-linked genetic predisposition
b is likely to be triggered by viral infection
c has a strong autoimmune aetiology
d has a higher prevalence in obese people
e is associated with resistance to insulin in the target tissue

1.64 *Renal glycosuria*

a occurs more commonly during pregnancy
b will almost inevitably progress to clinical diabetes
c is usually accompanied by ketonuria
d is usually associated with a suboptimal endocrine function of the pancreas
e is caused by injury to the renal tissues by diabetes

1.65 *Haemoglobin A_1 (Hb A_1)*

a is one of the components of haemoglobin A
b level is useful for assessing the overall blood glucose control in the past 2 weeks
c level is associated with the risk for vascular complications of diabetes
d a level of 17% is satisfactory in patients with well controlled diabetes
e measurement renders blood glucose monitoring unnecessary

1.66 *Causes of microcytic hypochromic anaemia include*

a menstruation
b gastrointestinal bleeding
c folate deficiency
d haemolysis
e β-thalassaemia minor

1.67 *Which of the following results are compatible with the diagnosis of pernicious anaemia?*

a low mean red cell volume (MCV)
b low red cell folate level
c megaloblastic bone marrow
d abnormal vitamin B_{12} absorption test corrected by addition of intrinsic factor
e presence of anti-intrinsic factor serum antibodies

1.68 *Recognized causes for secondary polycythaemia (erythrocytosis) include*

a polycythaemia rubra vera (primary proliferative polycythaemia)
b high altitude
c chronic obstructive airway disease
d congenital spherocytosis
e renal carcinoma

1.69 *Chronic lymphocytic leukaemia*

a is commoner in males than females
b is very common in Chinese people
c may present with painless lymphadenopathy
d is rapidly fatal in the elderly
e is characteristically associated with severe bleeding

1.70 *Which of the following results support the diagnosis of multiple myeloma*

a serum monoclonal immunoglobulin
b increased level of normal immunoglobulin
c Bence-Jones protein in urine
d translucencies in skull radiograph
e normal ESR

1.71 *Which of the following statements about acute gout is/are true?*

a the interphalangeal joint of the great toe is the commonest affected joint
b the affected joint is extremely tender to touch
c it may be precipitated by alcohol
d thiazide diuretics may relieve the symptoms
e non-steroidal anti-inflammatory drugs such as indomethacin are effective treatments

1.72 *Extra-articular manifestations of rheumatoid arthritis include*

a polycythaemia
b episcleritis
c peripheral neuropathy
d dry eyes
e erythema nodosum

1.73 *Recognized treatments for rheumatoid arthritis include*

a antimalarials
b oral gold
c non-steroidal anti-inflammatory drugs
d azathioprine
e penicillamine

1.74 *Which of the following statement about septic arthritis is/are true?*

a it is more common in patients with diabetes
b multiple joints are characteristically involved
c joint aspiration is essential if the diagnosis is suspected
d diagnosis can usually be made by its radiographic appearance
e intravenous antibiotics are acceptable treatments

1.75 *Clinical features of systemic lupus erythematosus include*

a nephrotic syndrome

b Raynaud's phenomenon
c psychosis
d alopecia
e a spontaneous abortion

1.76 *Predisposing factors for osteoporosis include*

a excessive exercise
b male sex
c obesity
d advanced age
e late menopause

1.77 *Recognized clinical features of Paget's disease of bone include*

a bowing of the femur
b spontaneous fracture
c deafness
d coldness of the affected parts
e headache

1.78 *Which of the following statements about pityriasis rosea is/are true?*

a it predisposes to malignancy
b a 'herald patch' often appears first
c a 'Christmas tree' distribution of lesions on the back is characteristic
d the diagnosis can be confirmed by a serum autoantibody test
e it should be treated by an antifungal agent

1.79 *Signs of an upper motor neurone lesions include*

a reduced tendon jerks
b extensor plantar response
c sustained clonus
d fasciculation of affected muscles
e severe muscle wasting

1.80 *Which of the following tendon reflexes and spinal segments are correctly paired?*

a	biceps jerk	cervical 3/4
b	supinator jerk	cervical 5/6
c	triceps jerk	cervical 7
d	knee jerk	lumbar 1/2
e	ankle jerk	sacral 1

1.81 *Frontal lobe lesions may cause*

a incontinence of urine

b apraxia
c persistent grasp reflex
d homonymous hemianopia
e agnosia

1.82 *Characteristic signs of Horner's syndrome include*

a ptosis
b exophthalmos
c loss of consensual pupillary reflex
d dilated pupil
e decreased sweating on the affected side of the face

1.83 *Causes of sensorineural deafness include*

a infection with mumps
b ear wax
c otosclerosis
d Menière's disease
e acoustic neuroma

1.84 *Which of the following statements about a transient ischaemic attack is/are true?*

a it usually lasts about 3–5 days
b the risk for a stroke is increased after a transient ischaemic attack
c carotid transient ischaemic attack is often associated with transient monocular blindness
d aspirin 300 mg daily is beneficial
e no investigations are indicated if the symptoms last less than 24 h

1.85 *Recognized treatments for idiopathic Parkinson's disease include*

a anticholinergic drugs
b phenothiazine drugs
c combination of L-dopa and carbidopa
d bromocriptine
e sterotactic thalamotomy

1.86 *Which of the following statements about multiple sclerosis is/are true?*

a it occurs more frequently in the tropical than temperate countries
b the natural history is usually that of progressive deterioration
c MRI scan of the brain shows abnormality in the majority of the cases
d optic neuritis is a recognized association
e abnormalities in the cerebrospinal fluid (CSF) may occur

1.87 *Causes of peripheral neuropathy include*

a excess alcohol intake
b diabetes mellitus
c vitamin B_{12} deficiency
d carpel tunnel syndrome
e cervical spondylosis

1.88 *Which of the following statements about myasthenia gravis is/are true?*

a the muscarinic acetylcholine receptors are abnormal
b it is sometimes associated with thymic abnormalities
c it is commoner in men than women
d the symptoms often improve an hour after an intravenous injection of edrophonium
e diplopia is a common symptom

1.89 *Which of the following statements about acute salicylate poisoning is/are true?*

a it is associated with metabolic acidosis
b it is associated with respiratory acidosis
c tinnitus is a common symptom
d gastric emptying is not indicated if the ingestion occurs more than 6 h previously
e forced alkaline diuresis is a recognized treatment if the salicylate level is very high

1.90 *Clinical features of systemic amyloidosis include*

a proteinuria
b hepatomegaly
c splenomegaly
d heart failure
e carpel tunnel syndrome

1.91 *Against which of the following liver infections is active immunization possible?*

a hepatitis A
b hepatitis B
c hepatitis C
d hepatitis D
e hepatitis E

1.92 *Which of the following disorders are autosomal dominant in inheritance?*

a Von Willebrand's disease

b Wilson's disease (hepatolenticular degeneration)
c adult polycystic disease
d hereditary haemorrhagic telangiectasia
e glucose-6-phosphate dehydrogenase deficiency

1.93 *Which of the following disorders occur more frequently in subjects with obesity?*

a osteoarthritis
b varicose veins
c ischaemic heart disease
d menorrhagia
e hyperthyroidism

1.94 *Which of the following statements about achalasia is/are true?*

a it is associated with degeneration of the ganglionic nerve plexus of the oesophagus
b the disease usually presents from childhood
c the characteristic symptom is dysphagia of solids but not liquids
d retrosternal chest pain is very rare
e oesophageal manometry can be diagnostic

1.95 *Neurological and psychiatric manifestations of acquired immunodeficiency syndrome (AIDS) include*

a cognitive impairment
b sensory neuropathy
c autonomic neuropathy
d depressive features
e psychotic features

1.96 *Recognized associations of Crohn's disease include*

a episcleritis
b erythema nodosum
c pericholangitis
d ankylosing spondylitis
e erythema marginatum

1.97 *Which of the following statements about descriptions of skin conditions is/are true?*

a a papule is a flat circumscribed area of discoloured skin
b petechiae are larger than ecchymoses
c a bulla is larger than a vesicle
d purpura blanch on pressure
e a vesicle is filled with pus

1.98 *Side-effects of topical steroids applied to the skin include*

a thickening of the skin
b spread of local skin infection
c telangiectasia
d striae
e formation of vesicles

1.99 *Psoriasis*

a characteristically affects the flexor surface of the elbows and knees
b occurs most frequently in African countries
c is commonly associated with pitting of the nails
d is characteristically associated with a positive Koebner phenomenon
e is associated with joint disease in more than 50% of the patients

1.100 *Recognized treatments of psoriatic skin lesions include*

a dithranol
b topical steroids
c retinoic acid derivatives
d miconazole
e psoralens with UVA therapy (PUVA)

1.101 *Which of the following statements about systemic lupus erythematosus (SLE) is/are true?*

a photosensitivity may be the presenting feature
b raynaud's phenomenon occurs more frequently in SLE than in systemic sclerosis
c the sex distribution is equal
d the cutaneous manifestations of SLE are significantly different from those of discoid lupus erythematosus
e hydroxychloroquine is a recognized treatment

1.102 *Basal cell carcinoma of the skin*

a occurs more frequently in black people
b occurs most frequently in young adults
c occurs most often in the arms
d frequently metastasizes
e is frequently associated with superficial dilated blood vessels over the surface

1.103 *Which of the following statements about vitiligo is/are true?*

a it is a rare condition affecting less than 1 in every 10 000 people
b serum antimelanocyte antibodies are sometimes detected
c it has an association with pernicious anaemia

d affected subjects sometimes have a positive family history
e the condition can be effectively treated in more than 90% of the patients

1.104 *Internuclear ophthalmoplegia*

a is caused by a lesion in the medial longitudinal fasciculus
b is almost pathognomonic of multiple sclerosis if bilateral
c is associated with the failure of the ipsilateral eye to abduct
d is associated with coarse nystagmus of the contralateral eye on abduction
e is associated with a constricted pupil on the ipsilateral eye

1.105 *Characteristic signs of a complete third cranial nerve palsy include*

a ipsilateral complete ptosis
b adduction of ipsilateral eye
c elevation of ipsilateral eye
d dilated ipsilateral pupil
e loss of pupillary reaction of the contralateral eye when light is shone onto the ipsilateral eye

1.106 *Causes of mononeuritis multiplex (multiple mononeuropathy) include*

a sarcoidosis
b malignancy
c rheumatoid arthritis
d diabetes mellitus
e amyloidosis

1.107 *Which of the following tendon reflexes are correctly matched to their spinal levels?*

a supinator C5–6
b biceps C7–8
c ankle S1
d knee L1–2
e triceps C7

1.108 *Signs of pseudobulbar palsy include*

a a wasted tongue
b dysarthria
c emotional lability
d absent jaw jerk
e dilated fixed pupils

1.109 *Signs of a lateral cerebellar lesion (i.e. lesion in a cerebellar lobe) include*

a impaired rapid alternating movements of the hand

b resting tremor
c horizontal nystagmus towards the side of the lesion
d ataxic gait with a tendency to fall towards the side of the lesion
e truncal ataxia

1.110 Complications of mitral stenosis include

a atrial fibrillation
b systemic embolism
c pulmonary hypertension
d arterial hypertension
e left ventricular hypertrophy

1.111 Clinical features of dystrophic myotonica include

a ptosis
b weakness confined to proximal muscles
c cataracts
d frontal balding
e cardiomyopathy

1.112 Diseases associated with exposure to asbestos include

a carcinoma of the bronchus
b pleural thickening
c progressive fibrosis
d mesothelioma
e sarcoidosis

1.113 Which of the following statements about chronic bronchitis and emphysema is/are true?

a it is commoner in women than in men
b the risk of the disease in a heavy smoker is less than twice that in a non-smoker
c α1-antitrypsin deficiency accounts for over 10% of the cases
d Streptococcus pneumoniae and Haemophilus influenzae are common organisms causing acute exacerbation
e a low haemoglobin level is characteristic

1.114 Causes of clubbing of the finger include

a idiopathic fibrosing alveolitis
b chronic bronchitis and emphysema
c subacute infective endocarditis
d inflammatory bowel disease
e carcinoma of the colon

1.115 Abnormal ECG feature of pulmonary embolism may include

a left axis deviation

b right bundle branch block
c sinus tachycardia
d T wave inversion in leads V4–6
e S wave in lead I, Q wave and inverted wave in lead III

1.116 *Which of the following investigative results support the diagnosis of nephrotic syndrome?*

a a low albumin level
b excessive 24 h urinary protein (6 g)
c a high cholesterol level
d abnormal liver function test
e a low triglyceride level

1.117 *Which of the following haematological results support the diagnosis of haemolysis?*

a increased conjugated bilirubin level
b reduced urinary urobilinogen
c increased reticulocyte count
d increased level of haptoglobin
e reduced red cell life-span demonstrated by ^{51}Cr-labelled red cells

1.118 *Which of the following statements about systemic sclerosis is/are true?*

a Raynaud's phenomenon occurs in the majority of the patients
b oesophageal involvement is less common than in systemic lupus erythematosus
c antinucleolar antibodies may be elevated
d corticosteroids provide an effective cure in more than half of the patients
e progressive fibrosis may occur in many different organs

1.119 *Which of the following statements about polymyalgia rheumatica is/are true?*

a the onset is characteristically acute
b the distal muscles are mostly affected
c the ESR level is characteristically elevated
d it affects men and women equally
e muscle stiffness is characteristically most severe in the evenings

1.120 *Which of the following statements about inappropriate antidiuretic hormone secretion (SIADH) is/are true?*

a it is often caused by squamous cell carcinoma of the lung
b it may present with confusion and irritability
c plasma sodium level is characteristically high
d urinary sodium excretion is characteristically excessive
e demeclocycline is a recognized treatment

1.121 *Which of the following are necessary criteria for the diagnosis of brain death?*

a complete loss of brain stem function
b the possibility of the effect due to drugs such as respiratory depressants must be excluded
c the possibility of the effect due to hypothermia must be excluded
d a flat EEG must be obtained
e cerebral blood flow must be performed

1.122 *Systemic sclerosis*

a is commoner than systemic lupus erythematosus
b occurs more frequently in males than in females
c frequently presents initially with Raynaud's phenomenon
d is frequently associated with a raised ESR
e is associated with reduced level of serum immunoglobulins

1.123 *Ankylosing spondylitis*

a is a chronic progressive condition
b tends to be more severe in women
c occurs in more than half of those with the HLA-B27 gene
d occurs more commonly in Japan
e seldom affects those less than 35 years

1.124 *Which of the following clinical features support a mechanical rather than an inflammatory cause of back pain?*

a gradual onset
b pain worse in the evening
c bilateral pain
d pain relief from exercise
e morning stiffness

1.125 *Which of the following hand abnormalities are characteristic of osteoarthritis?*

a Bouchard's nodes
b flexion of distal interphalangeal joints
c swan neck deformity
d Herberden's nodes
e ulnar deviation of the fingers at the metacarpal phalangeal joints

1.126 *Recognized causes for secondary osteoporosis include*

a untreated Turner's syndrome
b hyperthyroidism
c corticosteroid therapy

d chronic renal failure
e multiple myeloma

1.127 *Recognized clinical features of hypoparathyroidism include*

a circumoral numbness
b constipation
c polyuria
d drowsiness
e laryngeal stridor

1.128 *Clinical signs of infective endocarditis include*

a central cyanosis
b splenomegaly
c hepatomegaly
d splinter haemorrhages of the nails
e clubbing of the fingers

1.129 *Causes for sinus tachycardia include*

a anxiety
b hypothyroidism
c anaemia
d exercise
e Wolff–Parkinson–White syndrome

1.130 *Characteristic features of a right bundle block on the ECG include*

a absent p waves
b prolonged QRS interval
c RSR pattern in the leads V5 and V6
d progressive lengthening of PR interval on each successive beat
e T inversion in the leads V5 and V6

1.131 *Dilated cardiomyopathy*

a is the commonest form of cardiomyopathy
b occurs more frequently in male than female
c may be precipitated by a viral infection
d has an autosomal dominant pattern of inheritance
e frequently causes sudden death

1.132 *Corticosteroid is a recognized treatment for*

a relapse of multiple sclerosis
b Parkinson's disease
c myasthenia gravis

d dermatomyositis
e migraine

1.133 *Characteristic features of trigeminal neuralgia include*

a confinement to the supply of one division of the trigeminal nerve
b precipitation by wind or touch
c persistent and continuous facial pain
d a markedly raised ESR
e relief by carbamazepine

1.134 *Papilloedema is*

a characterized by a swollen pink optic disc
b associated with blurred optic disc margins
c usually unilateral
d associated with an enlarged blind spot
e most commonly caused by raised intracranial pressure

1.135 *Characteristic clinical features of idiopathic Parkinson's disease include*

a clasp-knife rigidity
b intention tremor
c loss of arm swing
d festinating gait
e micrographia

1.136 *Causes of transudative pleural effusion include*

a bacterial pneumonia
b cardiac failure
c bronchial carcinoma
d nephrotic syndrome
e rheumatoid arthritis

1.137 *Carcinoid syndrome*

a may occur with intestinal carcinoid tumour without metastases
b may present with constipation
c may present with attacks of wheezing
d may present with tricuspid stenosis
e is associated with reduced urinary excretion of 5-HIAA (5-hydroxyindole acetic acid)

1.138 *Recognized causes of cirrhosis of the liver include*

a hepatitis A infection
b hepatitis C infection
c hepatitis E infection

d Wilson's disease
e α1-antitrypsin deficiency

1.139 *Anion gap*

a is the difference between the sodium and the chloride concentration in the plasma
b is abnormal if it is over 4 mmol/litre
c is increased in lactic acidosis
d is increased in renal tubular acidosis
e is increased in hypercloraemic acidosis

1.140 *Causes of hypokalaemia include*

a spironolactone therapy
b corticosteroid therapy
c gastroenteritis
d Addison's disease
e villous adenoma of the rectum

1.141 *Characteristic biochemical findings of osteomalacia include*

a high serum calcium level
b low serum phosphate level
c high alkaline phosphatase level
d high parathyroid hormone (PTH) level
e high alanine aminotransferase (ALT) level

1.142 *Which of the following statements about adult polycystic disease of the kidneys is/are true?*

a it has an autosomal dominant inheritance with incomplete penetrance
b the cysts usually appear after the age of 45
c the cysts are in the renal medulla
d it may cause hypertension
e it has a recognized association with cerebral artery berry aneurysms

1.143 *Essential hypertension*

a affects less than 1% of the population
b is less common than secondary hypertension
c occurs more frequently and more severely in black people of African origin
d is associated with sodium retention
e predisposes to cerebrovascular accidents

1.144 *Causes of eosinophilia include*

a atopic asthma
b glandular fever
c Hodgkin's disease

d Legionnaire's disease
e parasitic infections

1.145 *Haematological findings characteristic of iron-deficiency anaemia include*

a a hypochromic macrocytic film
b a high MCV
c a high total iron binding capacity (TIBC)
d a high ferritin level
e abnormal haemoglobin electrophoresis

1.146 *Clinical features of hypothyroidism include*

a lethargy
b weight loss
c bradycardia
d diarrhoea
e delayed relaxation of tendon jerks

1.147 *Phaeochromocytoma*

a are sometimes associated with medullary carcinoma of the thyroid
b always arises from the adrenal medulla
c are always malignant
d may secreted noradrenaline and adrenaline
e should be treated with a combination of β- and α-adrenergic blocking drugs

1.148 *Causes of pathological gynaecomastia include*

a Leydig cell testicular tumour
b liver disease
c ranitidine therapy
d digoxin therapy
e Klinefelter's syndrome

1.149 *Clinical signs characteristic of hyperlipidaemia include*

a necrobiosis lipoidica
b corneal arcus
c Kayser-Fleischer ring
d lipaemia retinalis
e tendon xanthoma

1.150 *Recognized treatments for acne vulgaris include*

a topical benzoyl peroxide
b topical disinfectants
c topical dithranol
d oral erythromycin
e isotretinoin

Answers

1.1 a **False** b **True** c **True** d **True** e **False**
Hypothermia is defined as a fall of the *core* temperature to below 35°C, and the rectal temperature should be recorded using a low-reading thermometer or a thermocouple. Elderly, neonates, and alcohol abusers are especially vulnerable. It may also be secondary to hypothyroidism, phenothiazine overdose, and Addison's disease. Tiredness and stiff muscles are often the first symptoms. Both pulse and blood pressure may fall. Arrhythmia may occur, and a J wave in the ECG which occurs at the junction of the QRS complex and the ST segment is characteristic. Treatment should be gradual rewarming. Pupillary reflex and tendon reflexes are often absent in hypothermic patients, and death should not be diagnosed until the patient is rewarmed to at least 36°C and the neurological function reassessed.

1.2 a **False** b **True** c **True** d **False** e **True**
Symptoms of symptomatic HIV infection include fever, malaise, weight loss, and diarrhoea. Signs of symptomatic HIV infection include wasting, lymphadenopathy, and splenomegaly. Opportunistic infections such as oral candida, retinal cytomegalovirus (CMV) and histoplasmosis, perianal herpes, and pneumocystis may occur. Secondary neoplasms such as Kaposi's sarcoma and lymphoma may also occur.

1.3 a **False** b **False** c **True** d **True** e **False**
Typhoid fever is caused by *Salmonella typhi*, which is a gram negative bacillus. The incubation period is about 10–14 days. The symptoms in the first week are fever, muscle aches, headache, and constipation. By the beginning of the second week, diarrhoea, abdominal distension, and splenomegaly may occur, and a rash may appear on the abdomen which fades on pressure (rose spots). About 5% of patients become chronic carriers of *S. typhi*.

1.4 a **False** b **True** c **False** d **False** e **False**
The first heart sound originates from closure of the mitral and tricuspid valves, especially the mitral valve. It is best heard at the apex. The first heart sound is usually loud in hyperdynamic circulation (e.g. anaemia, hyperthyroidism) and in mitral stenosis. The first heart sound is soft in heart failure and in mitral regurgitation when the valve leaflets fail to close properly.

1.5 a **True** b **True** c **False** d **False** e **True**
An exercise ECG is performed with the subject progressively increasing exercise. The subject's symptoms and blood pressure should be closely monitored. It is contraindicated in unstable angina, severe heart failure, or hypertension, and severe outflow obstruction such as aortic stenosis. Exercise ECG can be used to detect stress-provoked arrhythmia and ischaemia which may not detected on a resting ECG.

1.6 a **False** b **True** c **True** d **True** e **False**
Pulmonary oedema is associated with increased pulmonary venous pressure. The

initial features of pulmonary oedema on a chest radiograph are distension of upper pulmonary veins, enlarged hilar vessels, and generalized increased pulmonary vascularity. Kerley 'B' lines are horizontal lines in the costophrenic angles caused by thickened interlobular septa and dilated lymphatics due to oedema. Pleural effusions may occur in severe pulmonary oedema. The cardiac size is often enlarged (increased cardiothoracic ratio).

1.7 a **False** b **True** c **True** d **True** e **True**
Acute pulmonary oedema should be treated by sitting the patient up, and administering high concentration oxygen, intravenous morphine to alleviate breathlessness, and diuretics such as frusemide. Vasodilators such as sublingual or intravenous nitrate may be used, but blood pressure should be closely monitored for hypotension. If these measures are ineffective, inotropic agents such as dopamine or dobutamine may be considered.

1.8 a **True** b **False** c **True** d **True** e **False**
Sinus bradycardia occurs if the pulse rate is sinus, but less than 60 beats/min. In sinus rhythms, P waves must be present. It may be physiological, as in some athletes or during sleep. Pathological causes include myocardial infarction, sick sinus syndrome, hypothyroidism drug therapy (e.g. beta-blockers) and hypothermia. Fever causes sinus tachycardia.

1.9 a **False** b **True** c **False** d **True** e **True**
In atrial fibrillation, the atria contract rapidly but ineffectively, and the ventricles respond at irregular intervals. Hence, the pulse is characteristically "irregular irregular". It is not uncommon in the elderly, and is often asymptomatic. Atrial fibrillation may be treated by drugs such as digoxin, beta-blockers, and verapamil. Alternatively, elective DC cardioversion may be used. Atrial fibrillation predisposes to thromboembolism, and anticoagulants are sometimes prescribed to those with other risk factors for thromboembolism.

1.10 a **False** b **False** c **True** d **True** e **False**
Ventricular tachycardia is a serious arrhythmia and is nearly always caused by serious heart disease. It may proceed to ventricular fibrillation, and hence treatment should be given promptly. Symptoms may include dizziness, shortness of breath, or syncope. Unlike in supraventricular tachycardia, the QRS complex is very broad, and there is no response to carotid sinus massage in ventricular tachycardia. Treatment is either DC cardioversion or intravenous lignocaine or other suitable type I anti-arrhythmic drugs.

1.11 a **True** b **True** c **False** d **False** e **True**
Possible immediate treatment of supraventricular tachycardia include vagal manoeuvre (e.g. carotid sinus massage, Valsalva manoeuvre), intravenous adenosine, DC cardioconversion, intravenous verapamil (but this should never be given if beta-blockers have recently been given). Other treatments include digoxin or amiodarone, and surgical ablation of aberrant pathways if they are demonstrated using electrophysiological studies.

1.12 a **False** b **False** c **False** d **True** e **False**
In third degree (complete) heart block, the atrioventricular conduction fails completely, and the atria and ventricles beat completely independently. The atrial rate is faster than the ventricular rate, and the pulse is slow and regular at the ventricular rate (about 30–50 beats/min). The Wenkebach phenomenon describes the progressive lengthening of the PR interval until a dropped beat occurs, and is a feature of second degree Mobitz type I heart block. In third degree heart block, the canon waves may be seen in the neck veins when the right atrium intermittently contracts with a closed tricuspid valve.

1.13 a **False** b **True** c **True** d **True** e **False**
Angina pectoris occurs when myocardial oxygen demand exceeds supply. The diagnosis is made mainly from the history. A sense of tightness or pain in the chest is often described, which may radiate to the neck, jaw, or left arm. Feeling of breathlessness is also common. It is characteristically precipitated by exercise, but meals and cold weather are also well-known precipitating factors. It is typically relieved by rest or sublingual nitrate. Physical examination and resting ECG often show no abnormality. However, the exercise ECG may show downsloping ST depression, and may provide a guide to the extent of coronary artery disease.

1.14 a **False** b **True** c **True** d **True** e **True**
Recognized treatments for acute myocardial infarction include bed rest, high flow oxygen, intravenous cannula for intravenous access, intravenous opiates with antiemetics, intravenous thrombolytics (e.g. streptokinase) in the absence of contraindications, and intravenous beta-blockers. Contraindications for intravenous thrombolytics include high risks of haemorrhage and uncontrolled hypertension. Early administration of beta-blockers has been shown to reduce mortality and complications such as arrhythmia.

1.15 a **True** b **True** c **True** d **False** e **False**
Most cases of hypertension are without specific underlying causes (i.e. essential hypertension). Secondary causes of hypertension include renal diseases (e.g. renal artery stenosis, chronic pyelonephritis, systemic lupus erythematosus, polycystic kidney disease); endocrine disorders (such as Cushing's syndrome, Conn's syndrome, and phaeochromocytoma), and drug therapy (e.g. corticosteroids, non-steroidal anti-inflammatory drugs). Coarctation of the aorta is a cardiac cause of secondary hypertension.

1.16 a **True** b **True** c **True** d **True** e **False**
Symptoms of a moderate-sized pulmonary embolus include shortness of breath, pleuritic chest pain, and haemoptysis. Common signs include pyrexia, pleural rub, or signs of a pleural effusion. In more severe cases, there may be cyanosis and a raised jugular vein pulse (JVP).

1.17 a **False** b **True** c **True** d **True** e **False**
Signs characteristic of mitral regurgitation include atrial fibrillation, displaced apex beat (due to left ventricular dilatation), a quiet first heart sound, and a pansystolic

murmur loudest at the apex radiating to the axilla which is best heard on lying the patient on the left side.

1.18 a **True** b **False** c **False** d **True** e **True**
Signs of aortic regurgitation include increased pulse pressure, which is reflected by a collapsing pulse and bounding peripheral pulses. An early diastolic murmur in the aortic area radiating to the carotids with the patient leaning forward in expiration is characteristic. However, there may be associated ejection systolic murmur or a soft mid-diastolic murmur (Austin Flint murmur). There may also be a thrusting apex due to left ventricular enlargement.

1.19 a **True** b **True** c **True** d **True** e **False**
Acute pericarditis is pericardial inflammation. The commonest causes are following an acute myocardial infarction, and viral infection (especially the coxsackie B virus). The characteristic symptom is retrosternal pain which radiates to the shoulders and the neck, and which is made worse by movement and deep breathing. The characteristic sign is the pericardial friction rub which is high-pitched scratching produced by movement of the inflamed pericardium. The pain is best treated with a non-steroidal anti-inflammatory drug such as indomethacin.

1.20 a **False** b **True** c **False** d **True** e **False**
Respiratory failure is divided into type I (when the carbon dioxide level is not increased) and type II (when the carbon dioxide level is increased). In chronic type II respiratory failure, the oxygen level is reduced in the presence of carbon dioxide retention. The kidneys conserve bicarbonate to maintain a normal range of pH. The commonest cause is chronic obstructive airway disease, but may also be caused by hypoventilation in severe kyphoscoliosis or ankylosing spondylitis. Asthma usually causes type I respiratory failure where hyperventilation causes a low carbon dioxide level. Only controlled low concentration of oxygen should be used in type II respiratory failure, as a high concentration may reduce respiratory drive further and induce severe hypercapnia.

1.21 a **False** b **False** c **True** d **False** e **False**
Unlike early onset asthma, late onset asthma is not usually associated with allergic disorders. Family history of allergic disorders is usually absent, and the skin tests are negative. During an attack, the chest is hyperexpanded. The presence of wheezing does not correlate with the severity of the attack. A silent chest is a sign of very poor air entry, and is a serious sign. The FEV_1 to VC ratio is low, characteristic of an obstructive lung defect. Inhaled sodium cromoglycate (which acts by stabilizing the mast cells), although effective in early onset asthma, is seldom effective in late onset asthma.

1.22 a **False** b **True** c **True** d **True** e **True**
Pneumococcus is the commonest identifiable organism found in pneumonia. It occurs in all age groups, but especially in younger adults. It occurs more frequently in winter. Common symptoms are high pyrexia, ache and pains, headache, productive cough,

and pleuritic chest pain. Signs of consolidation are frequently present 1–2 days after the onset of illness. The neutrophil count is characteristically increased markedly.

1.23 a **True** b **False** c **True** d **True** e **False**
Tuberculosis may affect tissues outside the lung. In the eyes, it may cause iritis, choriditis, or phyctenular conjunctivitis. It may cause osteomyelitis, and vertebral collapse in the bones and joints. It may be deposited in the adrenal gland to cause Addison's disease. It may invade the bone marrow and give rise to anaemia. It may cause meningitis or tuberculoma in the central nervous system. The typical skin lesions are lupus vulgaris and erythema nodosum. Erythema marginatum is characteristic of rheumatic fever.

1.24 a **True** b **False** c **True** d **True** e **False**

The most important predisposing factor for bronchial carcinoma is cigarette smoking. Other predisposing factors are asbestos exposure, atmospheric pollution (e.g. in urban dwellers), and possibly passive smoking. Bronchial carcinoma is the commonest cancer in men and the second commonest cause of cancer in women (the commonest cause being breast cancer). About half of bronchial carcinomas are of the squamous type, and about a quarter are of the small cell type.

1.25 a **True** b **True** c **True** d **True** e **True**
The two commonest clinical features caused by bronchial carcinoma are cough and haemoptysis. Breathlessness may occur if the carcinoma causes a collapse of a lobe of a lung or a large pleural effusion. Pleuritic chest pain may occur if the pleura are involved. If the intercostal nerves are involved, there may be pain in the distribution supplied by the dermatome. Invasion of the brachial plexus may cause pain in the upper limb. Carcinoma in the apex of the lung (Pancoast tumour) may cause pain in the upper limb and unilateral Horner's syndrome.

1.26 a **True** b **True** c **True** d **True** e **True**
Extrapulmonary manifestations of bronchial carcinoma which are not due to metastasis include clubbing with or without hypertrophic pulmonary osteoarthropathy, ectopic hormone secretion (ADH and ACTH secreted by small cell carcinoma and PTH secreted by squamous carcinoma); and neurological syndromes including polyneuropathy, cerebellar degeneration, and Eaton-Lambert myasthenia.

1.27 a **True** b **False** c **True** d **True** e **False**
Sarcoidosis is a multisystem granulomatous disease which may affect many organs in the body. It commonly gives rise to hilar lymphenopathy of the lung and interstitial lung disease. It also causes lymphanopathy, hepatosplenomegaly, and splenomegaly. In the central nervous system, it may cause meningitis, diabetes insipidus, and cranial nerve palsy. It may also cause peripheral neuropathy. The commonest associated skin lesion is erythema nodosum. The eye lesions may include iritis, uveitis, and keratoconjunctivitis. Calcium metabolism may be deranged causing hypercalcaemia and renal failure.

1.28 a **False** b **False** c **True** d **True** e **False**
Sarcoidosis is a granulomatous disease, and is distinguished from tuberculosis by its absence of caseation. Bilateral hilar lymphanopathy is often asymptomatic and detected on routine chest radiograph. Erythema nodosum, uveitis, and lung fibrosis may respond to corticosteroid treatment. The plasma level of angiotensin-converting enzyme is often raised, and is useful to monitor disease activity and response to treatment.

1.29 a **True** b **True** c **False** d **True** e **False**
Pleural effusion occurs when fluid accumulates between the pleural spaces. An exudate contains a high concentration of protein, and may be caused by bacterial pneumonia, tuberculosis, carcinoma, or pulmonary infarction. An transudate contains a low concentration of protein, and may be caused by heart failure or hypoproteinaemia. Pneumothorax and fibrosing alveolitis do not cause pleural effusions.

1.30 a **False** b **False** c **False** d **True** e **False**
Characteristic clinical features of a spontaneous pneumothorax are sudden onset of unilateral chest pain associated with breathlessness. Cyanosis may be present if the pneumothorax is of the open or tension type. Physical signs include deviation of trachea to the unaffected side, and reduced movement of chest wall, hyperresonance, diminished or absent breath sounds, and reduced vocal resonance on the affected side.

1.31 a **False** b **True** c **True** d **False** e **True**
Characteristic symptoms of peptic ulcer disease include well-localized epigastric pain which is aggravated by hunger. The patient often wakes up with pain in the middle of the night, and seeks relief by taking food, milk, or antacids. The pain is characteristically episodic, and feels perfectly well in between. Associated symptoms include heartburn, waterbrash, and occasional vomiting.

1.32 a **False** b **True** c **True** d **True** e **True**
Helicobacter pylori is a gram negative bacterium found in the mucous epithelial layer of the stomach. It has been shown to cause about 90% of duodenal ulcers and 75% of gastric ulcers. *H. pylori* may be detected by the ELISA test (by detecting antibodies to serum Helicobacter proteins), the urease breath test, and histology of peptic ulcer biopsy. Eradication can be achieved in the majority of cases either with bismuth and antibiotics, or with omperazole and two other antibiotics. The recommended regime for eradication is continually changing.

1.33 a **True** b **False** c **True** d **False** e **False**
Common drugs used in peptic ulcer diseases include antacids, H_2 antagonists (e.g. cimetidine and ranitidine), and proton pump inhibitors (e.g. omperazole). Bismuth is used both as part of triple therapy to eradicate *H. pylori* and on its own by its action in enhancing mucosal defence. Prostaglandin analogues (e.g. misoprostol) are used to protect against the action of non-steroidal anti-inflammatory drugs. Non-steroidal anti-inflammatory drugs and high dose corticosteroids are contraindicated in peptic ulcer disease.

1.34 a **True** b **True** c **False** d **False** e **False**
Both ulcerative colitis and Crohn's disease usually present as chronic disorders with exacerbation and remission. The characteristic symptoms of Crohn's disease are right iliac fossa peritoneal pain or colicky pain due to bowel obstruction. Diarrhoea may occur, but not as severely as in ulcerative colitis. The characteristic symptoms of ulcerative colitis are bloody diarrhoea with mucus and pus. Pain on defecation and tenesmus may also occur. Malabsorption is often a major feature of Crohn's disease due to the extent of small bowel disease, bowel resection, and bacterial colonization. Anal fissure, abscesses, and fistulas are commoner in Crohn's disease.

1.35 a **False** b **True** c **True** d **True** e **True**
Toxic dilatation of the colon commonly occurs in severe ulcerative colitis or Crohn's disease. The characteristic symptoms are profuse diarrhoea, pyrexia, dehydration, tachycardia, abdominal tenderness, and abdominal distension. This is a very serious condition, and the patient is at serious risk of colonic perforation.

1.36 a **False** b **True** c **True** d **False** e **True**
Patients with Crohn's disease usually have malabsorption and should be given a high energy high protein diet. Dietary supplementation may also be needed. Mild Crohn's disease can be treated by oral sulphasalazine and corticosteroid enema, and antidiarrhoeal drugs such as loperamide and codeine phosphate. Chronic Crohn's disease can be treated by oral corticosteroids or azathioprine. If medical treatment is ineffective, bowel resection may be required.

1.37 a **False** b **True** c **True** d **True** e **False**
Pseudomembranous colitis is caused by Clostridium difficile, which produces at least two exotoxins (A and B) to cause intestinal damage. It is commoner in elderly patients in hospital who are receiving broad-spectrum antibiotics. The characteristic symptoms are watery diarrhoea and lower abdominal pain. The treatments are oral metronidazole for mild disease and oral vancomycin for severe disease.

1.38 a **True** b **False** c **True** d **False** e **False**
Irritable bowel disease is a bowel dysfunction for which no organic causes can be found. It commonly occurs in women between the ages of 20 and 40. The characteristic symptoms are lower abdominal pain which may be precipitated by food and may be relieved by defecation. Pellet-like stools are characteristic. Either constipation or diarrhoea may occur. Diarrhoea typically occurs in the daytime, and it may be associated with psychological disturbances.

1.39 a **True** b **True** c **False** d **False** e **True**
Clinical features of portal hypertension include collateral circulation (oesophageal varices, haemorrhoids, and caput medusae), splenomegaly with hypersplenism, and ascites. Hypersplenism is associated with a reduced platelet count. Hepatic encephalopathy may be result from portasystemic shunting.

1.40 a **False** b **True** c **True** d **False** e **True**
Hepatic encephalopathy is a neuropsychiatric disorder associated with liver disease. Although the exact biochemical responsible is unknown, liver failure, increased protein digestion in the intestine, and portasystemic shunting are known precipitating factors. Hence, increased dietary protein, gastrointestinal bleeding, and constipation are known precipitating factors. Infection is also a known precipitating factor.

1.41 a **True** b **True** c **True** d **False** e **False**
Causes of acute hepatitis include all hepatitis viruses, cytomegalovirus, Epstein-Barr virus, drugs such as paracetamol, toxic substances such as carbon tetrachloride, and metabolic diseases such as Wilson's disease. Primary biliary cirrhosis and gallstones both cause cholestatic jaundice.

1.42 a **False** b **True** c **True** d **False** e **True**
Clinical signs of cirrhosis include clubbing, skin stigmata (e.g. spider naevi, liver palm), oestrogen effects (e.g. gynaecomastia, testicular atrophy), jaundice, hard irregular painless hepatomegaly, and signs of portal hypertension (splenomegaly, caput medusae, ascites).

1.43 a **True** b **True** c **True** d **False** e **True**
Predisposing conditions for hepatocellular carcinoma include chronic hepatitis B infection, chronic hepatitis C infection, alcohol liver disease, haemochromatosis, primary biliary cirrhosis, and α_1-antitrypsin deficiency.

1.44 a **True** b **False** c **True** d **True** e **False**
Deficiency of thiamine (vitamin B_1) may cause three possible clinical syndromes: dry beriberi, wet beriberi, and Wernicke-Korsakoff syndrome. The main clinical feature in dry beriberi is peripheral neuropathy. The clinical features of wet beriberi are those of high output cardiac failure. In Wernicke's encephalopathy, the clinical features the triad of mental confusion, ataxia, and ophthalmoplegia. If untreated, it may progress to Korsakoff's psychosis, characterized by memory deficits and confabulation. Night blindness is caused by vitamin A deficiency, and rickets is caused by vitamin D deficiency.

1.45 a **False** b **False** c **True** d **True** e **False**
Major causes for inappropriate ADH secretion are diseases of the central nervous system (e.g. cerebral tumour, head injury, meningitis) and small cell carcinoma of the bronchus. It also occurs postoperatively. In diabetes insipidus, there is a deficiency of ADH.

1.46 a **True** b **True** c **True** d **True** e **False**
Acute treatments for hyperkalaemia include intravenous calcium gluconate 10% to protect the heart against cardiac arrest; infusion of a mixture of dextrose and insulin; and oral ion exchange resin. The underlying cause should be treated, and metabolic acidosis should be corrected. If these measures are ineffective, peritoneal dialysis or haemodialysis may be required. Spironolactone increases the potassium level.

1.47 a **False** b **True** c **True** d **True** e **False**
Metabolic acidosis may be caused by excessive intake of acid, failure to excrete acid effectively, and loss of bicarbonate. Causes for excessive intake of acid include methanol poisoning and salicylate poisoning. Causes for failure to excrete acid effectively include acute and renal failure, and distal renal tubular acidosis. Causes for loss of bicarbonate include proximal renal tubular acidosis. Hypokalaemia and persistent vomiting are both associated with metabolic alkalosis.

1.48 a **True** b **False** c **True** d **True** e **False**
Characteristic features of acute glomerulonephritis include acute onset of haematuria (often with a smoky appearance), proteinuria, hypertension, oliguria, and very occasionally oedema. It may be preceded by streptococcal infection.

1.49 a **True** b **True** c **True** d **False** e **True**
Patients with chronic renal failure may have a variety of non-specific symptoms such as malaise, anorexia, nausea, headaches, pruritus, and pallor. Anaemia is common as a result of a number of factors, including reduced dietary intake, diminished erythropoiesis, and reduced red cell survival. Osteomalacia may result from failure to convert 25-hydroxycholecalciferol to 1,25-hydroxycholecalciferol. In addition, bone disease may result from increased PTH level. Peripheral neuropathy, myopathy, hypertension, and metabolic acidosis are also more common in patients with chronic renal failure.

1.50 a **True** b **False** c **True** d **False** e **True**
Huntington's chorea, congenital spherocytosis, and polyposis coli are autosomal dominant in inheritance. Almost all enzyme deficiencies (including α_1-antitrypsin deficiency) are autosomal recessive in inheritance. Haemophilia A is sex-linked recessive in inheritance.

1.51 a **False** b **False** c **True** d **True** e **False**
In sex-linked recessive disorders, the son receives the X chromosome from the mother and the Y chromosome from the father. He has the disorder if he receives the affected X chromosome from his mother. Hence, an affected father cannot transmit the disorder to his son. A carrier mother has one normal and one affected X chromosome, and has a 50% chance of transmitting it to her son. The daughter receives one X chromosome from each of her parents. An affected father will pass on the affected X chromosome to all his daughters. A carrier mother has one normal and one affected X chromosome, and will pass on the affected chromosome to half her daughters. An affected mother has two affected X chromosomes, and all her daughters will be carriers.

1.52 a **False** b **False** c **True** d **True** e **False**
The hormones secreted by the anterior pituitary gland are adrenocorticotrophic hormone (ACTH), growth hormone (GH), thyroid stimulating hormone (TSH), luteinizing hormone (LH), follicle stimulating hormone (FSH), and prolactin. Thyroxin is secreted by the thyroid gland, and oxytocin is secreted by the posterior pituitary gland.

1.53 a **False** b **True** c **True** d **True** e **True**
Symptoms of pituitary tumours may be classified into two groups: pressure effects on surrounding structures, and excessive or deficiency secretion of hormones from the pituitary glands. Pressure on optic nerves or optic chiasma may lead to optic atrophy and optic field defects. The characteristic field defect of pressure on optic chiasma is bitemporal hemianopia. Pressure on the third, fourth, or sixth cranial nerve may cause diploplia and paralysis of eye movements. Pressure on the dura may cause headache.

1.54 a **True** b **True** c **True** d **False** e **False**
Clinical features of acromegaly include soft tissue changes and enlargement of hands and feet and other bony enlargements. Soft tissue changes give rise to skin thickening, enlargement of lips and tongue, myopathy, and carpel tunnel syndrome. There may be impaired glucose tolerance or clinical diabetes mellitus.

1.55 a **False** b **True** c **False** d **True** e **False**
In diabetes insipidus there is a deficiency of antidiuretic hormone. Hence, the subject continues to pass diluted urine of low osmolality in spite of high plasma osmolality. The characteristic symptoms are polyuria and polydipsia. Whereas cranial diabetes insipidus is due to lack of production of ADH from the posterior pituitary gland, nephrogenic diabetes insipidus is due to the renal tubules being unresponsive to ADH. Hence, cranial diabetes insipidus (but not nephrogenic diabetes insipidus) responds clinically to treatment with desmopressin (DDVAP), a long-acting analogue of vasopressin.

1.56 a **False** b **True** c **True** d **False** e **True**
The physical features of hyperthyroidism include heat intolerance, sweating, fatigue, tremor, weight loss in spite of normal or increased appetite, diarrhoea, palpitations (due to sinus tachycardia or atrial fibrillation), shortness of breath on exertion, and brisk tendon jerks. In Graves' disease, there may be ocular signs (lid retraction, lid lag, and exopthalmos) and pretibial myxoedema. Psychological features include emotional lability, irritability, or even psychosis.

1.57 a **True** b **False** c **True** d **True** e **False**
In Graves' disease, usually both T_3 and thyroxine are elevated. The TSH level is very much reduced due to suppression by circulating thyroxine. There is little or no response of TSH to an intravenous injection of TRH. The presence of TSH-receptor antibodies (TRAb), IgG antibodies acting on the TSH receptors on the thyroid gland, causes excessive thyroid hormone production.

1.58 a **True** b **False** c **False** d **True** e **False**
Common causes for hypercalcaemia include primary and tertiary hyperparathyroidism, malignancy (causing ectopic PTH secretion or bone metastasis), chronic renal failure, and sarcoidosis (due to increased sensitivity to vitamin D). In secondary hyperparathyroidism, the parathyroidism partially compensates for a low serum calcium level by increasing PTH secretion. In osteomalacia, the calcium level is low.

1.59 a **False** b **False** c **True** d **True** e **True**

Treatment for hypercalcaemia depends on the underlying cause as well as the level of plasma calcium. The first step should be rehydration with saline, with or without intravenous frusemide. The plasma sodium, potassium, magnesium, and bicarbonate levels should be monitored and corrected if necessary. Intramuscular salmon calcitonin (salcatonin) injection three times daily lowers the calcium level by inhibiting the osteoclasts activity. Phosphate can be given either orally or intravenously. Intravenous bisphosphonate may be used especially if malignancy is the underlying cause.

1.60 a **False** b **True** c **True** d **True** e **True**

Cushing's syndrome comprises the clinical features associated with chronic inappropriate increase in corticosteroid level. The causes may be Cushing's disease (increased pituitary ACTH production), ectopic ACTH secretion (e.g. by small cell carcinoma of the bronchus), adrenal tumours, and prolonged steroid therapy. Conn's syndrome is associated with inappropriate increased production of aldosterone in the adrenals.

1.61 a **False** b **True** c **True** d **False** e **True**

In primary hyperaldosteronism, aldosterone level is increased due to either adrenal hyperplasia or adrenal adenoma. The raised aldosterone level leads to sodium retention which suppresses renin secretion. In secondary hyperaldosteronism, renin activity is increased which causes increased aldosterone secretion via angiotensin II release. The increased renin activity may be due to either physiological causes such as inadequate intake or excessive loss of sodium, or pathological causes such as diuretic therapy, congestive heart failure, cirrhosis with ascites, or renal artery stenosis.

1.62 a **True** b **False** c **True** d **True** e **False**

Clinical features of Addison's disease may be classified into those due to glucocorticoid deficiency, mineralcorticoid deficiency, and increased ACTH secretion. Clinical features due to glucocorticoid deficiency include weakness, nausea, vomiting, postural hypotension, and hypoglycaemia. Hypotension is due to mineralcorticoid deficiency. Pigmentation of skin and conjunctivae is due to excessive ACTH secretion.

1.63 a **False** b **False** c **False** d **True** e **True**

Insulin dependent diabetes mellitus (IDDM) has an HLA-linked genetic predisposition and an association with other autoimmune disorders, and circulating islet cell autoantibodies can often be detected in new cases. It may also be precipitated by viral infection such as coxsackie virus. Hence, IDDM appears to be an autoimmune disease. Non-insulin dependent diabetes mellitus (NIDDM), however, has no HLA-linked genetic predisposition or any other evidence of an autoimmune disorder. The monozygotic twin concordance rate is higher than IDDM, but the exact genetic nature is not understood. NIDDM occurs more commonly in subjects with obesity, hypertension, and hyperlipidaemia. Most subjects with NIDDM have insulin resistance in target tissues.

1.64 a **True** b **False** c **False** d **False** e **False**

Renal glycosuria is due to low renal threshold for glucose. Hence, glucose appears in the urine in spite of normal glucose tolerance. It commonly occurs transiently during pregnancy. However, all glycosuria during pregnancy should be investigated thoroughly as hyperglycaemia during pregnancy may cause increased perinatal mortality. Renal glycosuria is not related to diabetes mellitus.

1.65 a **True** b **False** c **True** d **False** e **False**
Haemoglobin A_1 constitutes about 7% of the total haemoglobin A, the rest being haemoglobin A_0. Haemoglobin A_1 is synthesized by the addition of a glucose group to haemoglobin A_0, and its concentration therefore reflects the mean blood glucose concentration within the half-life of the red blood cells of about 2 months. It has been shown to be closely associated with the risk of vascular complications and mortality rate. In well-controlled diabetes, the haemoglobin A_1 should be below 9%. Blood glucose levels should always be monitored.

1.66 a **True** b **True** c **False** d **False** e **True**
The two major causes for hypochromic microcytic anaemia are iron deficiency and haemoglobinopathies. Iron deficiency anaemia is most commonly due to menstruation in women of reproductive age. Gastrointestinal bleeding, malnutrition, and malabsorption are other causes. In tropical countries, hookworms, and schistosomiasis are common causes. Haemolysis and folate deficiency are associated with macrocytosis.

1.67 a **False** b **False** c **True** d **True** e **True**
Pernicious anaemia is an autoimmune disease associated with intrinsic factor deficiency. Anti-intrinsic factor antibodies can be detected in half of the cases. Intrinsic factor is secreted by gastric parietal cells, and it facilitates absorption of vitamin B_{12} from the distal ileum. Hence, pernicious anaemia is associated with reduced absorption of vitamin B_{12}, which is corrected by the addition of intrinsic factor. Macrocytic anaemia results from the vitamin B_{12} deficiency.

1.68 a **False** b **True** c **True** d **False** e **True**
Secondary polycythaemia is increased red blood cell production as a secondary phenomenon. This may be either as a response to hypoxia (e.g. high altitude, chronic obstructive airway disease, and congenital cyanotic heart disease) or excessive inappropriate erythropoietin production (e.g. renal, bronchial, or cerebellar carcinoma). Polycythaemia rubra vera is an example of primary polycythaemia.

1.69 a **True** b **False** c **True** d **False** e **False**
Chronic lymphocytic leukaemia usually occurs in patients over the age of 50. It is extremely rare in Chinese people. It is characterized by an accumulation of incompetent B cells which fail to produce antibodies. It may be asymptomatic. The common symptoms are tiredness and malaise, painless rubbery lymphanopathy, or increased susceptibility to infection. The platelet level is usually only mildly reduced, and severe bleeding is a very rare feature. The older patients generally die of other causes, and their life expectancy is not significantly diminished by the presence of the disease.

1.70 a **True** b **False** c **True** d **True** e **False**

Diagnosis of multiple myeloma can be made with at least two out of three of the following features:- monoclonal antibodies in serum or urine (as Bence Jones protein), infiltration of bone marrow with malignant plasma cells, or destructive bone lesions. The level of normal immunoglobulin is usually reduced. The ESR is usually over 100 mm in the first hour.

1.71 a **False** b **True** c **True** d **False** e **True**

The metatarsophalangeal joint of the great toe is the commonest affected joint in acute gout. The joint is usually red, swollen, and extremely tender. Gout may be precipitated by alcohol, dietary changes, and diuretics such as thiazides. Thiazide diuretics should be stopped. Non-steroidial anti-inflammatory drugs are the best immediate treatment. Colchicine is also effective, but may cause vomiting or diarrhoea.

1.72 a **False** b **True** c **True** d **True** e **False**

There are numerous extra-articular manifestations of rheumatoid arthritis. Eye complications include dry eyes, episcleritis, and scleritis. Vasculitis may be manifested by Raynaud's phenomenon, ulcers, or pyoderma gangrenosum. Cardiac manifestations include pericarditis and myocarditis. Pulmonary manifestations include pleural effusions, fibrosing alveolitis, and pulmonary nodules. Neurological manifestations include carpel tunnel syndrome, peripheral neuropathy, and mononeuritis multiplex. A normochromic normocytic anaemia is the commonest haematological manifestation.

1.73 a **True** b **True** c **True** d **True** e **True**

General management for rheumatoid arthritis includes education and simple analgesia such as aspirin or non-steroidal anti-inflammatory drugs. If these measures are ineffective, disease-modifying suppressive drugs can be used. These include antimalarials and sulphasalazine, gold, methotrexate, and penicillamine. If these drugs are also ineffective, immunomodulating drugs such as azathioprine and metrotrexate can be tried. Systemic corticosteroids are useful in treating acute severe exacerbation.

1.74 a **True** b **False** c **True** d **False** e **True**

Septic arthritis in adults are commonly caused by streptococcus or staphylococcus. Diabetes mellitus, immunosuppresion, joint trauma, and existing joint diseases especially rheumatoid arthritis are all predisposing factors. Although more than one joint may be involved, a single joint involvement is characteristic. Joint aspiration and blood culture should be immediately performed once the diagnosis is suspected. Radiographic changes are usually absent in the early stages. Appropriate intravenous antibiotics administered for several weeks are the usual treatment.

1.75 a **True** b **True** c **True** d **True** e **True**

Systemic lupus erythematosus is a multisystem autoimmune connective tissue disease, and may give rise to a wide variety of symptoms. The main features are photosensitive erythematous 'butterfly' rash across the face, alopecia, migratory polyarthritis, and polyarthralgia. The most serious feature is renal involvement which may result in nephrotic syndrome and renal failure. Cardiac manifestations include pericarditis and myocarditis. Pulmonary manifestations include pleurisy and fibrosing alveolitis. Psychiatric manifestations may include dementia, depression, or psychosis. Neurological complications include cerebellar ataxia, cranial nerve palsies, and peripheral neuropathy. Recurrent spontaneous abortions may be the presenting features.

1.76 a **False** b **False** c **False** d **True** e **False**
Internal predisposing factors for osteoporosis include female sex, short stature, advanced age, low body mass index, and early menopause. External predisposing factors include reduced physical activity, low calcium intake, cigarette smoking, and alcohol abuse. Predisposing diseases for osteoporosis include Cushing's syndrome and thyrotoxicosis.

1.77 a **True** b **True** c **True** d **False** e **True**
In Paget's disease of the bone, there is bowing, enlargement, and softening of the bones, with increased blood flow through them. As a result of enlargement of the skull bones, there may be headache or deafness due to compression of the auditory nerves. As a result of softening of the bone, there may be spontaneous fracture. As a result of the increased blood flow, the affected part feels warm. Rarely, the patient may be in high flow cardiac failure.

1.78 a **False** b **True** c **True** d **False** e **False**
Pityriasis rosea is a benign condition of unknown aetiology. Typically, a 'herald patch' about 4 cm in diameter appears first, followed by smaller plaques and a scaly 'Christmas-tree' distribution of lesions on the back. The lesions regress spontaneously after several weeks. The diagnosis can only be made clinically and require no treatment. Pityriasis vesicolor requires antifungal treatment.

1.79 a **False** b **True** c **True** d **False** e **False**
Signs of an upper motor neurone lesions include hypertonia (either spasticity or clasp-knife rigidity), extensor clonus, and tendon reflexes, extensor plantar response, and loss of abdominal reflex. There is no fasciculation and little or no muscle wasting.

1.80 a **False** b **True** c **True** d **False** e **True**
The correct segmental supply for the tendon reflexes are:

biceps	cervical 5/6
supinator	cervical 5/6
triceps	cervical 7/(8)
knee jerk	lumbar 3/4
ankle jerk	sacral 1/(2)

1.81 a **True** b **False** c **True** d **False** e **False**
Clinical features of frontal lobe lesions include lack of social inhibition, antisocial behaviour, impaired memory, loss of smell, loss of initiative, and incontinence of

urine or faeces. Apraxia and agnosia are both signs of dominant parietal lobe lesion. Homonymous hemianopia is a sign of occipital lobe lesion.

1.82 a **True** b **False** c **False** d **False** e **True**
The characteristic signs of Horner's syndrome are ptosis, small pupil, enopthalmos, and decreasing sweating on the same side of the face. All pupillary reflexes are normal.

1.83 a **True** b **False** c **False** d **True** e **True**
Conductive deafness is due to failure of conduction of sound from the external acoustic meatus to the cochlea. It may be caused by ear wax, otosclerosis, or middle ear disease. Sensorineural deafness is caused by failure to conduct sound signals from the cochlea to the brain. It may be caused by damage to the cochlear (e.g. Meniere's disease), auditory fibres of the eighth cranial nerve (e.g. mumps infection or acoustic neuroma).

1.84 a **False** b **True** c **True** d **True** e **False**
A transient ischaemic attack is an episode of cerebral ischaemia in which the symptoms last less than 24 h. It often results from the embolus of a thrombus from extracerebral arteries. As the risk factors for transient ischaemic attacks and strokes are similar, the risk of a stroke is increased in a person known to have a transient ischaemic attack. Hence, a transient ischaemic attack must be investigated thoroughly. Aspirin 300 mg daily is useful as an antiplatelet agent in reducing the incidence of strokes.

1.85 a **True** b **False** c **True** d **True** e **True**
Management of Parkinson's disease includes stopping drugs which may cause parkinsonism, such as phenothiazines (e.g. chlorpromazine) and butyrophenones (e.g. haloperidol). Physiotherapy may be given. Anticholinergic agents, amantidine, and selegiline may then be tried at an early stage. As the disease progress, a combination of L-dopa and peripheral decarboxylase inhibitor can be given. Unfortunately, side-effects such as orofacial dyskinesis and dystonia may occur after a few years. Low dose bromocriptine may also be used. In severe cases, sterotactic thalamotomy may be considered. The use of fetal midbrain implantation into the basal ganglia is under evaluation, but there are ethical issues relating to its use.

1.86 a **False** b **False** c **True** d **True** e **True**
Multiple sclerosis occurs more frequently in temperate than tropical countries, but the reason for this is unknown. The natural history is typically that of relapse and remission. In their first attack, patients usually recover from their symptoms within a few months. The optic nerve is often affected, and clinical optic neuritis may be the presenting symptoms. Even in patients without clinical optic neuritis, delayed visual evoked response is common. MRI scan is the most sensitive radiological investigation available for multiple sclerosis, and shows lesions in over 90% of patients with definite multiple sclerosis. However, the lesions may not be distinguishable from those of another disease such as cerebrovascular disease.

1.87 a **True** b **True** c **True** d **False** e **False**
The term peripheral neuropathy is used to denote a generalized neuropathy in which many peripheral nerves are affected. There are many causes: the commonest are excess alcohol, diabetes mellitus, renal failure, connective tissue disease, vitamin deficiencies, and bronchial carcinoma. Carpel tunnel syndrome is an entrapment neuropathy, and only the median nerve is affected.

1.88 a **False** b **True** c **False** d **False** e **True**
In myasthenia gravis, the nicotinic acetylcholine receptors at the postsynaptic receptors of the neuromuscular junctions are blocked or lysed by antibodies. Myasthenia gravis is commoner in women than in men. Ptosis, diplopia, and abnormal fatigue of head and neck muscles are common. The symptoms often temporarily improve within half a minute of an intravenous edrophonium chloride (Tensilon) injection, but this only lasts about 3 min.

1.89 a **True** b **False** c **True** d **False** e **True**
Salicylate poisoning causes metabolic acidosis, which is partially compensated by hyperventilation. Hence, a mixture of metabolic acidosis and respiratory alkalosis occurs. Tinnitus, deafness, and blurring of vision are common symptoms. In general, gastric lavage or induced vomiting is not indicated in overdoses of most drugs if ingestion has taken place more than 4 h previously. However, aspirin and tricyclic antidepressants are exceptions as they delay gastric emptying. In severe salicylate poisoning, forced alkaline diuresis (when saline, dextrose, and sodium bicarbonate are given in rotation) is the preferred treatment. If this is contraindicated, haemodialysis is an alternative treatment.

1.90 a **True** b **True** c **True** d **True** e **True**
Clinical features of systemic amyloidosis result from deposition of amyloid in various organs. For example, hepatosplenomegaly and macroglossia may occur. Amyloid may be deposited in the kidneys, causing nephrotic syndrome and renal failure. Deposition of amyloid in the heart may restrict heart movements and cause cardiac failure. Carpel tunnel syndrome results form compression of the median nerve.

1.91 a **True** b **True** c **False** d **True** e **False**
Live vaccines are available for hepatitis A and B. Hepatitis D is an incomplete RNA particle contained in a shell of hepatitis B antigen, and its replication is dependent on the presence of hepatitis B virus. Hence, hepatitis B vaccine is also protective against hepatitis D. No vaccines are available yet for hepatitis C or hepatitis E.

1.92 a **True** b **False** c **True** d **True** e **False**
Most disorders caused by enzyme deficiencies are inherited recessively. Wilson's disease is autosomal recessive in inheritance and glucose-6-phosphate dehydrogenase deficiency is sex-linked recessive in inheritance.

1.93 a **True** b **True** c **True** d **True** e **False**
obese people have an increased risk of a wide range of disorders. These include

psychological problems, ischaemic heart disease, hypertension, strokes, diabetes, varicose veins, hiatus hernia, gallstones, and osteoarthritis. Hyperthyroidism causes weight loss.

1.94 a **True** b **False** c **False** d **False** e **True**
Achalasia is a disease associated with lack of peristalsis of the oesophagus, and failure of the lower oesophageal sphincter to relax on swallowing. The characteristic symptoms are intermittent dysphagia of both solids and liquids; retrosternal chest pain sometimes occurs. Abnormalities may be detected on chest radiograph (showing a dilated oesophagus); a barium swallow (showing dilatation of oesophagus and lack of peristalsis) and oesophageal manometry may demonstrate both lack of peristalsis of the oesophagus and failure of the lower oesophageal sphincter to relax, and can be diagnostic.

1.95 a **True** b **True** c **True** d **True** e **True**
A wide range of neurological features occurs in people with AIDS, although the mechanism is not well understood. These include sensory or motor neuropathy, autonomic neuropathy, and dementia in the late stages. Depressive and psychotic features may occur. These may be either organic manifestations of AIDS or psychological reactions to the diagnosis.

1.96 a **True** b **True** c **True** d **True** e **False**
Crohn's disease is associated with HLA-B27. Hence, there is an increased risk of ankylosing spondylitis. Monoarticular arthritis may also occur. Skin manifestations include erythema nodosum and pyoderma gangrenosum, although the latter is commoner in ulcerative colitis than Crohn's disease. Erythema marginatum is a feature of rheumatic fever. Eye manifestations include uveitis and episcleritis. Hepatic and biliary manifestations include gallstones, pericholangitis, sclerosing cholangitis, and cirrhosis of the liver.

1.97 a **False** b **False** c **True** d **False** e **False**
A macule is a *flat* circumscribed area of discoloration of skin. A papule is a *raised* area of skin. A nodule is a raised palpable area of skin more than 1 cm in diameter. Petichiae are small bruises less than 3 mm in diameter. Ecchymoses are bruises more than 3 mm in diameter. Purpura are large extravasation of blood into the skin, and do not blanch on pressure. A vesicle is a fluid-filled blister. A bulla is a large fluid-filled blister. A pustule is a blister filled with pus.

1.98 a **False** b **True** c **True** d **True** e **False**
Long-term topical steroid should be avoided as far as possible, especially if applied to the face. The least potent steroid cream with the desired effect should be used. Side-effects include thinning of the skin, telangiectasia, striae, and spread of local unsuspected infection.

1.99 a **False** b **False** c **True** d **True** e **False**
Psoriasis is a chronic skin condition which remits and relapses in an unpredictable

manner. It occurs most frequently in temperate countries, and is relatively rare in black people. The aetiology is uncertain, although it has HLA associations with HLA-B13, B16, and DR7; it may be triggered by infection, or by emotional or mechanical trauma. The skin lesions can be induced in normal areas of skin by scratching when the disease is active. This is known as Koebner's phenomenon. Pitting of the nails is common. Other associated lesions are onycholysis (separation of the nail from the underlying nail bed) and fissured nails. Joint disease occurs in about 10% of the patients.

1.100 a **True** b **True** c **True** d **False** e **True**
Recognized treatments of psoriatic skin lesions include dithranol, coal tar, topical steroids, retinoic acid derivatives, and psoralens with UVA (PUVA). Dithranol acts by inhibiting DNA synthesis. Topical vitamin D_3, low dose tetracycline, and cytotoxic drugs may be of limited use.

1.101 a **True** b **False** c **False** d **False** e **True**
Systematic lupus erythematosus (SLE) occurs about 9 times more frequently in women than in men. Cutaneous manifestations of SLE include photosensitivity, butterfly rash on the cheeks, nailfold capillary dilatation, and Raynaud's phenomenon of the fingers. However, Raynaud's phenomenon occurs more frequently in systemic sclerosis than in SLE. The cutaneous manifestations of SLE closely resemble those of discoid lupus erythematosus. Treatment of the cutaneous manifestations of SLE and discoid lupus erythematosus include antimalarials (e.g. hydroxychloroquiine) and immunosuppressive drugs (e.g. steroids, azothhiaprine).

1.102 a **False** b **False** c **False** d **False** e **True**
Basal cell carcinoma of the skin are also known as rodent ulcers. They occur most frequently in fair-skinned middle-aged or elderly people, especially in tropical countries. They are located most frequently in sun-exposed areas, especially the side of the nose and around the orbit. The characteristic appearance is an ulcerated papule or nodule with a pearly edge, and with superficial dilated blood vessels over the lesion. Although they may be locally invasive, they very rarely metastasise.

1.103 a **False** b **True** c **True** d **True** e **False**
Vitiligo is a relatively common skin condition affecting about 1% of the population. The main pathology is loss of melanocytes from the affected areas of skin. It is thought to be an autoimmune disease. Antimelanocyte antibodies are sometime detected in the blood, and there is an association between vitiligo and other autoimmune disorders such as thyroid diseases and pernicious anaemia. Affected subjects often have a positive family history. Unfortunately, none of the treatments available is particularly effective.

1.104 a **True** b **True** c **False** d **True** e **False**
The horizontal eye movements are coordinated by the 'centre for lateral gaze' in the brain stem on each side. Impulses from the centres pass to the ipsilateral lateral rectus via the sixth nerve, and the contralateral medial rectus via the medial longitudinal fasciculus and the third nerve. Hence, a lesion on the medial longitudinal fasciculus

would result in failure of the ipsilateral eye to adduct. It is also associated with coarse nystagmus of the contralateral eye on abduction. The pupil size is normal.

1.105 a **True** b **False** c **False** d **True** e **False**

Characteristic signs of a complete third cranial nerve palsy include unilateral complete ptosis, abduction and depression of the ipsilateral eye ('down and out'), and a fixed dilated pupil. However, the contralateral pupil constricts when light is shone onto the ipsilateral eye, as the ipsilateral optic nerve is intact.

1.106 a **True** b **True** c **True** d **True** e **True**

Causes of mononeuritis multiplex include diabetes mellitus, connective tissue disease such as polyarteritis nodosa, sarcoidosis, malignancy, drugs, toxin, alcohol, and amyloidosis. Leprosy is the commonest cause worldwide.

1.107 a **True** b **False** c **True** d **False** e **True**

The spinal levels of the tendon jerks are:

biceps and supinator jerks	C5–6
triceps jerk	C7
knee jerk	L3–4
ankle jerk	S1

1.108 a **False** b **True** c **True** d **False** e **False**

Signs of pseudobulbar palsy are upper motor neurone lesions of the lower cranial nerves. They include a stiff, spastic, and weak tongue, dysarthria, difficulties with swallowing, and emotional lability. It is distinguished from bulbar palsy (a lower motor neurone lesion) in that the jaw jerk is characteristically exaggerated, and that the tongue is not wasted.

1.109 a **True** b **False** c **True** d **True** e **False**

Signs of a lateral cerebellar lesion include ataxic gait (with a tendency to fall towards the side of the lesion), intention tremor with past pointing, clumsy rapid alternating movements (dysdiadochokinesis), and horizontal nystagmus towards the side of the lesion. Truncal ataxia is a symptom of mid-line cerebellar lesions.

1.110 a **True** b **True** c **True** d **False** e **False**

Mitral stenosis results in increase in left atrial pressure, left atrial pressure hypertrophy, and dilatation. This in turn causes increase in the pulmonary hypertension and pulmonary oedema, and right ventricular hypertrophy. Systemic embolization may occur with atrial fibrillation.

1.111 a **True** b **False** c **True** d **True** e **True**

Dystrophic myotonica is an autosomal dominant condition. The main clinical features are distal muscle weakness, myotonia, ptosis, frontal balding, cataracts, cardiomyopathy, and glucose intolerance.

1.112 a **True** b **True** c **True** d **True** e **False**

Diseases associated with exposure to asbestos include pleural plaques, bilateral diffuse pleural thickening, asbestosis (progressive fibrosis of the lung usually after 5 years of exposure), and mesothelioma (usually after more than 20 years of exposure). Asbestos exposure and cigarette smoking have an additive effect in the increase of the risk of bronchial carcinoma.

1.113 a **False** b **False** c **False** d **True** e **False**
Chronic bronchitis and emphysema (or chronic obstructive airway disease) occurs more frequently in men than women. Cigarette smoking is the most important aetiological factor, and the risk of a heavy smoker developing the disease is more than 15 times that of a non-smoker. α_1-Antitrypsin deficiency only accounts for about 2% of all cases. *Streptococcus pneumoniae* and *Haemophilus influenzae* are the commonest organisms causing acute exacerbation. A high haemoglobin level is characteristic as a response to chronic hypoxaemia.

1.114 a **True** b **False** c **True** d **True** e **False**
Causes of clubbing can be broadly classified as respiratory, cardiovascular, gastrointestinal, and congenital. Respiratory causes include carcinoma of the bronchus, lung abscess, bronchiectasis, pulmonary fibrosis, and pleural tumours (e.g. mesothelioma). Cardiovascular causes include subacute infective endocarditis and congenital cyanotic heart disease. Gastrointestinal causes include inflammatory bowel disease and cirrhosis of the liver.

1.115 a **False** b **True** c **True** d **False** e **True**
Small or moderate size pulmonary embolus may either produce no abnormal ECG changes, or only sinus tachycardia. In the presence of a large embolus, there may be right atrial dilatation, right ventricular dilatation, or right ventricular hypertrophy. Right atrial dilatation is associated with tall peaked P waves in lead II. Right ventricular dilatation and hypertrophy may produce right axis deviation, T wave inversion in V1–3, and partial or complete right bundle branch block. The S1–Q3–T3 pattern is due to right ventricular strain.

1.116 a **True** b **True** c **True** d **False** e **False**
In nephrotic syndrome, there is excessive excretion of protein in urine, a low serum albumin level, oedema, and a high cholesterol level. Abnormal liver function tests may indicate liver disease as the cause for the low albumin level. The triglyceride level is often high.

1.117 a **False** b **False** c **True** d **False** e **True**
Haemolysis causes breakdown of red cells and a reduced red cell life span. The bone marrow compensates by increasing red cell production. Hence, the reticulocyte count is raised. The haemoglobin released is initially bound to heptoglobin. Hence, the heptoglobin level is reduced. When this is saturated, the haemoglobin is broken down into haem and globin molecules. Unconjugated bilirubin is formed from the haem molecules, which also increases the urinary urobilinogin.

1.118 a **True** b **False** c **True** d **False** e **True**
Systemic sclerosis is a condition that affects many different systems. The skin,

oesophagus, and lungs are most frequently affected. The kidneys are affected in about a third of patients, and this may lead to renal failure and malignant hypertension. Antinucleolar and anticentromere antibodies are specifically elevated, and are found in more than 50% of patients. Unfortunately, there are currently no effective treatments to halt the progress of the disease.

1.119 a **False** b **False** c **True** d **False** e **False**
The aetiology of polymyalgia rheumatica is unknown, although it may be associated with malignancy. It is part of the spectrum of conditions with giant cell arteritis as the basic pathological lesion. It occurs most frequently in the elderly, with women affected 3 times more frequently than men. The characteristic symptoms are pain and stiffness of proximal muscles, especially in the morning. Common associated symptoms include anorexia, malaise, weight loss, and low grade fever. The ESR is characteristically elevated. The treatment is oral corticosteroid, which should be reduced very gradually and continue for at least about 18 months.

1.120 a **False** b **True** c **False** d **True** e **True**
There are numerous causes for inappropriate ADH secretion, including carcinoma, lung, and central nervous system (CNS) lesions. Small cell carcinoma of the lung is a frequent cause, but squamous cell carcinoma often secretes inappropriate PTH. The symptoms are due to a low plasma sodium level, and include confusion, irritability, and fits. The low plasma osmolality is associated with an inappropriately high level of urinary sodium excretion. The treatment is fluid restriction. If this is not tolerated, or if this is ineffective, demeclocycline may be used to inhibit the action of ADH on the kidney.

1.121 a **True** b **True** c **True** d **False** e **False**
For a diagnosis of brain death in the UK, there must be an irreversible condition causing severe structural brain damage, and a positive diagnosis must be obtained. There must be complete loss of brain stem function, as evidenced by lack of papillary response, lack of spontaneous eye movements or response to caloric testing, absent corneal, blink and cough reflex, and absent response to deep painful stimuli. There must be no respiratory effort on removal of ventilatory support and with a sufficiently high partial pressure of carbon dioxide in the blood. Any possible effects due to hypothermia or drugs must be excluded. However, there are no requirements to perform a EEG or cerebral blood flow study.

1.122 a **False** b **False** c **True** d **False** e **False**
Systemic sclerosis is a multisystem syndrome with inflammation, fibrosis, and vasculitis. It is very uncommon, with an incidence of about 1 in 100,000, and occurs more commonly in women and in those with a positive family history. It includes a wide range of disease spectrum ranging from Raynaud's phenomenon, localized scleroderma (skin thickening), to diffuse systemic sclerosis with cardiac, renal, and pulmonary involvement. It is associated with positive ANA in some patients. Anti-Scl–70/DNA topoisomerase-1 enzyme is quite specific, although it is present

in only a fifth of the patients. The ESR is usually normal, and the serum immunoglobulins level is usually increased.

1.123 a **True** b **False** c **False** d **False** e **False**
Ankylosing spondylitis is a chronic progressive disease affecting the axial skeleton and proximal large joints. It occurs more frequently in those between 20 and 40 years of age and in those with the HLA–B27 gene. Although over 90% of those with ankylosing spondylitis have the HLA–B27 gene, only about 5% of those with the gene develop the disease. The gene has a equal sex distribution, but the disease tends to be more severe in men than in women.

1.124 a **False** b **True** c **False** d **False** e **False**
Compared with inflammatory back pain, mechanical back pain is more likely to be of sudden onset, precipitated by movement, unilateral, worse in the evenings, and aggravated by exercise. Morning stiffness usually suggests an inflammatory cause.

1.125 a **True** b **True** c **False** d **True** e **False**
Osteoarthritis particularly affects the distal interphalangeal joints (DIP), and may cause either flexion or lateral deviation. Enlargements of the distal and proximal interphalangeal joints are known as Herberden's and Bouchard's nodes respectively, and are characteristic of osteoarthritis. Subluxation of the carpometacarpal joint of the thumb is also common. Rheumatoid arthritis typically affects the metacarpophalangeal joints (MCP) and the proximal interphalangeal joints (PIP). Swan neck deformity, boutonniäre deformity, and Z-shaped deformity are characteristic of rheumatoid arthritis. Swan-neck deformity is due to hyperextension of the PIP joint with flexion at the DIP joint.

1.126 a **True** b **True** c **True** d **True** e **True**
Osteoporosis is a reduction of the quantity of bone per unit volume, and predisposes to fractures. Idiopathic osteoporosis commonly occurs in postmenopausal women. Secondary osteoporosis may be due to endocrine abnormalities (e.g. sex hormone deficiency such as untreated Turner's syndrome, hyperthyroidism, and excessive glucocorticoids), malignancies (e.g. multiple myeloma), chronic renal failure, alcoholism, and hereditary causes such as osteogenesis imperfecta.

1.127 a **True** b **False** c **False** d **False** e **True**
Recognized clinical features of hypocalcaemia include neurological and cardiovascular symptoms. Neurological symptoms include peripheral parathesiae and circumoral numbness, tetany, laryngeal stridor, and convulsions. Positive Chvostek's sign (twitching of the facial muscle on gentle tapping of the facial nerve) and Trousseau's sign (tetanic spasm of the hand caused by inflation of the sphygmomanometer cuff at the arm) may also occur. Cardiovascular symptoms may include arrhythmia. Polyuria, constipation, and drowsiness are features of hypercalcaemia.

1.128 a **False** b **True** c **False** d **True** e **True**
Clinical signs of infective endocarditis include fever, anaemia, clubbing of the finger,

changing heart murmurs, splenomegaly, and signs of infarcts due to embolism (e.g. splinter haemorrhages, Osler's nodes on the finger pads, Roth spots in the retina, and haematuria).

1.129 a **True** b **False** c **True** d **True** e **False**
Sinus tachycardia is a heart rate of over 100 beats/min in sinus rhythm. Causes for sinus tachycardia include fever, anaemia, exercise, anxiety, and thyrotoxicosis. Hypothyroidism causes sinus bradycardia, and Wolff-Parkinson-White syndrome characteristically causes supraventricular tachycardia.

1.130 a **False** b **True** c **False** d **False** e **False**
Characteristic features of right bundle block on the ECG include prolonged QRS interval, RSR pattern in the right ventricular leads (V1 and V2), and other abnormalities in the ST segments in the right ventricular leads (e.g. late S waves, T inversion). Absent P waves are characteristic of atrial fibrillation. RSR pattern in the V5 and V6 leads may be caused by left bundle branch block. Progressive lengthening of PR interval on each successive beat is characteristic of Mobitz 1 second-degree heart block.

1.131 a **True** b **True** c **True** d **False** e **False**
Dilated cardiomyopathy is characterized by dilatation of the ventricles, and is the commonest form of cardiomyopathy. It occurs more frequently in middle-aged men. In many cases, the aetiology is unknown. However, previous viral infection and alcoholism are thought to be important causes. Relevant family history is usually absent. The characteristic clinical presentation is progressive cardiac failure, mitral, and tricuspid regurgitation due to ventricular dilatation and atrial fibrillation. A family history and sudden death frequently occurs in hypertrophic cardiomyopathy.

1.132 a **True** b **False** c **True** d **True** e **False**
Corticosteroids have non-specific immunosuppressive properties, and are used in the treatment of neurological diseases mediated by immune responses such as cerebral lupus, other cerebral vasculitis, myasthenia gravis, dermatomyositis, and relapses of multiple sclerosis.

1.133 a **True** b **True** c **False** d **False** e **True**
Trigeminal neuralgia characteristically occurs in those above the age of 40. The pain is brief but very severe, and is characteristically confined to one division of the supply of the trigeminal nerve. It is often precipitated by touch and wind, and patients may avoid washing. It is occasionally associated with other neurological disorders such as multiple sclerosis or acoustic tumour, and they must be excluded. Carbamazepine is the treatment of choice. A markedly raised ESR in the presence of headache or facial pain suggests temporal arteritis.

1.134 a **True** b **True** c **False** d **True** e **True**
Papilloedema is characterized by a swollen pink optic disc, blurred disc margins, and haemorrhages at the disc margins. It is usually bilateral. As the blind spot corresponds with the optic disc, papilloedema results in an enlarged blind spot. The

commonest cause for papilloedema is increased intracranial pressure due to either space-occupying lesions or hydrocephalus. Rarer causes include benign intracranial hypertension, Guillain–Barré syndrome, and sarcoidosis.

1.135 a **False** b **False** c **True** d **True** e **True**
The cardinal clinical features of Parkinson's disease include bradykinesia, resting tremor, lead-pipe or cogwheel rigidity, and loss of postural reflexes. Bradykinesia and rigidity lead to the characteristic festinating gait. Other classical features include reduced blinking, positive persistent glabella tap, blepharospasm, loss of arm swing, soft monotonous voice, and micrographia.

1.136 a **False** b **True** c **False** d **True** e **False**
Transudative pleural effusion is clear watery fluid in the pleural space with a low protein content. They generally result from increased hydrostatic pressure across the pulmonary capillaries (e.g. cardiac failure) or hypoproteinaemia (e.g. nephrotic syndrome, cirrhosis of the liver). Exudative pleural effusion is generally caused by primary lung disease with pleural inflammation.

1.137 a **False** b **False** c **True** d **True** e **False**
Carcinoid syndrome occurs only in the presence of carcinoid tumour with hepatic metastases, as the secretory products from carcinoid tumours are inactivated on reaching the liver. The source of carcinoid tumour is usually from APUD cells in the small intestine. The products secreted by carcinoid tumours consist of mainly serotonin (5-hydroxytryptamine), but also include kinins, histamines, and prostaglandins. The clinical features include facial flushing, diarrhoea, attacks of wheezing, and right-sided cardiac lesions such as tricuspid or pulmonary stenosis. The diagnosis is confirmed by increased 24 h urinary excretion of 5-HIAA (a breakdown product of serotonin).

1.138 a **False** b **True** c **False** d **True** e **True**
Common causes of cirrhosis of the liver include alcohol and hepatitis B and C infections. Rarer causes include metabolic disorders (e.g. Wilson's disease, haemochromatosis, α_1-antitrypsin deficiency, galactosaemia), drugs (e.g. methyldopa) and autoimmune disease (e.g. primary biliary cirrhosis). Hepatitis A may cause viral hepatitis with jaundice, but it does not lead to cirrhosis. Hepatitis E is water-borne or spread by the faecal-oral route and does not lead to cirrhosis.

1.139 a **False** b **False** c **True** d **False** e **False**
The anion gap is equal to $[(Na^+ + K^+)-(Cl^- + HCO_3^-)]$. The normal value is below 20 mmol/litre, and this reflects the concentration of phosphates, sulphates, and normal level of organic acids. It is useful in classifying metabolic acidoses into those which are predominantly due to addition to organic acids, and those which are due to loss of bicarbonate. Metabolic acidosis due to addition of organic acids (e.g. lactic acids) is associated with increased anion gap. Those which are due to loss of bicarbonate (e.g. renal tubular acidosis) are associated with normal anion gap, as the lost bicarbonate ions are replaced by chloride ions (hyperchloraemic acidosis).

1.140 a **False** b **True** c **True** d **False** e **True**
Hypokalaemia is mainly caused by either increased output from the kidneys (e.g. proximal renal tubular acidosis, hyperaldosteronism, or steroid therapy), or from the gastrointestinal tract (e.g. gastroenteritis, villous adenoma of the rectum). Spironolactone is a potassium-sparing diuretic. Addison's disease is associated with a lack of mineralcorticoids and a high potassium level.

1.141 a **False** b **False** c **True** d **True** e **False**
Osteomalacia is characterized by vitamin D deficiency. This is associated with a low serum calcium, high serum phosphate, and a high alkaline phosphatase level. There is often compensatory secondary hyperparathyroidism. Hence, the PTH level is high. The alanine aminotransferase (ALT) level is normal.

1.142 a **False** b **False** c **False** d **True** e **True**
Adult polycystic kidney disease has an autosomal dominant inheritance with complete penetrance, and is commoner than the autosomal recessive infantile polycystic disease. The cysts are usually present by early adulthood in the renal cortex. As the cysts enlarge, they compress and destroy normal renal tissues, resulting in steady decline of renal function. It may present with hypertension, haematuria, or end-stage renal failure. It is associated with cysts in other organs, including berry aneurysms in the cerebral arteries, liver, pancreas, and spleen. Patients with berry aneurysms are susceptible to subarachnoid haemorrhage, especially in the presence of hypertension.

1.143 a **False** b **False** c **True** d **True** e **True**
Essential hypertension affects more than 5% of the population, and is commoner than secondary hypertension. It usually presents at 25–55 years of age, and occurs more frequently and severely in black people of African origin. It is associated with sodium retention, and it is thought that elevated levels of natriuretic hormone inhibit sodium/potassium ATPase, and increase renal sodium excretion. Essential hypertension predisposes to increased risk of ischaemic heart disease and cerebrovascular accidents.

1.144 a **True** b **False** c **True** d **False** e **True**
Causes of eosinophilia include allergy (e.g. atopic asthma, allergic rhinitis), parasitic infections (e.g. schistosomiasis), and haematological malignancies (e.g. Hodgkin's disease). Atypical lymphocytosis is characteristic in glandular fever, and neutrophilia is characteristic in legionnaire's disease.

1.145 a **False** b **False** c **True** d **False** e **False**
Haematological findings characteristic of iron-deficiency anaemia include a hypochromic microcytic blood film, a low mean cell volume (MCV) and a low mean corpuscular haemoglobin concentration (MCHC), reflecting small red cells with low haemoglobin concentration. The serum iron concentration is low, the total iron binding capacity is high. The serum ferritin level correlates with the total body iron, and

is low. Haemoglobin electrophoresis is normal. An abnormal haemoglobin electrophoresis would indicate thalassaemia.

1.146 a **True** b **False** c **True** d **False** e **True**
Characteristic symptoms of hypothyroidism include lethargy, weight gain, cold intolerance, dry skin, husky voice, constipation, and occasionally depression. Characteristic signs include myxodema facies, bradycardia, and delayed relaxation of tendon jerks. Occasionally, a goitre is palpable.

1.147 a **True** b **False** c **False** d **True** e **True**
Phaeochromocytoma are tumours arising from the sympathetic chains. Although the majority (90%) arise from the adrenal medulla, they may arise outside. Only about 10% are malignant. Tumours from the adrenal medulla secrete both noradrenaline and adrenaline, but those arising from outside secrete only noradrenaline. Once the tumour is diagnosed, it should be treated by an α-receptor blocking agent (e.g. phenoxybenzamine) followed by a β-receptor blocking agent (e.g. propranolol) to prevent hypertensive crises.

1.148 a **True** b **True** c **False** d **True** e **True**
Gynaecomastia may be physiological (e.g. in the newborn, at puberty). Pathological causes of gynaecomastia may be due to excess oestrogen production (e.g. Leydig cell testicular tumour, liver disease, adrenal tumour), testosterone failure (e.g. testicular failure, Klinefelter's syndrome), and drugs such as digoxin, spironolactone, and cimetidine. Ranitidine does not have this side-effect.

1.149 a **False** b **True** c **False** d **True** e **True**
Clinical signs characteristic of hyperlipidaemia include corneal arcus, xanthelasma, tendon or palmar xanthomata, and lipaemia retinalis (cholesterol crystals seen in the retinal arteries). Necrobiosis lipoidica is characteristic of diabetes mellitus, and Kayser-Fleischer ring is characteristic of Wilson's disease due to deposition of copper on the cornea.

1.150 a **True** b **True** c **False** d **True** e **True**
A wide range of treatments for acne vulgaris is available. In mild disease, topical disinfectants (e.g. betadine, chlorhexadine), keratolytic (e.g. benzoyl peroxide, salicylic acid) or antibiotics (e.g. erythromycin) should be used. If the disease is moderately severe, a combination of topical and systemic (e.g. oral erythromycin, cyproterone acetate, or the contraceptive pill for women) could be used. Isotretinoin should be considered only for those with severe acne which fails to respond to other treatments.

2 *Surgery*

Questions

2.1 *Fibroadenomas*

a characteristically occur in postmenopausal women
b are usually firmly attached to the underlying tissues
c progress to carcinoma in about 50% of the cases
d do not usually cause pain
e sometimes disappear spontaneously

2.2 *Risk factors for the development of carcinoma of the breast include*

a a positive family history
b increased age
c early menopause
d delayed menarche
e nulliparity

2.3 *Which of the following factors in breast carcinoma indicate a favourable prognosis?*

a high oestrogen receptor (ER) activity
b smooth contour
c presence of undifferentiated cells
d reactive hyperplasia in the regional lymph nodes
e large size

2.4 *A goitre*

a may be visible
b appears in the upper part of the neck
c characteristically moves downwards on swallowing
d may occur physiologically during pregnancy
e may cause dysphagia

2.5 *Primary hyperthyroidism (Graves' disease)*

a is the commonest cause of hyperthyroidism
b occurs more frequently in males
c is usually associated with loss of appetite
d may be associated with pretibial myxoedema

e is associated with an exaggerated increase in TSH in response to intravenous TRH injection

2.6 *Postoperative complications of thyroidectomy include*

a hypercalcaemia
b stridor
c hoarse voice
d asphyxia
e hypothyroidism

2.7 *Which of the following statements about thyroid cancers is/are true?*

a follicular carcinoma is the commonest type
b papillary carcinoma has the best prognosis
c medullary carcinoma is associated with increased calcitonin secretion
d anaplastic carcinoma is commonest below the age of 45
e Horner's syndrome may result from anaplastic thyroid carcinoma

2.8 *Parathyroid adenoma*

a is the commonest cause of primary hyperparathyrodism
b affects males more than females
c may cause renal calculi
d may cause chronic pancreatitis
e is associated with a high phosphate level

2.9 *Recognized treatment of acromegaly include*

a bromocriptine
b tamoxifen
c external radiation
d trans-spheonoidal surgical removal
e radioactive pituitary

2.10 *Coronary artery bypass grafting*

a may be performed without coronary angiography
b is usually performed using a synthetic graft
c has a mortality rate of about 1–2%
d is indicated for angina pectoris caused by triple vessel disease which does not respond to drug treatment
e results in complete relief of symptoms in less than a third of the patients

2.11 *Risk factors for peripheral vascular disease include*

a smoking
b diabetes
c hypertension
d beta blocker medication
e tall stature

2.12 ***Which of the following statements about peripheral vascular disease of the lower limbs is/are true?***

a the symptoms characteristically deteriorate steadily
b rest pain is relieved by raising the legs
c rest pain of the legs at rest is common in pure aorto-iliac disease
d impotence may be a symptom of aorto-iliac disease
e the commonest site of occlusion is the superficial femoral artery

2.13 ***Signs of chronic ischaemia of the lower limbs include***

a warmth
b brittle nails
c marked pallor on elevation of the legs
d leg ulcers
e dependent rubor

2.14 ***Which of the following statements about arterial bypass graft is/are true?***

a a synthetic graft gives a better outcome than a autogenous vein graft
b it is possible to construct a femoro-peroneal bypass
c it is the treatment of choice for a short femoral occlusion
d patency rate is higher for aorto-iliac segment reconstruction than femoral popliteal bypass
e if a saphenous vein graft is used a femoral popliteal bypass, the vein should either be reversed or the valves of the vein damaged

2.15 ***Which of the following are common causes for failure of the flap to heal following amputation?***

a a level of amputation higher than the optimal
b haematoma formation
c inadequate blood supply
d insufficient tension on the stitch line
e infection

2.16 ***Recognized treatment for acute thrombotic arterial occlusion of the lower limbs include***

a systematic antihypertensive drug
b systemic heparin
c streptokinase delivered into the thrombus
d emergency thrombectomy
e a bypass operation

2.17 ***Which of the following statements about abdominal aortic aneurysms is/are true?***

a they occur above the level of the renal arteries in more than 50% of the cases

b they are associated with hypertension
c aneurysms are more likely to rupture the larger their sizes
d elective repair is indicated for aortic aneurysms of 6cm in diameter
e they may be asymptomatic

2.18 *Varicose veins*

a are more common in men than women
b is more common in those whose jobs require prolonged standing
c should be examined with the patient lying down
d may be familial
e may be secondary to deep vein thrombosis

2.19 *Thyroglossal cysts*

a may be acquired
b usually present in the first year of life
c are often nodular
d characteristically move upwards on tongue protrusion
e commonly present as right-sided neck swelling

2.20 *Sebaceous cysts*

a rarely occur on the scalp
b characteristically possess a punctum on careful examination
c may be excised under local anaesthetic
d contain cheesy white debris
e should be excised immediately if they are infected

2.21 *Common causes of bilateral painful parotid swelling include*

a acute parotitis
b parotid calculi
c mumps
d Sjîgren's syndrome
e parotid neoplasia

2.22 *Which of the following statements regarding salivary gland tumours is/are true?*

a neoplasia in the submandibular gland is more common than in the parotid gland
b more than 50% of the sublingual gland tumours are benign
c a parotid mass associated with facial nerve palsy is strongly suggestive of malignancy
d most parotid tumours are pleomorphic adenoma
e surgical removal is mandatory for all pleomorphic salivary adenoma

2.23 *Clinical features of acute peritonitis include*

a guarding

b increased bowel sound
c deep breathing
d tachycardia
e agitation

2.24 *The indirect inguinal hernia*

a is the commonest type of abdominal wall hernias
b passes above the pubic tubercle
c passes lateral to the pubic tubercle
d cannot be controlled by placing a finger at the internal inguinal ring
e results from the failure of obliteration of the processus vaginalis

2.25 *Which of the following statements about achalasia is/are true?*

a dysphagia is the cardinal symptom
b swallowing solids is often more difficult than swallowing liquid
c it predisposes to carcinoma
d barium swallow often shows constriction above the lower oesophageal sphincter
e it predisposes to aspiration pneumonia

2.26 *Which of the following statements about carcinoma of the oesophagus is/are true?*

a adenocarcinoma are the commonest
b most carcinoma occur at the middle third of the oesophagus
c it has an overall 5 year survival of more than 30%
d it is commoner in Western countries than the Far East
e hoarseness is a late manifestation

2.27 *Which of the following statements about perforated peptic ulcers is/are true?*

a perforated gastric ulcer is more common than perforated duodenal ulcer
b the typical presentation is sudden onset of severe abdominal pain
c absence of free air under the diaphragm on erect abdominal radiograph excludes the diagnosis
d a nasogastric tube should be inserted as soon as possible
e perforated gastric ulcer is best treated by simple closure

2.28 *Recognized complications of surgical treatment for peptic ulcer include*

a the dumping syndrome
b reactive hypoglycaemia
c diarrhoea

d anaemia
e vomiting

2.29 *Diverticular disease of the colon*

a occurs most commonly in the transverse colon
b is commoner with increasing age
c is associated with high roughage in the diet
d is associated with muscle thickening on barium enema
e may be asymptomatic

2.30 *Complications of diverticular disease of the colon include*

a pericolic abscess
b colovesical fistula
c faecal peritonitis
d intestinal obstruction
e malignant changes

2.31 *Which of the following features are more common in ulcerative colitis than in Crohn's disease?*

a fistula formation
b continuous colonic lesions
c full thickness bowel involvement
d colonic carcinoma
e anal lesions

2.32 *Adenomatous polyp of the colon*

a is the commonest type of colonic polyp
b almost always causes rectal bleeding
c may be removed colonoscopically
d often causes excessive mucus discharge
e predisposes to malignancy

2.33 *Which of the following are predisposing factors for large-bowel carcinoma?*

a negroes
b family history of large-bowel carcinoma
c villous adenoma
d high fibre diet
e ulcerative colitis

2.34 *Which of the following symptoms and signs are frequently found in the early stages of carcinoma of the caecum?*

a severe rectal bleeding

b constipation
c abdominal distension
d weight loss
e anaemia

2.35 *Which of the following statements about acute appendicitis is/are true?*

a it begins with well-localized para-umbilical pain
b the pain shifted to the right iliac fossa after some time
c anorexia is frequently present
d diarrhoea may be a symptom of pelvic appendicitis
e rectal examination is unnecessary if there is no right iliac fossa tenderness

2.36 *Which of the following clinical features are common in the early stages of a high small bowel obstruction?*

a abdominal distension
b vomiting
c constipation
d low abdominal pain
e dehydration

2.37 *Which of the following statements about haemorrhoids is/are true?*

a they are said to be of first degree if they prolapse during defaecation but return spontaneously afterwards
b they are said to be of third degree if they prolapse during defaecation and remain prolapsed
c they often cause bright red rectal bleeding
d symptomatic first degree haemorrhoids may be treated by injection sclerotherapy
e immediate haemorrhoidectomy is mandatory for thrombosed haemorrhoids

2.38 *Which of the following conditions may predispose to ano-rectal abscess formation?*

a Crohn's disease
b AIDS
c tuberculosis
d rectal carcinoma
e past history of anorectal abscess

2.39 *Pilonidal sinus*

a may occur on the hands of barbers
b usually occurs anterior to the anus
c characteristically contains hairs

d occurs more commonly in the elderly
e is best drained under local anaesthetic

2.40 *Venous portosystematic anastamosis occurs*

a at the junction between the oesophagus and the stomach
b at the junction between the stomach and the jejunum
c in the periumbilical area
d at the caecum
e in the anorectal area

2.41 *The Minnesota tube (used in the treatment of acute oesophageal bleeding)*

a has three lumina
b is usually left in place for at least 3 days
c allows aspiration of the stomach content
d allows aspiration of the pharyngeal content
e may be used to directly compress both the oesophagogastric junction and the oesophageal varices

2.42 *Treatments which may be used to prevent further bleeding from oesophageal varices include*

a injection sclerotherapy
b ventriculo-peritoneal shunt
c peritoneo-venous shunt
d endoscopic banding
e highly selective vagotomy

2.43 *Gallstones*

a are commoner in females
b are commoner in Asian countries
c are visible on plain radiograph in over 50% of the cases
d may cause acute cholecystitis
e may cause obstructive jaundice

2.44 *Which of the following statements about acute cholecystitis is/are true?*

a it often precedes biliary colic
b severe right hypochondrial pain radiating to the right subscapsular region is a characteristic feature
c it usually settles within 36 h
d Murphy's sign may be presente
e Jaundice may be present during an acute attack

2.45 *Which of the following statements about cholecystectomy is/are true?*

a it can be performed laparoscopically
b an operative cholangiography is indicated in a patient with previous history of jaundice
c cholecystectomy is indicated if gallstones are demonstrated on ultrasound
d postoperative complication includes biliary peritonitis
e postoperative complication includes bile duct stricture

2.46 *Which of the following measures are appropriate in the management of acute pancreatitis?*

a opiate injection
b increase oral fluid intake
c urine output monitoring
d resection of the pancreas
e intravenous steroid

2.47 *Common clinical features of carcinoma of the head of the pancreas include*

a weight loss
b dark urine
c dark stool
d palpable gallbladder
e abdominal distension

2.48 *Symptoms of benign prostatic hyperplasia include*

a urinary frequency
b nocturia
c poor stream or urine
d postmicturition dribbling
e urinary urgency

2.49 *A stone in the right lower ureter*

a typically causes pain which occurs in waves
b may cause haematuria
c may be disintegrated with laser lithothripsy
d requires open surgery for removal in more than 90% of the cases
e can be demonstrated by intravenous urogram (IVU)

2.50 *Which of the following statements about renal carcinoma is/are true?*

a it is commoner in women than men
b it commonly secrete calcitonin

c polycythaemia is a recognized associated feature
d it may present with fever of unknown origin
e chemotherapy is the main treatment

2.51 *Diverticular disease*

a most commonly occurs in the ascending colon
b is synonymous with diverticulitis
c may be associated with colicky abdominal pain relieved by defaecation
d should be treated with a low-fibre diet
e may cause rectal bleeding

2.52 *Which of the following scrotal lumps may be felt separately from the testis?*

a epididymal cyst
b hydrocoele
c testicular tumour
d orchitis
e epididymitis

2.53 *Torsion of the testis*

a is commonest in the elderly
b is rarely associated with vomiting
c should be treated conservatively if the diagnosis is uncertain
d causes sudden onset of testicular pain
e may require bilateral fixation procedure

2.54 *Which of the following situations constitute sufficient consent for treatment?*

a consent from the wife of a 60 year old patient requiring inguinal hernia repair
b consent from a 9 year old boy for a squint operation
c consent from a 34 year old schizophrenic patient for an inguinal hernia repair
d consent from the mother of a 12 year old girl for appendectomy
e consent from the mother of a 20 year old mentally handicapped man (with a mental age of 3) for sterilization

2.55 *Which of the following presenting features of acute pancreatitis are associated with increased mortality risk?*

a Age less than 55 years
b white cell count of 20×10^9/litre
c glucose level of 6 mmol/litre
d serum amylase > 1000 U/ml
e haemoglobin of 14 g/litre

2.56 *A ganglion*

a arises from the underlying bone
b commonly appears on the dorsum of the wrist
c contains clear fluid
d is premalignant
e may be removed under regional anaesthesia

2.57 *Causes of faecal incontinence include*

a rectal prolapse
b faecal impaction
c dementia
d multiple sclerosis
e obstetric tears

2.58 *Which of the following statements about cancer of the prostate is/are true?*

a it has a peak incidence at 50 years of age
b it commonly metastasizes to bone
c PSA (prostatic specific antigen) can be used to monitor disease progression
d it is commoner in China and Japan than in the United Kingdom
e an irregular nodular hard prostate felt on rectal examination is diagnostic

2.59 *Malignant melanomas*

a are commoner in black people than in white people
b have become more common in the last decade
c are highly associated with exposure to sunlight
d seldom spread via the bloodstream
e should all be excised with a 2 mm clearance margin

2.60 *Which of the following statements about testicular tumour is/are true?*

a it occurs mainly in the elderly
b yolk cell tumour is the commonest type
c alfafetoprotein (AFP) and β-human chorionic gonadotropin (HCG) are useful tumour markers
d the 5 year survival rate for seminomas is less than 20%
e it may present with a painless testicular mass

2.61 *Recognized indications for CSF examination by lumbar puncture include suspected*

a meningitis
b intracranial space-occupying lesion

c subarachnoid haemorrhage
d subdural haemorrhage
e extradural haemorrhage

2.62 *Which of the following statements true about MRI compared to CT scanning, in the investigation of neurosurgical conditions?*

a it has a higher resolution
b it is more readily available
c it gives rise to a higher dose of ionizing radiation to the patient
d it is less suitable for visualizing structures neurological structures near bones
e it is more effective in the diagnosis of cervical disc prolapse

2.63 *Recognized causes for communicating hydrocephalus include*

a occlusion of the aqueduct of Sylvius by a tumour
b bacterial meningitis
c acoustic neuroma
d subarachnoid haemorrhage
e choroid plexus papilloma

2.64 *Recognized indications for admission to hospital after a history of head injury in a 40 year old male include*

a persistent and increasing drowsiness
b blood pressure 140/100 mm Hg
c generalized hyperreflexia
d left sided muscle weakness in the limbs
e skull fracture demonstrated on radiography

2.65 *Which of the following statements about extradural haematoma is/are true?*

a it occurs more frequently above the age of 45
b posterior fossa is the commonest site
c it is almost always associated with a clinical detectable skull fracture
d increasing drowsiness after a 'lucid' interval is characteristic
e a ventriculo-peritoneal shunt should be inserted

2.66 *Characteristic clinical features of subarachnoid haemorrhage include*

a a long history of frontal headache
b wavy lines across the visual fields
c neck stiffness
d photophobia
e increasing drowsiness following the headache

2.67 *Characteristic signs for L4/L5 prolapsed intervertebral disc include*

a wasting of the quadriceps muscles
b weakness of dorsiflexion of the foot
c numbness of the dorsum of the dorsum
d reduced knee jerk
e reduced ankle jerk

2.68 *Which of the following operations can be performed by laparoscopy?*

a cholecystectomy
b appendicectomy
c repair of an aortic aneurysm
d inguinal hernia repair
e closure of anterior perforation of duodenal ulcers

2.69 *Physical signs which suggest visceral injury after a closed abdominal injury include*

a unexplained hypertension
b abdominal distension
c lower rib fractures
d abominal guarding and rigidity
e blood at the urethral meatus

2.70 *In the presence of abdominal distension, which of the following physical signs is/are consistent with ascites as the cause of distension?*

a dullness to percussion over the umbilical area in the supine position
b dullness to percussion over the flank in the supine position
c dullness to percussion over the umbilical area when rolled in the lateral position
d the presence of fluid thrill
e increased high pitched bowel sounds

2.71 *Biliary colic*

a occurs more commonly in the female than the male
b may be caused by sudden occlusion of the cystic duct
c characteristically lasts for over 72 h
d nearly always requires hospital admission
e may be confirmed by ultrasound examination

2.72 *Side-effects of partial gastrectomy include*

a inability to take a normal size meal
b fainting and sweating soon after eating

c vitamin B_{12} deficiency
d iron deficiency
e severe chronic constipation

2.73 *Sliding hiatus hernia*

a is less common than the rolling (para-oesophageal) type
b is associated with oesophageal reflux
c is usually small
d may be associated with Barrett's oesophagus
e requires fundoplication in most cases

2.74 *Chronic pancreatitis*

a characteristically presents with abdominal guarding and rigidity
b can be excluded by a normal amylase level
c is likely if pancreatic calcification is seen on the CT scan
d predisposes to the development of diabetes mellitus
e predisposes to malabsorption

2.75 *Which of the following statements about Crohn's disease is/are true?*

a the initial presentation is usually after the age of 40
b the jejunum is the commonest affected site
c it may mimic appendicitis in its presentation
d surgery is more often required than for ulcerative colitis
e it is associated with a higher risk of malignancy than ulcerative colitis

2.76 *Bladder tumours*

a are mostly squamous cell tumours
b occur more frequently in women than in men
c occur more frequently in smokers
d characteristically present with painless haematuria
e are usually treated by radiotherapy

2.77 *Wound dehiscence after an abdominal operation*

a occurs most frequently 24 h postoperatively
b is usually accompanied by excruciating pain
c often accompanies inadequate abdominal wall repair
d is often associated with wound infection
e should be repaired by tension sutures through the whole thickness of the abdominal wall

Answers

2.1 a **False** b **False** c **False** d **True** e **True**

Fibroadenomas are benign tumours, and usually occur in young women. They are characteristically smooth firm mobile masses, commonly known as 'breast mice'. They may occur singly or in multiples. If left untreated, they usually grow in size to about 3–4 cm in diameter and then form a calcified mass in the long term, although they may occasionally disappear spontaneously. Treatment is usually by surgical removal to avoid long-term changes and patient's anxiety, although conservative treatment with careful follow-up may be adopted if no malignant cells are seen in the aspiration cytology.

2.2 a **True** b **True** c **False** d **False** e **True**

The risk of developing breast carcinoma appears to be related to the exposure to the effects of the functioning ovaries. Hence, early menarche, late menopause, and nulliparity are all risk factors. Increased age and a positive family history in the near relative are also risk factors. More controversially, high social class is thought to be associated with increased risk, and combined oral contraceptives are thought to be protective.

2.3 a **True** b **True** c **False** d **True** e **False**

Clinical factors indicating a favourable prognosis of breast cancer include small size, smooth contour, little or no lymph node involvement, and early staging. Histological factors include high differentiation, presence of lymphocytic infiltration, and reactive hyperplasia in regional nodes. A high oestrogen receptor activity indicates a good response to ovarian ablation in the premenopausal women or tamoxifen in the postmenopausal women, and is a good prognostic factor.

2.4 a **True** b **False** c **False** d **True** e **True**

A goitre is a visible or palpable enlargement of the thyroid gland. The swelling is in the lower part of the neck, and characteristically moves upwards on swallowing. It may be present physiologically and transiently in puberty and pregnancy. A goitre may enlarge and cause tracheal compression causing stridor and dyspnoea, or oesophageal compression causing dysphagia.

2.5 a **True** b **False** c **False** d **True** e **False**

Primary hyperthyroidism accounts for about three-quarters of all cases of hyperthyroidism. The other causes are non-toxic goitres and toxic adenoma. It usually occurs in young female. The thyroid gland is diffusely enlarged and highly vascular, and a bruit may be audible. It is usually associated with eye signs (exophthalmos, lid retraction, and lid lag), pretibial myxoedema, and acropachy (which resembles clubbing of the fingers). The T_3 and T_4 levels are high, suppressing the production of TSH from the pituitary gland. The TSH response to intravenous TRH injection is often absent.

2.6 a **False** b **True** c **True** d **True** e **True**
Common postoperative complications of thyroidectomy include haemorrhage, damage to the pairs of parathyroid glands at the back of the thyroid gland, damage to superior laryngeal nerve or recurrent laryngeal nerve, excess removal of the thyroid gland, and a keloid scar. Postoperative haemorrhage may cause venous congestion and tracheal compression causing asphyxia. Damage to the parathyroid glands may cause hypocalcaemia and tetany. Damage to the external branch of the superior laryngeal nerve may cause weakness in adduction of the vocal cords, resulting in a weak, hoarse voice. Damage to one recurrent laryngeal nerve causes the vocal cord on that side to be in the mid-abducted position, and results in an altered, weak voice. Damage to both recurrent laryngeal nerves result in stridor, and is usually immediately recognizable postoperatively after extubation. Excess removal of the thyroid gland may result in hypothyroidism.

2.7 a **False** b **True** c **True** d **False** e **True**
Papillary carcinoma accounts for about 50% of thyroid carcinoma. It occurs in relatively young people, and usually presents as a solitary slow-growing thyroid nodule. It has the best prognosis, with a 10 year survival rate of over 80%. Anaplastic carcinoma is the next commonest, and mainly occurs in older patients. It rapidly spreads locally to involve recurrent laryngeal nerve causing hoarseness, the trachea causing stridor, the oesophagus causing dysphagia, and cervical sympathetic nerves causing Horner's syndrome. Follicular carcinoma usually presents as a solitary thyroid nodule at age 25–50, and has a prognosis between that of papillary and follicular carcinoma. Medullary carcinoma secretes calcitonin and may be part of the multiple endocrine neoplasia II syndrome. Prognosis is poor.

2.8 a **True** b **False** c **True** d **True** e **False**
In primary hyperparathyroidism, there is oversecretion of PTH in spite of a normal level of calcium. The commonest cause is an adenoma (about 90%), parathyroid hyperplasia, and parathyroid carcinoma. It is more common in women than men. It may affect the urinary tract, causing nephrocalcinosis and urinary calculi. It may also affect the bone, causing demineralization. Other features include acute and chronic pancreatitis, weakness, peptic ulceration, or even psychosis. The serum calcium and chloride level are typically high and the phosphate level low. The PTH is usually high but may be normal.

2.9 a **True** b **False** c **True** d **True** e **True**
Acromegaly results from excess secretion of growth hormone from an anterior pituitary gland tumour. Bromocriptine or somastostatin analogues may be used to lower growth hormone level. Tamoxifen is used for breast cancer and not for pituitary tumour. Small pituitary adenomas are usually treated by trans-sphenoidal surgical removal, but radioactive pituitary implants or occasionally external radiation are used for larger adenomas.

2.10 a **False** b **False** c **True** d **True** e **False**
Coronary heart disease is the commonest cause of death in developed countries, and

the number of coronary artery bypass grafting operations is increasing. It has been shown to be cost-beneficial especially in those with two- or three-vessel disease, and is indicated for those with angina symptoms who have persistent symptoms despite medical treatment. The purpose is to form a conduit to deliver arterial blood into normal coronary arterial tree beyond atheromatous or thrombotic obstructions shown on coronary angiography. Hence, coronary angiography must be first performed. The graft may be obtained from the patient's saphenous vein or internal mammary artery. Complete relief of symptoms is achieved in about two-thirds of patients. However, the operation carries a 1–2% mortality risk, and the symptoms may return some years later due to obstruction of thrombus in the grafted vein or progression of the coronary artery disease.

2.11 a **True** b **True** c **True** d **True** e **False**
Coronary artery disease, stroke, mesenteric ischaemia, and peripheral vascular disease of the lower limbs are all due to ischaemia caused by atherosclerosis. Hence, their risk factors are similar and include smoking, hypercholesterolaemia, hypertension, obesity, and diabetes. Beta-blockers may cause peripheral vasoconstriction and exacerbates peripheral vascular disease of the lower limbs.

2.12 a **False** b **False** c **False** d **True** e **True**
The superficial femoral artery is the commonest site of obstruction. However, the symptom is initially minimal if there are patent collateral vessels (profunda). Claudication occurs when they are blocked. Elevation of the legs would diminish its arterial supply and exacerbate rest pain. Pure aorto-iliac obstruction may cause calf pain and pain in the buttock and thighs. In men, impotence may result from internal iliac arteries occlusion (Leriche's syndrome), but rest pain of the legs is unusual.

2.13 a **False** b **True** c **True** d **True** e **True**
Signs of chronic limb ischaemia include pale cold atrophic skin, brittle nails, and absent peripheral pulses. On elevation of the leg, there is marked pallor, but the foot becomes bright red on hanging the leg down. This is known as dependent rubor. In severe femorodistal diseases, there may be leg ulcers and gangrene.

2.14 a **False** b **True** c **False** d **True** e **True**
An arterial bypass graft is usually the treatment of choice if the arterial occlusion is extensive. A femoral stenosis or short occlusion is best treated by percutaneous angioplasty. A balloon catheter is introduced into the femoral artery under local anaesthetic to the stenotic site, and the balloon is inflated to enlarge the arterial lumen. For arterial reconstruction surgery, an autogenous vein graft has a higher patency rate and lower sepsis rate than a synthetic graft. The patency rate is also higher the wider the vessel lumen being reconstructed. If a venous graft is used, the vein should either be reversed, or the valves of the vein damaged by valvulotome, as otherwise the valves would prevent flow of arterial blood through the graft. The femoral popliteal bypass is frequently performed, but it is also possible to construct a femorotibial or a femoroperoneal bypass graft. Using microsurgical techniques, it is possible to take the graft down even further towards the ankle or the foot.

2.15 a **False** b **True** c **True** d **False** e **True**
Common causes for failure of the flap to heal after amputation include infection, excessive tension on the stitch line, haematoma formation, or inadequate blood supply. Failure to heal is commoner if the level of amputation is too low (e.g. below-knee amputation if above-knee amputation is indicated).

2.16 a **False** b **True** c **True** d **True** e **False**
Acute thrombotic ischaemia of the lower limbs is often triggered by a fall in blood pressure, and it is important to maintain a reasonable blood pressure (by volume repletion, inotropic agents, and treatment of heart failure) to maintain the blood flow once the thrombus is cleared. Systemic heparin should be started to prevent further spread of the thrombus. Treatment by either thrombolytic therapy (e.g. streptokinase) delivered into the thrombus by percutaneous catheter, or emergency thrombectomy (by a Fogarty catheter through the common femoral artery under local anaesthesia) are required in most cases.

2.17 a **False** b **True** c **True** d **True** e **True**
Abdominal aortic aneurysms are more likely to occur in men, in the elderly, and in those with hypertension. The vast majority of aneurysms occur below the level of the renal arteries. Those which occur above the level of the renal arteries are more difficult to repair surgically. Abdominal aortic aneurysms may be asymptomatic and detected routinely on physical or ultrasound examination. They may present with back pain, central abdominal pain, or loin pain. Finally, they may leak or rupture giving rise to severe back or abdominal pain with hypovolaemic shock. Large aneurysms are more likely to rupture than small ones (Laplace's law). Hence, abdominal aortic aneurysms over 5 cm in diameter should be repaired electively.

2.18 a **False** b **True** c **False** d **True** e **True**
Varicose veins are caused by incompetence of the valves at the junction between the superficial veins and the deep veins. This results in excessive pressure on the superficial veins, which therefore become dilated and tortuous. The condition may be primary or secondary to deep vein thrombosis or trauma. Primary varicose veins are more common in women, in those with a family history, in the obese, in those who stand for prolonged periods of time, and during pregnancy. The patient with varicose veins should be examined standing, as this makes the varicose veins more prominent.

2.19 a **False** b **False** c **False** d **True** e **False**
Thyroglossal cysts are developmental in origin, and result from the persistence of the thyroglossal duct. Embryologically, the thyroglossal duct is a midline tubular structure from the foramen caecum at the base of the tongue to the embryological isthmus and lobes of the thyroid gland. Hence, the cysts characteristically moves upwards on tongue protrusion. Although they are developmental in origin, they frequently present in adolescence or early adult life as a smooth, painless, midline swelling. It may also get infected and presents as a discharging sinus.

2.20 a **False** b **True** c **True** d **True** e **False**
Sebaceous cysts are thought to arise from blockage of hair follicles, which gives rise to the characteristically small surface punctum. They commonly occur in hair-bearing areas such as the scalp. They lie within the skin, and contain cheesy white debris and sebum. They can be excised with an elliptical skin incision under local anaesthetic. However, if they are infected, they should first be incised to release the infected material, and excision should be performed at a later date.

2.21 a **False** b **False** c **True** d **True** e **False**
Mumps and autoimmune diseases such as Sjîgren's syndrome are the main causes of bilateral painful parotid swellings. Acute parotitis is usually unilateral and is caused by ascending infection due to poor oral hygiene. Salivary calculi are most common in the submandibular gland, and usually occur unilaterally. Parotid neoplasm are usually unilateral and painless.

2.22 a **False** b **False** c **True** d **True** e **False**
More than three-quarters of salivary gland tumours occur in the parotid gland. Most parotid gland tumours are pleomorphic salivary adenoma affecting the superficial portion of the gland. Pleomorphic salivary adenoma are very slow growing. They do not invade surrounding tissues or metastasize. Hence, if the diagnosis is confirmed by fine needle aspiration cytology, surgical removal is not mandatory. Most tumours of the minor salivary glands are malignant. A parotid mass associated with facial palsy is usually due to invasion of the facial nerve by a anaplastic carcinoma of the parotid gland.

2.23 a **True** b **False** c **False** d **True** e **False**
Clinical features of acute peritonitis partly depend on whether it is localized or generalized. Respiration and movement aggravate the pain, and the patient usually breathes shallowly and lies still. The abdomen may be scaphoid. There is tenderness on palpation, guarding, and rebound tenderness. Bowel sounds are reduced and the abdomen may become silent. The inflammation and infection of the peritoneum result in pyrexia and tachycardia. Profuse vomiting, severe dehydration, hypovolaemia, and septic shock may supervene in late stages, and the patient may become toxic and confused.

2.24 a **True** b **True** c **False** d **False** e **True**
Indirect inguinal hernia results from the failure of obliteration of the processus vaginalis, and accounts for 60% of all abdominal wall hernias overall. The processus vaginalis is the peritoneum which the testis drags during its descent through the inguinal canal. The opening of the canal lies 1 cm above the midpoint between the pubic symphysis and the anterior superior iliac spine, and pressure at this point would control a reduced indirect inguinal hernia. The indirect inguinal hernia passes above and medial to the pubic tubercle, in contrast to the femoral hernia which passes below and lateral to the pubic tubercle. The direct inguinal hernia results from weakness of the abdominal wall, and occurs from middle age.

2.25 a **True** b **False** c **True** d **False** e **True**
Achalasia is an oesophageal motility disorder probably caused by degeneration of the nerve plexus (Auerbach's plexus). Dysphagia is the cardinal symptom, with taking liquids more difficult than solids. Retrosternal pain may occur, and regurgitation may lead to aspiration pneumonia. Carcinoma may develop in chronic achalasia. Barium swallow shows gross dilatation of the oesophagus above the lower oesophageal sphincter. Treatment is either by hydrostatic balloon dilatation, or cardiomyotomy. Cardiomyotomy involves a longitudinal incision through the musculature of the oesophagus without breaching the mucosa.

2.26 a **False** b **True** c **False** d **False** e **True**
The vast majority of oesophageal tumours are malignant, and more than 90% of oesophageal carcinomas are squamous carcinomas. Most squamous carcinomas occur in the middle third of the oesophagus. Oesophageal carcinomas are more common in the Far East and African countries, in men, and in older people. Risk factors include smoking, alcohol, betel nut chewing, achalasia, and Plummer-Vinson syndrome. Dysphagia and weight loss are the main symptoms. Hoarseness may be due to recurrent laryngeal nerve involvement and is a late manifestation. Squamous carcinomas may be radiosensitive. Generally speaking, carcinomas at the upper third of the oesophagus may be treated by radiotherapy, and those at the lower third treated by resection. However, just less than half are resectable, and the overall prognosis is poor with 5 year survival rates about 5%.

2.27 a **False** b **True** c **False** d **True** e **False**
About 90% of perforated peptic ulcers are perforated duodenal ulcers. Patients may or may not have previous history of peptic ulcer disease, but they usually present with sudden onset of severe abdominal pain which rapidly becomes generalized. There is often signs of peritonism (marked rigidity, guarding, tenderness, and rebound tenderness). Free air can be seen in only about 60% of the erect abdominal radiograph. If the diagnosis is suspected but free air cannot be seen on the erect abdominal radiograph, a gastrogarafin meal can be performed. Insertion of nasogastric tube to empty the gastric content is important to prevent further leakage into the peritoneal cavity. About a fifth of patients with perforated gastric ulcers have gastric carcinoma, and partial gastrectomy would be a more appropriate procedure.

2.28 a **True** b **True** c **True** d **True** e **True**
Long term complications of peptic ulcer surgery include recurrence of the ulcers, vomiting food or bile, the dumping syndrome, reactive hypoglycaemia, diarrhoea, and malabsorption. Food vomiting may be due to narrowing of a stoma or inappropriate gastrojejunostomy site. The dumping syndrome consists of epigastric fullness associated with sweating, flushing, and borborygmi within 30 min of a meal, which resolves within an hour. It is due to rapid emptying of hyperosmolar solution into the small bowel, resulting in large osmotic shift of fluid into the bowel and extracellular volume depletion. Reactive hypoglycaemia may occur within 2 h of a meal, and is due to initial hyperglycaemia due to rapid absorption of glucose from the upper small

bowel followed by excessive insulin secretion as a response. Anaemia may be due to a combination of malabsorption of iron and postoperative blood loss.

2.29 a **False** b **True** c **False** d **True** e **True**
Diverticular disease is more common with increasing age, and is most common in the sigmoid colon. A high fibre diet appears to protect from the disease. It may be asymptomatic, or may present with lower abdominal pain, change in bowel habit, or minor rectal bleeding. Diverticula and muscle thickening may be seen on barium enema.

2.30 a **True** b **True** c **True** d **True** e **False**
Complications of diverticular disease include bleeding, inflammation, perforation of a diverticular or an pericoloic abscess, intestinal obstruction, and fistula formation. Inflammation may result in pericolic abscess. Perforation of a diverticular would result in faecal peritonitis, while perforation of a pericoloic abscess would result in purulent peritonitis. Intestinal obstruction may result from oedema or fibrosis of the colon. Diverticular disease is the commonest cause of fistula formation with the bladder.

2.31 a **False** b **True** c **False** d **True** e **False**
Ulcerative colitis typically affects the large bowel only, whereas Crohn's disease may involve the whole gastrointestinal tract. Crypt abscesses in the mucosa are characteristic in ulcerative colitis, whereas the full thickness of the bowel is affected in Crohn's disease. Anal lesions and fistula formation are more common in Crohn's disease than in ulcerative colitis. Ulcerative colitis has a higher risk of malignant changes than Crohn's disease.

2.32 a **True** b **False** c **True** d **False** e **True**
Adenomatous polyps account for almost 90% of all colonic polyps, while villous adenomas account the majority of the rest. Adenomatous polyps vary in size from 1 mm in diameter to a pedunculated mass. Most polyps are symptomless, although they may bleed or intussuscept. They may be diagnosed by colonoscopy and removed via a diathermy snare. Villous adenoma (but not adenomatous polyps) cause excessive mucus secretion. The loss of potassium in mucus from villous adenoma may cause hypokalaemic alkalosis. Both villous adenoma and adenomatous polyps predispose to carcinoma.

2.33 a **False** b **True** c **True** d **False** e **True**
Large-bowel carcinomas are more common with increasing age. They are rare in black people and in the Far East. A low fibre, high fat diet, adenomatous polyps (including the familial adenomatous polyposis), villous adenoma, and inflammatory bowel disease are all known predisposing factors for large-bowel carcinomas.

2.34 a **False** b **False** c **False** d **True** e **True**
The contents of the caecum and ascending colon are mostly fluid. Hence, carcinoma at this site seldom leads to change in bowel habit. Rectal bleeding and intestinal obstruction are common for colonic carcinoma of the right colon (rectum, sigmoid

colon, and descending colon), but not for carcinoma of the caecum. Common symptoms for carcinoma of the caecum are non-specific symptoms and signs such as weight loss, loss of appetite, and iron-deficiency anaemia due to chronic blood loss. Occasionally, there may be right iliac fossa discomfort, and right iliac fossa mass may be palpable in the late stages.

2.35 a **False** b **True** c **True** d **True** e **False**
Acute appendicitis typically begins with ill-localized periumbilical pain. This is visceral pain, and reflects the fact that the appendix is a midline embryological structure. After a few hours, the pain may shift to the right iliac fossa. This is due to irritation of the parietal peritoneum, and the pain is sharp and well-localized. Anorexia is almost always present. Nausea and vomiting may occur. Diarrhoea may be due to irritation of the rectum by pelvic appendicitis. Rectal examination must be performed if acute appendicitis is suspected, but no signs are found in the abdomen. There are often no signs to be found on the abdomen in the presence of pelvic appendicitis, but tenderness may be elicited on rectal examination.

2.36 a **False** b **True** c **False** d **False** e **True**
The clinical features of uncomplicated intestinal obstruction depend on the level of the obstruction. In high small-bowel obstruction, vomiting, dehydration, and epigastric pain are common in the early stages, the onset is sudden, but abdominal distension and constipation are not present. Conversely, in low large-bowel obstruction, the onset is slow, abdominal distension and constipation are common, and the pain is central or low abdominal. Vomiting does not occur until the late stages.

2.37 a **False** b **True** c **True** d **True** e **False**
Haemorrhoids originate from the internal haemorrhoidal plexus in the upper anal canal, and they lie in the left lateral, right anterior, and right posterior positions of the anal canal. First-degree haemorrhoids are those which do not prolapse through the anus. Second-degree haemorrhoids are those which prolapse during defecation but return spontaneously afterwards. Third-degree haemorrhoids remain prolapsed after defecation, but may be returned manually. Fourth-degree haemorrhoids are those which cannot be returned to the anal canal. Bright red bleeding and prolapse are the commonest symptoms. Mucus discharge may sometimes occur. Thrombosed haemorrhoids may cause severe pain. Treatment for uncomplicated first-degree haemorrhoids may be simple advice about taking a high fibre diet and avoiding constipation. Treatment of higher-degree haemorrhoids includes injection sclerotherapy, rubber band ligation, and haemorrhoidectomy. Thrombosed haemorrhoids are now usually treated conservatively initially by bed rest, analgesia, and local dressing until resolution. Haemorrhoidectomy may be carried out at a later date.

2.38 a **True** b **True** c **True** d **True** e **True**
There are no predisposing causes in most cases of anorectal abscesses. However, known predisposing causes include previous history of anorectal abscess, rectal carcinoma, Crohn's disease, ulcerative colitis, HIV infection, and active tuberculosis.

2.39 a **True** b **False** c **True** d **False** e **False**
Pilonidal sinus typically starts posterior to the anus and extends caudally. It is commonest between 20 and 40 years of age, and may occur in the hands of barbers. It is thought to be caused by penetration of hair, with subsequent infection. A pilonidal sinus typically contains hairs. Treatment may consist of either primary suturing or marsupialization (laying it open and excising the skin edges) under general anaesthetic.

2.40 a **True** b **False** c **True** d **False** e **True**
Portal hypertension may cause collateral vessels to develop in the areas where portosystemic anastamosis occurs, resulting in portosystemic shunting. Portosystematic anastamosis occurs in the veins at the junction between the oesophagus and the fundus of the stomach; in the periumbilical areas; and in the anorectal region. They may cause oesophageal varices, caput medusae, and ano-rectal varices respectively.

2.41 a **False** b **False** c **True** d **True** e **True**
The Minnesota tube has four lumina: for aspiration of pharynx and oesophagus above the varices; to allow inflation of the oesophageal balloon to compress the varices (to prevent aspiration pneumonia); to allow inflation of the gastric balloon to compress the oesophagogastric junction; and to allow aspiration of gastric contents. It is now used in preference to the three-lumen Sengstaken-Blakemore tube. The tube should not be left for more than 36 h, as oesophageal necrosis may occur.

2.42 a **True** b **False** c **True** d **True** e **False**
Treatments which may be used to reduce oesophageal varices include injection sclerotherapy, endoscopic banding, and elective portosystemic shunting procedures. Transhepatic insertion of portosystemic shunts is currently under research. Ventriculoperitoneal shunting is a procedure for hydrocephalus, and highly selective vagotomy is used for treating peptic ulcers.

2.43 a **True** b **False** c **False** d **True** e **True**
Gallstones are commoner in developed countries, in females, and with increasing age. Most gallstones in developed countries are of the mixed type. Only a fifth of patients with gallstones can be detected by radiography. The majority of patients are asymptomatic, but gallstones may cause a variety of symptoms such as dyspepsia, biliary colic (transient obstruction of the gallbladder), acute cholecystitis (unrelieved obstruction of the neck of the gallbladder or the cystic duct), obstructive jaundice (obstruction of the bile duct), and gallbladder carcinoma.

2.44 a **False** b **True** c **False** d **True** e **True**
Acute cholecystitis usually follows an attack of biliary colic. The characteristic symptoms are right hypochondrial pain radiating to the right subscapsular region. Pyrexia, nausea, and vomiting are usually present. There is usually general abdominal tenderness and rigidity, especially in the right hypochondrium. Catching of breath at inspiration when the gallbladder is palpated is known as Murphy's sign, and is often present in acute cholecystitis. Jaundice may develop during an attack of cholecystitis.

2.45 a **True** b **True** c **False** d **True** e **True**
Cholecystectomy is generally indicated only for symptomatic gallstones. Either open or laparoscopic cholecystectomy may be performed. In the past, an operative cholangiography was always performed to detect stones in the bile ducts. Some surgeons now only perform cholangiography in those with a higher risk of ductal stones (e.g. those with a past history of obstructive jaundice). Postoperative complications include infection, leakage of bile causing biliary peritonitis, retained stones, bleeding, and bile duct stricture.

2.46 a **True** b **False** c **True** d **False** e **False**
The management of acute pancreatitis involves both supportive treatment and removal of gallstones if they are the cause of pancreatitis. Supportive treatment includes strong analgesia by opiates injection, nil by mouth, replacement of plasma volume by plasma or crystalloid infusion, and monitoring of vital signs and urine output. Treatments such as peritoneal lavage, antibiotics, and somastatin analogues are debatable. If the condition is caused by gallstones, consideration should be given to their removal by endoscopy (ERCP) or by surgery.

2.47 a **True** b **True** c **False** d **True** e **False**
Carcinoma of the head of the pancreas commonly presents with weight loss and symptoms of obstructive jaundice (dark urine, pale stool, pruritus). According to Courvoisier's law, the gallbladder is often palpable in patients with obstructive jaundice due to carcinoma of the head of the pancreas. Abdominal distension is very uncommon.

2.48 a **True** b **True** c **True** d **True** e **True**
Benign prostatic hypertrophy may result in bladder neck irritation and obstruction. Bladder neck irritation symptoms include frequency, nocturia, urgency, and dysuria. Obstructive symptoms include poor urinary stream and postmicturition dribbling.

2.49 a **True** b **True** c **True** d **False** e **True**
A stone in the right ureter typically causes ureteric colic which is severe and occurs in waves. Other symptoms are haematuria and those of urinary tract infection. It can be seen on IVU. If it is small, it usually passes spontaneously. Available treatment include disintegration by laser, pneumatic, or electrohydraulic lithotripsy. The stone can be visualized through a ureteroscope. Open surgery is seldom required.

2.50 a **False** b **False** c **True** d **True** e **False**
Renal tumour is commonly malignant. It is more common in men than in women. In the early stages, the clinical features are non-specific such as fever of unknown origin, weight loss, and raised ESR. It may secrete hormonal products such as renin and erythropoietin. Erythropoietin secretion may cause polycythaemia. Radical nephrectomy with or without postoperative radiotherapy is the main treatment.

2.51 a **False** b **False** c **True** d **False** e **True**
Diverticular disease is the presence of diverticula which are symptomatic. Diverticulitis means inflammation within diverticula. Diverticula occur most commonly in

the colon, and especially in the sigmoid colon. They are common in the elderly in developed countries. The aetiology appears to be lack of dietary fibre, leading to increased intraluminal pressure and herniation of mucosa through muscle walls of the bowel. The commonest symptoms are change in bowel habit, left-sided abdominal pain which is relieved by defecation, nausea, and flatulence. Diverticula may be inflammed, and the colon is then very tender with signs of peritonitis. Painless rectal bleeding may occur.

2.52 a **True** b **False** c **False** d **False** e **True**
In diagnosing a scrotal lump, the first question is whether one can get above the lump. If not, it may be an indirect inguinal hernia. If it is possible, the second question should be whether the scrotal lump is separate from the testis. Masses which arise from the testis itself (e.g. testicular tumours, orchitis) cannot be felt separately. However, masses which arise from the epididymis (e.g. epididymal cyst, epididymitis) can be felt separately. Hydrocoele is cystic and cannot be felt separately from the testis.

2.53 a **False** b **False** c **False** d **True** e **True**
Torsion of the testis occurs commonly between the ages of 15 and 30. It usually presents with sudden onset of severe testicular or abdominal pain associated with vomiting or nausea. On examination, the testis is hot, swollen, and tender. The testis may lie transversely. Doppler ultrasound may demonstrate the degree of blood flow to the testis. This is an emergency and must be surgically explored immediately. If the testis is viable, fixation (orchidopexy) may be performed on both sides to prevent torsion of the other testis in future.

2.54 a **False** b **False** c **True** d **True** e **False**
Generally speaking, consent for medical treatment for all adults above 18 years of age must be given by the person receiving treatment. In the case of mentally handicapped adults who cannot understand the nature of the treatment, neither the patient nor any one else can give consent. For elective procedures such as sterilization, consent from the High Court may be sought. For emergency procedures, the treatment may be legally given by the doctors out of necessity, but good practice dictates that at least two doctors should agree that the treatment is appropriate. All procedures on children below the age of 16 require the consent of one person with parental responsibility.

2.55 a **False** b **True** c **False** d **False** e **False**
According to Ronson's criteria, factors associated with increased mortality at presentation are increased age (>55 years), high white cell count ($>16\times10^9$/litre), high glucose level (>11 mmol/litre), high LDH level (>350 IU/litre), and high AST level (>60 IU/litre). Factors during the first 48 h associated with increased mortality are rapid haematocrit fall (>10%), rapid urea increase (>10 mmol/litre), low serum calcium level (<2 mmol/litre), acidotic (base excess greater than –4), hypoxic (PaO_2 < 8 kPa), and excessive fluid sequestration (>6 litres).

2.56 a **False** b **True** c **False** d **False** e **True**
A ganglion arises from the fibrous capsule of a joint or tendon sheath. It commonly appears on the dorsum of the wrist or foot. In contrast to a bursa, it contains mucoid material. It is not premalignant. It may be removed either under regional or general anaesthesia.

2.57 a **True** b **True** c **True** d **True** e **True**
The causes of faecal incontinence include neurological or psychiatric disorders, trauma (e.g. obstetric tears, surgical trauma), anorectal disease (e.g. rectal prolapse, anorectal cancer), and congenital abnormalities.

2.58 a **False** b **True** c **True** d **False** e **False**
The incidence of cancer of the prostate increases with age, and is uncommon before the age of 60. It is common in northern Europe and the UK but is rare in China and Japan. It may present as an incidental finding on histological examination after prostatectomy, with urinary obstructive symptoms, or with symptoms from metastasis. Although an irregular nodular hard prostate felt on rectal examination is characteristic of prostate cancer, the diagnosis should not be made on clinical examination alone. The PSA level is typically high, and may be used to monitor both disease progression and response to treatment.

2.59 a **False** b **True** c **True** d **False** e **False**
Malignant melanomas are commoner in those with fair skin and are rare in black people. They have become more common in the last decade. Exposure to sunlight is the most important aetiological factor. They spread rapidly by both lymphatic system and the blood stream. Lymph node and distant metastases are associated with poor prognosis. The width of the clearance excision margin depends on the depth of the lesion. Generally speaking, 1 cm of clearance for every millimetre of depth should be allowed.

2.60 a **False** b **False** c **True** d **False** e **True**
Testicular tumours commonly occur in men aged between 20 and 40. The commonest types are seminomas and teratomas. Painless testicular mass should always be investigated for testicular tumours, but sometimes pain may be present. It may also present as a hydrocoele. AFP and β-HCG are useful tumour markers, and should be performed *before* orchidectomy. Testicular tumours can be treated by combining orchidectomy with radiotherapy (for seminomas) or chemotherapy (for teratomas). The prognosis is good compared with other cancers. The 5 year survival rate for seminomas is over 90%, and about 75% for teratomas.

2.61 a **True** b **False** c **True** d **False** e **False**
The most frequent indications for diagnostic examination of the CSF by lumbar puncture include suspected meningitis and subarachnoid haemorrhage. Other less frequent indications include neurological diseases such as multiple sclerosis, cytological examination for neoplastic disease, and radiological imaging. Lumbar puncture is absolutely contraindicated if there is any clinical evidence of raised

intracranial pressure or suspected intracranial space occupying lesions, as this may lead to brain herniation (coning) and death.

2.62 a **True** b **False** c **False** d **False** e **True**
In general, MRI is much more effective in diagnosing neursosurgical conditions than CT scan. The advantages include the lack of ionizing radiation, high resolution, and the absence of bone artefact. Therefore, it is much more effective in the visualization of the structure around the skull base and the vertebral column. The only disadvantage is that it is not readily available in many hospitals.

2.63 a **False** b **True** c **False** d **True** e **True**
Hydrocephalus is an enlargement of the ventricles of the brain dure to excessive accumulation of CSF. It is usually classified into two types, obstructive and communicating hydrocephalus. Obstructive hydrocephalus is caused by obstruction to the flow of CSF through the ventricular system. This includes obstruction in the lateral ventricle, the third ventricle (due to colloid cyst or glioma), the aqueduct of sylvius (e.g. through stenosis or tumour) and the fourth ventricle (e.g. by posterior fossa tumour or acoustic neuroma). Communicating hydrocephalus may be due to failure of absorption of CSF from the arachnoid granulations (e.g. increased viscosity of CSF in bacterial, tuberculous, or carcinomatous meningitis, and subarachnoid haemorrhage); or due to excessive production of CSF due to a chorioid plexus papilloma.

2.64 a **True** b **False** c **False** d **True** e **True**
Opinions regarding indications for admission to a hospital after a head injury may vary. Persistent or increasing reduction in the level of consciousness, focal neurological deficits, persistent vomiting or nausea, a proven skull fracture, and adverse social circumstances are all recognized indications. A blood pressure of 140/100 may be usual for that individual. Generalized hyperreflexia is likely to be due to anxiety.

2.65 a **False** b **False** c **True** d **True** e **False**
Extradural haematoma occurs more frequently in younger people, as the dura is less adherent to the underlying bone. It most frequently occurs in the temporal region, and results from bleeding form the middle meningeal artery. Although it may be associated with severe head injury with obvious skull fractures, the preceding head injury is often mild and trivial. Focal neurological signs may or may not be present. Increasing drowsiness after a 'lucid' interval is characteristic. An urgent CT scan should be performed, and an urgent craniotomy with evacuation of the clot is indicated. Occasionally, the deterioration is so rapid that a craniectomy needs to be performed without a CT scan.

2.66 a **False** b **False** c **True** d **True** e **True**
The classical presentation of subarachnoid haemorrhage is sudden onset of severe headache followed by meningism (e.g. neck stiffness, photophobia, vomiting) and increasing drowsiness. Wavy lines across the visual fields suggest the diagnosis of migraine.

2.67 a **False** b **True** c **True** d **False** e **False**
A prolapsed intervertebral disc causes compression of the nerve that runs under the pedicle of the verbetra below. Hence, a L4/L5 prolapsed intervertebral disc is likely to compress the L5 nerve root. Characteristic signs include weakness of the dorsiflexflexion of the foot, numbness, and paraesthesia of the dorsum of the foot, and pain along the posterolateral aspect of the calf and the dorsum of the foot. Weakness of the quadriceps and reduced knee jerks usually results from L3/L4 prolapsed intervertebral disc, while absent ankle jerks usually result from L5/S1 prolapsed intervertebral disc.

2.68 a **True** b **True** c **False** d **True** e **True**
Laparoscopy has been widely used by gynaecologists for over 25 years in the diagnosis of pelvic disorders and for tubal ligation. Since then, it has been adopted by the general surgeons in the diagnosis and management of a wide range of conditions. Indications for diagnostic laparoscopy in general surgery may include the diagnosis of ascites of unknown cause, evaluation of the aetiology of abdominal pain, staging of intra-abdominal malignancies, and assessing whether internal injuries have occurred in following abdominal trauma with a positive peritoneal lavage. Common indications for therapeutic laparoscopy in general surgery include cholecystectomy, appendicetomy, repair of an inguinal or femoral hernia, and closure of anterior duodenal perforation. Other possible indications for therapeutic laparoscopy include bowel resection, division of symptomatic adhesions, and the treatment of oesophageal reflux, and are currently under evaluation. Repair of aortic aneurysms currently cannot be performed laparoscopically.

2.69 a **False** b **True** c **True** d **True** e **True**
Visceral injuries must be excluded after a severe closed abdominal injury either by a diagnositc peritoneal lavage. If this is positive, a diagnostic laparoscopy, or immediate laparotomy should be performed. Physical signs which suggest visceral injury include tachycarida and hypotension (suggesting concealed haemorrhage), abdominal distension (from accuumlating blood or urine) and abdominal tenderness, rigidity, and guarding. Fractures of the lower ribs may be associated with injury to the liver or spleen. Blood at the urethral meatus and inability to pass urine may suggest rupture of the urethra.

2.70 a **False** b **True** c **True** d **True** e **False**
In the presence of ascites, the gas-filled bowel loops float on the top and the fluid is at the bottom. Hence, in the supine position, there is resonance over the umbilical area and dullness at the flanks. When the patient rolled on his/her side, there is dullness over the umbilical area, but resonance over the flank at the top. Fluid thrill is characteristic of ascites. It can be detected by flicking over one flank and detecting a 'splash' on the opposite side of the abdomen while an assistant steadies the centre of the abdomen with the side of the hand. Increased high-pitched bowel sounds indicate the presence of intestinal obstruction.

2.71 a **True** b **True** c **False** d **False** e **True**
Biliary colic is due to sudden and complete cystic duct or common bile duct

obstruction by gallstones. It occurs more frequently in female. Symptoms include severe colicy upper abdominal pain, often associated with vomiting. It characteristically lasts less than 24 h, and symptoms which persist beyond 24 h are more likely to be due to acute cholecystitis. In most cases, it can be managed at home, although hospital admission is required for severe cases. Ultrasound should be the initial investigation, and often demonstrates the presence of gallstones. The treatment is a planned cholecystectomy.

2.72 a **True** b **True** c **True** d **True** e **False**

There are potentially many possible side-effects of varying severity following partial gastrectomy. Inability to eat a normal-sized meals due to reduced gastric capacity is common. Dumping syndrome describes vasomotor symptoms such as fainting, sweating, pallor, and tachycardia after a meal. There are two causes for this: early dumping is due to transient hypovalaemia resulting from influx of a large volume of fluid into the stomach due to its osmotic pressure; and late dumping is due to an excessive insulin response from a steep rise in blood glucose level after a meal. Malabsorption and weight loss may occur. Iron deficiency anaemia may result from reduced absorption, and vitamin B_{12} deficiency may result from loss of intrinsic factor production from the stomach. There is a tendency to short transit time and diarrhoea after partial gastrectomy.

2.73 a **False** b **True** c **True** d **True** e **False**

Hiatus hernia occurts when the proximal part of the stomach passes through the diaphragm to the chest. It is divided into two types. The sliding type is commoner, and the gastro-oesophageal junction is drawn up into the chest. For the rolling type, the gastro-oesophageal junction remains below the diaphragm. The sliding type may become very large, disrupt the physiological antireflux mechanism, and is associated with oesophageal reflux. On the other hand, the rolling type is usually very small, and is not associated with oesophageal reflux. Chronic oesophageal reflux due to sliding hiatus hernia may lead to Barrett's oesophagus, with the metasplastic gatric glandular epithelium replacing the oesophageal epithelium, and is pre-malignant. Most cases of hiatus hernia respond to medical treatment with drugs such as histamine antagonists, proton pump antagonist, and agents which stimulate motility. Surgery is rarely required.

2.74 a **False** b **False** c **True** d **True** e **True**

Chronic pancreatitis characteristically presents with severe and persistent upper abdominal pain, but physical signs are usually absent. Amylase level may be moderately raised or normal. Pancreatic calcification demonstrated radiologically is almost diagnostic, but it is rarely present. Hence, the condition may often be misdiagnosed. Chronic pancreatitis eventually leads to pancreatic atrophy, and predisposes to both malabsorption (due to lack of pancreatic enzymes) and the development of diabetes mellitus.

2.75 a **False** b **False** c **True** d **True** e **False**

Crohn's disease usually first presents before 30 years of age. The terminal ileum is the commonest affected site, and may mimic appendicitis. Whilst the drugs used for ulcerative colitis and Crohn's disease are similar, long-term maintainence drugs for Crohn's disease is often ineffective. Surgery is more often required. Although there is a slightly increased risk of malignancy, the risk is much less than for ulcerative colitis.

2.76 a **False** b **False** c **True** d **True** e **False**
Bladder tumours are usually transitional cell carcinoma. Risk factors include advancing age, male sex, smokers, and exposure to industrial carcinogens such as dyes. They characteristically present with painless haematuria, and they are sometimes associated with urinary tract infection. The usual treatment is complete resection under cystoscopy. If they are too widespread to be resected, topical chemotherapy may be performed.

2.77 a **False** b **False** c **True** d **True** e **True**
Wound dehiscence after an abdominal operation usually occurs 5–8 days after an operation. It is mainly due to inadequate abdominal wall repair, but other factors such as infection, obesity, or chronic cough may be present. Pain associated with wound dehiscence is usually mild. The patient should be returned to theatre, and the wound repaired with tension sutures through the whole thickness of the abdominal wall.

3 *Pharmacology*

Questions

3.1 Compared with younger adults, the elderly

a have a higher incidence of drug interactions
b have a faster rate of renal drug clearance
c generally require a larger dose of drugs
d have a faster rate of drug metabolism
e have a higher incidence of drug side-effects

3.2 Muscarinic antagonist may be used clinically in

a inducing paralysis during anaesthesia
b dilating the pupils for ophthalmic examination
c counteracting phenothiazine-induced Parkinsonism
d treating asthma by inhalation
e treating glaucoma

3.3 Metoclopramide

a is a dopamine agonist
b stimulates gastric emptying
c increases oesophageal sphincter contraction
d may cause acute dystonic reactions (extrapyramidal side effects) in children
e is an anti-emetic

3.4 Which of the following drugs or class of drugs is/are used in the management of peptic ulcers?

a H_2 antagonist
b prostaglandin analogues
c proton pump inhibitors
d codeine phosphate
e corticosteroids

3.5 Which of the following statements about laxatives is/are true?

a bulk-forming laxatives should be taken with adequate intake of fluid
b lactulose is an example of faecal softener
c osmotic laxatives are useful in the treatment of hepatic encephalopathy

d stimulant laxatives are particularly useful in the presence of hard stools
e laxatives should be commenced in the absence of bowel motion for 3 days

3.6 *Digoxin*

a acts by inhibiting the sodium/potassium pump
b increases the conductivity at the atrioventricular node
c may be used in the treatment of heart failure
d has a wide therapeutic window
e is more likely to cause toxicity in the presence of hyperkalaemia

3.7 *Pancreatic enzyme supplements (pancreatin)*

a can be given intramuscularly
b should be taken on an empty stomach
c may be inactivated by gastric acid
d is used in the treatment of cystic fibrosis
e may cause nausea and vomiting

3.8 *Diuretics liable to cause hypokalaemia include*

a spironolactone
b bendrofluazide
c frusemide
d amiloride
e ethacrynic acid

3.9 *Recognized management for paroxysmal supraventricular tachycardia include*

a valsalva manoeuvre
b intravenous adenosine
c intravenous lignocaine
d direct current cardioconversion
e intravenous verapamil

3.10 *Amiodarone*

a is a class IV anti-arrhythmic drug
b has a half-life of 8 h
c is useful in treatment of arrhythmia associated with Wolff-Parkinson-White syndrome
d may cause photosensitive rash
e may be complicated by corneal deposits

3.11 *β-adrenoceptor antagonists may be used in the management of*

a asthma
b hypertension
c peripheral vascular disease

d angina
e thyrotoxicosis

3.12 *Which of the following statements about treatment of hypertension is/are true?*

a the aim should be to keep the diastolic blood pressure below 70 mm Hg
b drug therapy is indicated by one blood pressure reading of 160/90
c initial treatment should constitute a combination of two types of drugs
d methyldopa should be the first line hypertensive treatment
e antihypertensive therapy is never indicated in those over the age of 75

3.13 *Which of the following types of drugs is/are used in the treatment of hypertension?*

a thiazide diuretic
b calcium-channel blocking agent
c angiotensin-converting enzyme inhibitor
d β-adrenoceptor agonist
e α-adrenoceptor antagonist

3.14 *Angiotensin converting enzyme inhibitors*

a inhibit the conversion of angiotensin I to angiotensin II
b may be complicated by hypokalaemia
c may cause severe hypotension when the initial dose is given
d are effective in the treatment of heart failure
e are particularly suitable for those with some degree of renal failure

3.15 *Drugs used in the treatment of or prophylaxis against angina include*

a glyceryl trinitrate
b isosorbide dinitrite
c nifedipine
d verapamil
e atenolol

3.16 *Which of the following statements about anticoagulant drugs is/are true?*

a heparin antagonizes the effect of vitamin K
b heparin has a longer duration of action than warfarin
c heparin must be stopped before starting warfarin in the treatment of deep vein thrombosis
d a specific antidote exists to reverse the effect of heparin
e warfarin can be safely taken by pregnant women

3.17 *Fibrinolytic (thrombolytic) drugs include*

a tranesamic acid

b streptokinase
c aprotinin
d alteplase
e urokinase

3.18 Recognized immediate management of acute asthmatic attack in adults include

a nebulized salbutamol
b intravenous diazepam
c nebulized ipratropium
d nebulized sodium cromoglycate
e oral prednisolone

3.19 Treatments for acute anaphylactic shock include

a intravenous propranolol
b intramuscular adrenaline
c intravenous chlorpheniramine
d intravenous hydrocortisone
e intravenous ranitidine

3.20 Prescription of diazepam to the elderly may be complicated by

a ataxia
b amnesia
c confusion
d physical dependence
e psychological dependence

3.21 Recognized side effects of antipsychotic drugs include

a parkinsonian symptoms
b drowsiness
c excitement
d hypoprolactinaemia
e tardive dyskinesia

3.22 Lithium

a may be used for the treatment of mania
b may be used for the prophylaxis of recurrent depression
c it has a wide therapeutic window (i.e. the difference between toxic dosage and therapeutic dosage is large).
d dose should be increased if the patient has vomiting and diarrhoea
e is safe to use during pregnancy

3.23 Side effects of amitriptyline include

a drowsiness

b blurred vision
c retention of urine
d hypertension
e hyponatraemia

3.24 *Classes of antidepressant drugs include*

a monoamine oxidase inhibitors
b reversible monoamine oxidase type A inhibitors
c benzodiazepines
d barbiturates
e serotonin re-uptake inhibitors

3.25 *Aspirin is useful in management*

a immediately after an acute myocardial infarct
b of pyrexia due to a viral illness in a 2 year old child
c of dysmenorrhoea
d of musculoskeletal pain
e of peptic ulcers

3.26 *Side-effects of opioid analgesia (e.g. morphine) include*

a vomiting
b diarrhoea
c agitation
d respiratory depression
e hypertension

3.27 *Which of the following statements about the use of analgesia in terminal care is/are true?*

a opiates are always needed
b non-steroidal anti-inflammatory drugs are ineffective for pain due to bone secondaries
c opiate doses should not be increased by more than about 20% every week to prevent dependence
d opiates are generally more preferable to be given intravenously or intramuscularly than orally
e analgesics should be prescribed on a 'on request' basis (i.e. only when the patient experiences pain)

3.28 *Drugs useful in the prophylaxis of migraine include*

a pizotifen
b β-adrenoceptor antagonists
c ergotamine
d sumatriptan
e tricyclic antidepressants

3.29 *Carbamazepine is effective in the treatment of*

a absence seizures (petit mal)
b temporal lobe epilepsy
c trigeminal neuralgia
d prophylaxis of manic depressive illness unresponsive to lithium
e first line treatment of status epilepticus

3.30 *Side-effects of sodium valproate include*

a gum hypertrophy
b gastric irritation
c hirsuitism
d megaloblastic anaemia
e impaired liver function

3.31 *The plasma half-life of a drug ($t_{1/2}$)*

a is midway between the initial concentration and the steady-state concentration
b is longer the faster the drug reaches its steady state concentration
c increases as plasma concentration falls for a zero-order elimination process
d is constant if the elimination process is first-order
e is an important factor in determining the steady-state plasma concentration level if the rate of administration is altered

3.32 *Which of the following drugs act by enzyme inhibition?*

a salbutamol
b tolbutamide
c allopurinol
d enalapril
e acetazolamide

3.33 *Which of the following antibacterial agents act by inhibiting nucleic acid synthesis?*

a benzylpenicillin
b tetracycline
c ciprofloxacin
d co-trimoxazole
e chloramphenicol

3.34 *Side-effects of isoniazid include*

a liver toxicity
b red discolourization of urine
c peripheral neuropathy
d hyperuricaemia
e renal toxicity

3.35 *Recognized indications for non-steroidal anti-inflammatory drugs include*

a fever
b primary dysmennorrhoea
c induction of labour
d patent ductus arteriosus in neonate
e peptic ulcer

3.36 *Recognized indications for benzodiazepines include*

a sedation for short medical procedures
b emergency treatment of status epilepticus
c obsessive compulsive disorder
d alcohol withdrawal
e animal phobia

3.37 *Sulphonyureas*

a increase the production of insulin from the pancreas
b is most useful in patients with no normal pancreatic beta cell function
c frequently cause lactic acidosis
d may cause hypoglycaemia in normal subjects
e frequently cause weight gain

3.38 *Glucagon*

a is physiologically released in response to hyperglycaemia
b increases the synthesis of glucagon in the liver
c may be given orally to treat hypoglycaemia
d has a half-life of about 1 h
e nearly always render intravenous glucose unnecessary in the treatment of hypoglycaemia

3.39 *Treatments effective in terminating an acute attack of gout include*

a colchicine
b allopurinol
c indomethacin
d probenecid
e bendrofluazide

3.40 *Recognized indications for opiates include*

a persistent cough with no serious underlying pathology
b premedication for surgery
c constipation
d acute asthmatic attack
e acute left ventricular failure

3.41 *Compared to morphine, pethidine*

a is more likely to cause constipation
b has more hypnotic effect
c has a longer duration of analgesia
d is a more potent analgesia
e is more likely to prolong labour

3.42 *Levodopa*

a is a precursor of noradrenaline
b is used in the treatment of Parkinson's disease
c can pass through the blood-brain barrier
d is usually prescribed together with dopa decarboxylase
e may cause postural hypotension

3.43 *Recognized treatments for Parkinson's disease include*

a bromocriptine
b selective monoamine oxidase type A (MAO-A) inhibitors
c antimuscarinic agents
d antinicotinic agents
e amantidine

3.44 *Frusemide*

a acts on the ascending limb of the loop of Henle
b is an osmotic diuretic
c decreases the renal excretion of sodium
d has a low ceiling diuretic effect
e can be used to treat acute hypercalcaemia

3.45 *Which of the following antiviral agents is a recognized treatment for the virus with which it is paired here?*

a HIV	zidovudine
b amantidine	measles
c ganciclovir	cytomegalovirus
d acyclovir	respiratory syncytial virus
e interferon	hepatitis B

3.46 *Which of the following statements about aminoglycosides is/are true?*

a they are bacteriostatic
b they interfere with bacterial nucleic acid synthesis
c they can easily pass through the normal meninges to the blood-brain barrier
d monitoring only the trough plasma concentration is sufficient when they are used
e the dose should be increased in those with renal impairment

3.47 *Methotrexate*

a is an inhibitor of dihydrofolate reductase
b is a recognized treatment of choriocarcinoma
c is a recognized treatment of psoriasis
d may be administered intrathecally
e is contraindicated in renal failure

3.48 *Tetracycline*

a is bacteriostatic
b can pass through the placenta to reach the fetus
c is excreted unchanged in the urine
d is effective against chlamydiae
e is ineffective against pneumococcus

3.49 *Naloxone*

a is a partial agonist of the opiod receptors
b may induce an acute withdrawal reaction in opiate dependent patients
c may be used in the diagnosis of respiratory depression from opiate overdose
d is useful in the resuscitation of neonates whose mother received pethidine in the second stage of labour
e is usually given orally

3.50 *Nitrous oxide*

a is flammable
b is a strong respiratory drive depressant
c can be used as an analgesia during labour
d should be used with 21% oxygen
e has a recovery time of about 45 minutes

3.51 *Which of the following are legal requirements in a prescription for a controlled drug?*

a it must be dated in the prescriber's own handwriting
b it must order the total quantity of the drug to be dispensed at the same time
c it must contain the address of the patient
d the total quantity of the drug must be written in both words and figures
e it must state why the prescription is necessary

3.52 *Recognized treatments for hyperlipidaemia include*

a a low fat diet
b statins
c anion-exchange resins
d nicotinic acid derivatives
e fibrates

3.53 *Side-effects of theophylline include*

a tachycardia
b nausea
c diarrhoea
d convulsion
e insomnia

3.54 *Suxamethonium*

a is a pure competitive antagonist at the neuromuscular junction
b may cause transient muscular fasciculation
c usually has a paralysis recovery time of about 40 min
d readily crosses the placenta
e may cause prolonged paralysis in individuals with hereditary low plasma cholinesterase activity

3.55 *Side-effects characteristic of phenytoin include*

a gingival hyperplasia
b hyperkinesia in children
c fatal hepatic failure
d hirsuitism
e coarsening of facial features

3.56 *Which of the following drugs are liable to cause constipation?*

a morphine
b orphenadrine (antimuscarinic drug for Parkinson disease)
c senna
d lithium
e amitriptyline

3.57 *Which of the following drugs are best avoided if possible for mothers who are breast-feeding?*

a theophylline
b ibuprofen
c erythromycin
d doxepin
e chloramphenicol

3.58 *Tardive dyskinesia*

a usually occurs within 6 months of starting a neuroleptic drug
b is due to reduced dopamine activity
c is particularly prone to occur in the elderly
d is less likely to occur if antimuscarinic drugs are prescribed with the neuroleptic drug
e is less likely to occur if clozapine rather than chlorpromazine is used

3.59 Which of the following statements about anticholinesterase agents is/are true?

a pesticides sometimes contains irreversible anticholinesterase agents
b short acting anticholinesterase drugs are useful in the diagnosis of myasthenia gravis
c they are more effective in the treatment of Lambert-Eaton myasthenic syndrome than myasthenia gravis
d an excessively high dose of anticholinesterase drug may exacerbate the weakness in myasthenia gravis
e Alzheimer dementia is a recognized indication for anticholinesterase drugs

3.60 Pharmacological effects of calcium channel blocking agents may include

a venoconstriction
b arteriodilatation
c hypotension
d positive ionotropic effect
e increase the conduction at the sinoatrial and atrioventricular nodes

Answers

3.1 a **True** b **False** c **False** d **False** e **True**
Elderly people are more likely to have multiple symptoms and diseases and receive multiple drug therapy. This greatly increases the likelihood of drug interactions. Elderly people also have a lower renal clearance and metabolism of drugs. Generally speaking, the therapeutic doses are lower than in younger adults. Elderly people also have a greater proportion of fat. Hence, the volume of distribution is increased for fat-soluble drugs, but reduced for water-soluble drugs. Elderly people are also more susceptible to side-effects than younger adults owing to impaired physiological function of organs such as kidneys, central nervous system, and autonomic nervous system.

3.2 a **False** b **True** c **True** d **True** e **False**
Muscarinic receptors are responsible for parasympathetic effects, and are present in the heart, in the bronchioles, in the ciliary muscles in the eye, and in the central nervous system. Muscarinic antagonists may be used clinically to treat bradycardia (e.g. by intravenous atropine), to treat asthma by inhalation (e.g. ipatropium), to dilate the pupils (e.g. tropicamide, cyclopentolate), to treat Parkinsonism (e.g. orphenadrine or benzhexol), to treat motion thickness (e.g. hyoscine) and to treat irritable bowel disease, or dyspeptic symptoms (e.g. dicyclomine). Pilocarpine, one of the drugs used to treat glaucoma, is a muscarinic agonist. Drugs used to induce paralysis during anaesthesia are neuromuscular blocking agents, and the postsynaptic neuromuscular receptor is nicotinic.

3.3 a **False** b **True** c **False** d **True** e **True**
Metoclopramide is a dopamine antagonist. It decreases oesophageal sphincter contraction and stimulates gastric emptying. Hence, it is used to prevent vomiting and as accessory treatment for oesophageal reflux. It also increases intestinal transit time, and is used in barium follow-through examination. However, as a dopamine antagonist (like phenothiazines), it may cause extrapyramidal side-effects, including acute dystonic reaction and oculogyric crises, especially in children and young adults. Hence, it must be used with caution in these age groups.

3.4 a **True** b **True** c **True** d **False** e **False**
Drugs used in the management of peptic ulcers include antacids (e.g. magnesium trisilicate); histamine (H_2) antagonist (e.g. cimetidine, ranitidine); proton pump inhibitors (e.g. omperazole), prostaglandin analogues (e.g. misoprostol) and bismuth (alone or in conjunction with antibiotics). Codeine phosphate is sometimes used for symptomatic treatment of cough or diarrhoea. Corticosteroids may delay the healing of peptic ulcers.

3.5 a **True** b **False** c **True** d **False** e **False**
Laxatives are often used unnecessarily owing to lack of awareness of the wide variability of the frequency of bowel motions. Constipation is best defined as the passage of hard stool less often than the normal pattern of the individually concerned. Bulk-forming laxatives are especially suitable in the presence of hard stools. They are not digested in the alimentary tract, and act by retaining water in the bowel lumen to promote peristalsis. Hence, their use must be accompanied by adequate fluid intake. They should be used only if the patient is unable to increase intake of dietary fibre. Stimulant laxatives (e.g. docussate sodium) act by increasing intestinal motility, and may cause abdominal cramps. They are best avoided. Lactulose, a semisynthetic disaccharide of fructose and galactose, is an osmotic laxative. It increases the volume of fluid in the bowel lumen by osmosis. It is useful in the treatment of hepatic encephalopathy by reducing the absorption of proteins from the bowel.

3.6 a **True** b **False** c **True** d **False** e **False**
Digoxin is a cardiac glycoside, and acts by inhibiting the sodium/potassium pump. This causes an increase in intracellular sodium, which in turn causes an increase in sodium/calcium exchange. The resulting rise in calcium level causes an increase in the force of cardiac contraction. Digoxin is therefore used in the treatment of cardiac failure. It also reduces the conductivity of the heart. It is used in the treatment of atrial fibrillation by slowing the ventricular response to the fast atrial rate. Unfortunately, it has a narrow therapeutic window (i.e. the difference between toxic dosage and therapeutic dosage is small). Hence, blood digoxin level needs to be carefully monitored. Digoxin toxicity is especially likely to occur in the presence of hypokalaemia and renal impairment.

3.7 a **False** b **False** c **True** d **True** e **True**
Pancreatin is a pancreatic enzyme supplement given to compensate for reduced or

absent enzyme secretion in the pancreas. It is useful for cystic fibrosis, following pancreatectomy or chronic pancreatitis. It can only be given orally. It is inactivated by gastric acid, and may be inactivated before reaching the duodenum. Hence, it is best taken with food, and histamine antagonists may be given to inhibit gastric acid secretion. It is prone to cause gastrointestinal symptoms such as nausea, vomiting, and abdominal discomfort.

3.8 a **False** b **True** c **True** d **False** e **True**
Both the thiazide diuretics (e.g. bendrofluazide, chlorothiazide) and loop diuretics (e.g. frusemide, ethacrynic acid) are potassium losing, and hypokalaemia frequently occurs unless potassium supplements are given. Potassium-sparing diuretics act on the collecting tubules, and include aldosterone antagonist such as spironolactone, and sodium channel blockers such as amiloride.

3.9 a **True** b **True** c **False** d **True** e **True**
Initial management for paroxysmal supraventricular tachycardia is usually reflex vagal stimulation by Valsalva manoeuvre, or carotid sinus massage. If this is ineffective, intravenous adenosine may be given. The half-life of adenosine is only a matter of seconds, and it may be given even if the patient has been previously given β-antagonists. Intravenous verapamil may be given only if the patient is not currently receiving β-antagonists. Serious side-effects such as hypotension and asystole may occur if they are given together. Direct current cardioversion may be used if drug treatment is ineffective. Lignocaine and most class 1 anti-arrhythmic drugs are used for the treatment of ventricular tachycardia.

3.10 a **False** b **False** c **True** d **True** e **True**
Amiodarone is a class III anti-arrhythmic drug, and increases the refractory period of the cardiac muscle. It is therefore especially suitable for arrhythmia associated with Wolff-Parkinson-White syndrome. However, it has a very long half-life of over 10 days, and is liable to accumulate in the body. Other side-effects include photosensitive rash and either hypo- or hyperthyroidism (due to its iodine content), corneal deposits, and slow progressive pulmonary fibrosis. Hence, although they are also effective in other types of arrhythmias, much caution is required.

3.11 a **False** b **True** c **False** d **True** e **True**
β-adrenoceptors occur in the heart, the bronchi, the peripheral vasculature, and the central nervous system. The actions of β-adrenoceptor antagonists on the cardiovascular system include slowing the heart, reduction of cardiac load, and constriction of peripheral vessels. Hence, they are used in hypertension, angina, after myocardial infarct, and in ventricular arrhythmias. They protect the heart in thyrotoxicosis, but may exacerbate cardiac failure. They constrict bronchioles and may exacerbate asthma. They also reduces tremor and palpitations and can be used for anxiety.

3.12 a **False** b **False** c **False** d **False** e **False**
The aim of antihypertensive therapy should be to keep the systolic pressure to below 160 mm Hg and the diastolic pressure to below 90 mm Hg. Treatment should not

be started without abnormal values being detected on at least three occasions. If the diastolic pressure is above 140 mm Hg, the patient should be admitted to hospital. If the diastolic pressure is consistently above 110 mm Hg or the systolic is consistently above 200 mm Hg on three readings over a period of about 2 weeks, treatment should be commenced. If the systolic pressure is 160–200 mm Hg and the diastolic pressure is 90–109 mm Hg, the decision to treat depend on whether there are other pathologies such as diabetes, renal impairment, or left ventricular failure. The initial treatment is usually a diuretic, and other drugs (e.g. beta-blockers, calcium-channel blockers, angiotensin converting enzyme inhibitors) being added or substituted. There should be no age limit for antihypertensive treatment.

3.13 a **True** b **True** c **True** d **False** e **True**
Drugs commonly used in the treatment of hypertension include thiazide diuretics (e.g. bendrofluazide), β-adrenoceptor blocking agents (e.g. atenolol), calcium-channel blocking agents (e.g. nifedipine), and angiotension converting enzyme (ACE) inhibitors (e.g. captopril). If they are ineffective, vasodilators (e.g. hydralazine), α-adrenoceptor blocking agent (e.g. prazosin) and centrally acting drugs (e.g. methyldopa) may be used.

3.14 a **True** b **False** c **True** d **True** e **False**
ACE inhibitors (e.g. captopril) inhibit the conversion of angiotensin I to angiotensin II, and are useful in the treatment of hypertension and heart failure. ACE inhibitors are useful for hypertension if diuretics and β-blockers are ineffective. However, they may cause profound hypotension when the initial dose is given. Hence, diuretics and β-blockers are best discontinued before starting ACE inhibitors, and ACE inhibitors are best started in hospital. ACE inhibitors are liable to cause hyperkalaemia, and all potassium supplements and potassium-sparing diuretics should be stopped. ACE inhibitors may cause renal impairment, and should be used with extreme caution in people with limited renal reserves.

3.15 a **True** b **True** c **True** d **True** e **True**
Drugs used in the treatment of and prophylaxis against angina include nitrates, β-adrenoceptor antagonists, and calcium-channel blockers. Short acting nitrates (e.g. glyceryl trinitrate) may be given sublingually for rapid symptomatic relief of symptoms, whereas longer acting nitrates (e.g. isosorbide dinitrate) may be given orally for prophylaxis. Verapamil, but not nifedipine, is effective in the treatment of supraventricular tachycardia, but both verapamil and nifedipine are effective in the treatment of angina.

3.16 a **False** b **False** c **False** d **True** e **False**
Heparin inhibits blood clotting by binding with antithrombin III, which inhibits the action of thrombin. Hence, the onset of action is rapid, but its duration is short. Warfarin antagonises the effect of vitamin K. It takes 2–3 days to act, and its effect lasts for days. Hence, if a definitive diagnosis of deep vein thrombosis is made, both heparin and warfarin may be started simultaneously, and heparin is usually discontinued after a few days when the INR has reached a satisfactory level. In case of

heparin overdose, protamine sulphate is a specific antidote. Warfarin may cause congenital abnormality of the fetus. Placental or haemorrhage may also occur. Hence, warfarin should be used great caution during pregnancy.

3.17 a **False** b **True** c **False** d **True** e **True**
Fibrinolytic drugs activates plasminogen to form plasmin. Hence, they break down fibrin and dissolve thrombi. They are used in the emergency treatment of life-threatening deep vein thrombosis and pulmonary embolus, and in the management in the first 12 h of an acute myocardial infarction. Streptokinase, alteplase, and anistreplase are examples of fibrinolytic drugs. Urokinase is also used in thrombolysis in the eye. Antifibrinolytic drugs prevent the dissolution of fibrin. They are used in haemorrhage when it cannot be stopped by other means, such as after prostatectomy, dental haemorrhage, or menorrhagia. Examples of antifibrinolytc drugs include desmopressin, aprotinin, and ethamsylate.

3.18 a **True** b **False** c **True** d **False** e **True**
Immediate treatment of acute asthmatic attacks in adults may include high flow oxygen, nebulized β-adrenoceptor agonist (e.g. salbutamol), nebulized ipratropium, and corticosteroids (oral prednisolone or intravenous hydrocortisone). If these measure are ineffective, intravenous aminophylline may be used, providing that the patient is not already taking an oral theophylline. Sodium cromoglycate is used for prophylaxis, but is ineffective for treatment of an acute attack. Benzodiazepines (e.g. diazepam) must never be given, as they may cause respiratory depression and precipitate respiratory arrest.

3.19 a **False** b **True** c **True** d **True** e **False**
Anaphylactic shock is associated with respiratory obstruction (due to laryngeal oedema and bronchospasm) and hypotension. The most important treatment is a β-adrenoceptor agonist, usually intramuscular adrenaline. There are cardiovascular risks associated with intravenous adrenaline, and it should only be given very slowly with great caution if the anaphylaxis is very severe. Oxygen should be administered. An intravenous H_1 antagonist (e.g. chlorpheniramine) should be administered. Intravenous hydrocortisone takes several hours to act, but is useful to prevent further deterioration. Ranitidine is a H_2 antagonist, and is used for suppression of acid secretion in the stomach.

3.20 a **True** b **True** c **True** d **True** e **True**
Until recently, benzodiazepines were inappropriately but widely prescribed for minor symptoms such as transient insomnia and mild anxiety. However, it is now known that both physical and psychological dependence on benzodiazepines occurs, and tolerance to their effects develops. Hence, benzodiazepines should not be prescribed for more than 4 weeks for severe distress caused by anxiety or insomnia. Other side-effects in the elderly include ataxia, confusion, amnesia, and paradoxical excitement, or even aggression.

3.21 a **True** b **True** c **False** d **False** e **True**
Although there are many types of antipsychotic drugs, phenothiazines

(e.g. chlorpromazine) and butyrophenones (e.g. haloperidol) are the most commonly used for the treatment of psychosis, especially schizophrenia and manic depressive psychosis. Most of these drugs are dopamine antagonists, although the pharmacology of the newer types of antipsychotic drugs (atypical neuroleptics) are more complicated. The antidopamine actions give rise to extrapyramidal symptoms and hyperprolactinaemia. Extrapyramidal symptoms are the most troublesome side-effects. These include parkinsonian symptoms (e.g. rigidity, tremor), akathisia (restlessness of the legs), dystonia, and tardive dyskinesia if the drugs are used for a long period of time. Other side-effects are due to their cholinergic actions, and include drowsiness and dry mouth.

3.22 a **True** b **True** c **False** d **False** e **False**
Lithium salts are effective in the treatment and prophylaxis of mania, and in the prophylaxis of bipolar or unipolar depression. Unfortunately, lithium has a narrow therapeutic window (i.e. the difference between toxic dosage and therapeutic dosage is small). Toxicity is more likely in the presence of hyponatraemia due to reduced excretion, as sodium competes with lithium for reabsorption in the renal tubules. Hence, the dose should be reduced in the presence of vomiting and diarrhoea. There is a significant risk in congenital cardiac abnormalities in the fetus if lithium is taken during pregnancy.

3.23 a **True** b **True** c **True** d **False** e **True**
Amitriptyline is a sedative tricyclic antidepressant. The side-effects include muscarinic cholinergic effects such as dry mouth, blurred vision, and retention of urine. Postural hypotension and arrhythmia may occur, and ECG monitoring is essential in the management of amitripyline overdose. Other side-effects include drowsiness, confusion, and weight gain. Hyponatraemia may occur with all types of antidepressants due to inappropriate secretion of antidiuretic hormone, which may also cause drowsiness confusion and convulsions.

3.24 a **True** b **True** c **False** d **False** e **True**
The most commonly used antidepressants are tricyclics (e.g. amitriptiline) and serotonin re-uptake inhibitors (e.g. fluoxetine, paroxetine). MAO inhibitors (e.g. phenelzine) are particularly effective in patients with atypical or phobic symptoms. However, they interact with many types of food (e.g. cheese, yeast extract) and drugs (e.g. sympathomimetics in cough mixtures) to potentiate the pressor effect of tyramine, and may cause dangerous degree of hypertension. These side-effects are due to MAO type B inhibition. However, this side-effect is much less likely for mobenclamide, a reversible MAO type A inhibitor. Benzodiazepines are hypnotics and anxiolytics, and must not be used as antidepressants. Barbiturates are major tranquillizers.

3.25 a **True** b **False** c **True** d **True** e **False**
Aspirin is mainly used for its anti-inflammatory and antiplatelet actions. Its anti-inflammatory actions are due to inhibition of arachidonic acid cyclo-oxygenase, and decrease prostaglandin production. It is effective in the treatment of pyrexia,

musculoskeletal pain, arthritic pain, and dysmenorrhoea. Unless the circumstances are exceptional (e.g. Still's disease), it must not be used in children below the age of 12, as its use is associated with Reye's syndrome. Aspirin is also used as an antiplatelet agent immediately after a myocardial infarct, and in the prevention of strokes in high risk patients.

3.26 a **True** b **False** c **False** d **True** e **False**
The main effects of opiates are on the central nervous system and the gastrointestinal tract. The therapeutic effects on the central nervous system are analgesia and euphoria. However, they may also cause respiratory depression, especially when large doses are used and in accidental overdose. They may also cause hypotension. They suppress cough, and are often used as cough suppressants. Nausea and vomiting are common owing to action on the chemoreceptor trigger zone. In the gastrointestinal tract, opiates reduce motility, and constipation is often a troublesome side-effect.

3.27 a **False** b **False** c **False** d **False** e **False**
In terminal care, analgesics are more effective in preventing pain than treating established pain. Hence, they should be given regularly at the lowest dose possible to prevent pain. Oral analgesics should be given unless the patient either cannot swallow or vomits excessively. Non-steroidal anti-inflammatory drugs are often effective in keeping the patient pain free in the early stages, and are especially useful for pain due to bone secondaries. Although tolerance to opiates may develop, the aim of terminal care is to keep the patient comfortable. Hence, a certain dose of opiates is ineffective in preventing pain, this should be increased by 50%.

3.28 a **True** b **True** c **False** d **False** e **True**
First line treatment of *acute* migraine attacks include analgesics such as paracetamol and aspirin, and antiemetics such as metoclopramide. If this is ineffective, ergotamine may be used. However, there are several side-effects such as vomiting, abdominal pain, and muscle cramps. Sumatriptan, a new serotonin agonist, may also be used. Drugs used for *prophylaxis* of migraine include pizotifen, β-adrenoceptor antagonists (e.g. propranolol), and tricyclic antidepressants. Clonidine has not been found to be effective. Methysergide is effective, but unfortunately has serious side-effects such as retroperitoneal fibrosis and fibrosis of heart valves and pleura. Hence, it should only be used by specialists and require hospital supervision.

3.29 a **False** b **True** c **True** d **True** e **False**
Carbamazepine is useful in the treatment of most types of epilepsy except absence seizures (petit mal). It is especially effective in the treatment of temporal lobe epilepsy. It is also used for trigeminal neuralgia, and in the prophylaxis of manic depressive illness if lithium is ineffective. Intravenous diazepam is usually the first line treatment of status epilepticus.

3.30 a **False** b **True** c **False** d **False** e **True**
The side-effects of sodium valproate include gastric irritation, nausea, increased appetite and weight gain, and transient hair loss. It may also cause metabolic

abnormalities such as hyperammonaemia and impaired liver function tests. Rarely, this may progress to fatal hepatic failure. Pancreatitis may also occur. Gum hypertrophy and megaloblastic anaemia are side-effects of phenytoin.

3.31 a **False** b **False** c **False** d **True** e **False**
The plasma half-life of a drug is the time it takes for the plasma concentration of a drug to fall by half when it is discontinued. Hence, the half-life is shorter the faster the drug reaches its steady-state concentration. In a first-order elimination process, the rate of elimination is proportional to the plasma concentration. Hence, the plasma half-life is constant. In a zero-order elimination process (e.g. for alcohol above 100 mg/litre), the rate of elimination is constant (about 8 g/h). Hence, the half-life decreases as the plasma concentration falls. Whilst the plasma half-life is an important in determining the *time* it takes to reach steady-state concentration, it does not affect the actual steady-state concentration level, which is dependent only on the rate of administration relative to the rate of elimination.

3.32 a **False** b **False** c **True** d **True** e **True**
Salbutamol acts as a β-adrenergic agonist. Tolbutamide is one of the sulphonylureas, which act by activating receptors on the β cells of the pancreatic islets to release stored insulin. Allopurinol prevents gout by inhibiting xanthine oxidase. Enalapril acts by inhibiting ACE, and is used in the treatment of heart failure and hypertension. Acetazolamide inhibits carbonic anhydrase, and is used in the treatment of glaucoma.

3.33 a **False** b **False** c **True** d **True** e **False**
Antibiotics act generally via one of three mechanisms: inhibition of bacterial cell wall synthesis (e.g. penicillins, cephalosporins), inhibition of protein synthesis (e.g. tetracyclines, aminoglycosides, erythromycin, chloramphenicol), and inhibition of nucleic synthesis (e.g. sulphonamides, quinolones such as ciprofloxacin, and axoles such as metronidazole).

3.34 a **True** b **False** c **True** d **False** e **False**
The main side-effects of isoniazid are liver toxicity and peripheral neuropathy. Liver damage may range from mild elevation of liver enzymes to severe hepatitis. Peripheral neuropathy is caused by increased excretion of pyridoxine, owing to the structural similarity between isoniazid and pyridoxine. It occurs more commonly in slow acetylators and in those with liver disease. It may be prevented by prescribing pyridoxine with isoniazid. Other side-effects include optic neuritis and mental disturbances. Red discolourization of urine is a side-effect of rifampicin. Hyperuricaemia is a side-effect of pyrazinamide, and renal toxicity is a side-effect of streptomycin.

3.35 a **True** b **True** c **False** d **True** e **False**
Non-steroidal anti-inflammatory drugs all inhibit cyclo-oxygenase, although each individual agent has a variety of effects on other enzymes in prostaglandin synthesis. In general, they are anti-inflammatory (e.g. used in rheumatoid arthritis, juvenile chronic arthritis, pericarditis), antipyretic, and analgesic; they have a tendency to reduce platelet adhesiveness (e.g. aspirin used for prevention of vascular occlusion);

close ductus arteriosus in neonates (e.g. used in patent ductus arteriosus); and prolong gestation (although they are not often used in premature labour owing to risk of premature closure of ductus arteriosus). Non-steroidal anti-inflammatory drugs must be used with caution if there is a past history of peptic ulcers. Gastric mucosal prostaglandin inhibits acid secretion and promotes secretion of mucus. Inhibition by non-steroidal anti-inflammatory drugs may precipitate a recurrence of peptic ulcers.

3.36 a **True** b **True** c **False** d **True** e **False**
Benzodiazepines act by attaching to a specific site on the GABA receptor/chloride channel complex. There are three subtypes of benzodiazepine receptors, although the benzodiazepines currently available act on all three subtypes. Clinical effects include anxiolytic, sedative, hypnotic, and muscle relaxant properties. Hence, their anxiolytic effects are used for anxiety states and panic attacks, but should not be used for depression, obsessive compulsive disorders, or phobic anxiety confined to specific situations. Their sedative effects are used before short medical procedures such as endoscopies. Their hypnotic properties are used as a short-term measure to treat insomnia, but must not be used for longer than about 4 weeks to avoid tolerance and dependence. Their muscle relaxant properties are used to treat muscle spasm. Diazepam is used to treat status epilepticus. Benzodiazepines (e.g. reducing doses of chlordiazepoxide over a week) can be used to treat alcohol withdrawal.

3.37 a **False** b **False** c **False** d **True** e **True**
There are two main types of oral hypoglycaemic agents: sulphonylureas and biguanides. Sulphonyureas (e.g. tolbutamide, chlorpropamide) act by releasing stored insulin in the pancreatic β cells, but do not increase insulin formation. Hence, they are only useful in those with some normal β cell function. They may also cause hypoglycaemia in both normal and diabetic patients. They frequently cause weight gain. Biguanides (e.g. metformin) probably act by reducing the production of glucose from the liver and increasing the sensitivity of peripheral tissues to insulin. They do not cause hypoglycaemia by themselves. Biguanides may cause lactic acidosis.

3.38 a **False** b **False** c **False** d **False** e **False**
Glucagon is a polypeptide hormone which is physiologically released from the a islet cells of the pancreas in response to hypoglycaemia. It increases plasma glucose level by breakdown of liver glucagon to form glucose. Glucagon injection may be used to treat hypoglycaemia (e.g. due to insulin overdose in diabetic patients), and may be given by members of the patient's family in an emergency. It has a short half-life (about 5 min), and the effect is rapid. However, it is not effective if the liver glucagon is already depleted. Hence, intravenous glucose is still often necessary in the treatment of hypoglycaemia.

3.39 a **True** b **False** c **True** d **False** e **False**
Gout is associated with hyperuricaemia, through either overproduction or underexcretion of urate. Anti-inflammatory drugs (e.g. non-steroidal anti-inflammatory drugs such as indomethacin or colchicine) are effective in terminating an acute attack

of gout. Colchicine is highly effective, and appears to be specific for gout. Drugs used to prevent future attacks of gout include allopurinol (which inhibits xanthine oxidase and hence uric acid synthesis) and uricosurics such as probenecid (which increases the urate excretion in urine). However, both allopurinol and uricosurics are ineffective in an acute attack. Bendrofluazide may precipitate gout, and should be avoided.

3.40 a **True** b **True** c **False** d **False** e **True**
Pharmacological effects of opiates include analgesia, drowsiness, respiratory depression and depression of cough reflex, antiemesis, constipation, and dilatation of both arterioles and venules. Hence, they are indicated for the treatment of chronic pain in terminal illness, premedication before surgery, cough suppression, diarrhoea, and in left ventricular failure. They should never be given in an acute asthmatic attack because of their effects of respiratory depression and bronchoconstriction.

3.41 a **False** b **False** c **False** d **False** e **False**
Compared to morphine, pethidine has both a shorter duration and less potency as an analgesic. However, it also has less hypnotic, constipation, urinary retention, labour-prolonging effects. Hence, pethidine is widely used for moderately intense pain, and during labour.

3.42 a **False** b **True** c **True** d **False** e **True**
Levodopa is a natural precursor of dopamine. It is used in the treatment of Parkinson's disease which is due to degeneration of the nigrostriatal dopaminergic neurones. Levodopa can easily pass the blood-brain barrier. However, as it is decarboxylated peripherally by the enzyme dopa decarboxylase, a large dose is needed if it is used on its own. Hence, levodopa is usually prescribed with a peripheral decarboxylase inhibitor (e.g. carbidopa in the combination Sinemet) which inhibits the conversion of levodopa to dopamine peripherally. Common side-effects include postural hypotension, nausea, and involuntary movements.

3.43 a **True** b **False** c **True** d **False** e **True**
Parkinson's disease is due to degeneration of the dopaminergic nigrostriatal neurones, resulting in an imbalance between the cholinergic neurones and dopaminergic neurones. Drug used in treament of Parkinson's disease include those which increases dopaminergic stimulation (e.g. levodopa with peripheral decarboxylase inhibitors, bromocriptine, and amantidine), selective MAO-B inhibitors (e.g. selegiline), and antimuscarinic agents. Selective MAO-A inhibitors (e.g. moclobemide) are used in the treatment of depression. The brain cholinergic receptors are of the muscarinic type. Nicotinic receptors are situated in the neuromuscular junctions and some post-ganglionic endings.

3.44 a **True** b **False** c **False** d **False** e **True**
Frusemide acts on the ascending limb of the loop of Henle, and increases the sodium excretion. It impairs the urine-concentrating mechanism, and is a very effective diuretic. Increase in the dose of frusemide is accompanied by increased diuresis (i.e. it

has a high ceiling effect). It also increases the calcium excretion, and can be used to treat acute hypercalcaemia.

3.45 a **True** b **False** c **True** d **False** e **True**
Zidovudine inhibits reverse transcriptase, and causes premature chain termination in the replication of the single-stranded RNA of the HIV virus into double stranded DNA. Hence, zidovudine is used to treat human immunodeficiency virus. Amantidine has proved to be effective against influenza A only. Both acyclovir and ganciclovir inhibit viral DNA synthesis. Acyclovir is used to treat herpes virus (e.g. herpes simplex and herpes zoster). Ganciclovir is excreted unchanged in the urine, and is used to treat life- or sight-threatening cytomegalovirus.

3.46 a **False** b **False** c **False** d **False** e **False**
Aminoglycosides (e.g. gentamicin, neomycin) act by interfering with the bacterial protein synthesis through binding to the ribosomes so that the incorrect amino acid sequences are produced. Hence, they are bactericidal. They do not pass through normal or inflamed meninges, and hence should not be used in the treatment of bacterial meningitis. As they are excreted unchanged by the kidneys, a abnormally high plasma concentration can be nephrotoxic. Hence, the dose should be reduced in the presence of renal impairment, and monitoring of both the peak and trough concentrations is required to ensure that a therapeutic but not toxic dose has been achieved.

3.47 a **True** b **True** c **True** d **True** e **True**
Methotrexate is an inhibitor of dihydrofolate reductase, and prevents the synthesis of tetrahydrofolic acid which is essential for the synthesis of nucleic acids. It is a cytotoxic agent, and used in the treatment of a variety of malignancies including childhood acute lymphoblastic leukaemia, choriocarcinoma, non-Hodgkin's lymphomas, and metastatic breast cancer. As methotrexate also suppress epidermal activity, it is also used to treat psoriasis. Methotrexate may be administered orally, intramuscularly, intravenously, or intrathecally. It is administered intrathecally as a central nervous system prophylaxis of childhood acute lymphoblastic leukaemia. As it is excreted by the kidneys, it is contraindicated in the presence of significant renal impairment.

3.48 a **True** b **True** c **True** d **True** e **False**
Tetracyclines (e.g. tetracycline, doxycycline) are broad-spectrum antibiotics, and are active against nearly all gram positive and gram negative bacteria. They are specifically used to treat chlamydiae and mycoplasma pneumonia. As tetracycline is excreted unchanged in the urine, it should be avoided in the presence of significant renal impairment. It should be avoided in pregnancy and for children under 12 years of age, as they are taken up by the teeth and growing bones of the fetus or children, and causes discoloration.

3.49 a **False** b **True** c **True** d **True** e **False**
Naloxone is a pure antagonist at all opioid receptors. Hence, it temporarily reverses, and is diagnostic of, respiratory depression due to opiate overdose. However, it may

induce an acute withdrawal reaction in opiate-dependent patients. It is also routinely used to treat respiratory depression in neonates whose mother received pethidine in the second stage of labour. It can only be given by injection, as only a small proportion of the oral dose reaches the blood stream.

3.50 a **False** b **False** c **True** d **False** e **False**
Nitrous oxide is a colourless non-flammable gas with slightly sweetish smell. Since it has a strong analgesic effect without depressing the respiratory drive, it is widely used for its analgesic effect in equal proportion with oxygen (as Entenox) during labour. It is also used together with other anaesthetic agents for surgical anaesthesia. As nitrous oxide has a low solubility in blood, it has both a short induction and recovery time (<5 min).

3.51 a **True** b **False** c **True** d **True** e **False**
The principle legal requirements in a prescription for a controlled drug are that it must contain the patient's name and address; the form and strength of the preparation should be stated; the total quantity of the preparation should be written in both words and figures, and the dose and frequency of administration should be specified. The prescription should be in the prescriber's own handwriting unless exemption has been obtained by the prescriber, but in any event, the date and the signature must be in the prescriber's handwriting. It may order the prescription to be dispensed by instalments.

3.52 a **True** b **True** c **True** d **True** e **True**
Management of hyperlipidaemia involves diagnosis and treatment of any underlying disorders, appropriate dietary advice, and drug treatments if necessary. Available drug treatments include anion-exchange resins (e.g. cholestyramine), fibrates (e.g. bezafibrate), nicotinic acid derivatives (e.g. acipimox), and statins (e.g. simvastatin). Statins inhibit HMG CoA in cholesterol synthesis, and have recently been shown in several studies to be effective both in primary and secondary prevention of ischaemic heart disease in hypercholestolaemic patients.

3.53 a **True** b **True** c **True** d **True** e **True**
Theophylline is a bronchodilator, and is used to treat asthma. It is a competitive inhibitor of adenosine receptors as well as a phosphodiesterase inhibitor. However, it has a low therapeutic window, and the plasma concentration should be monitored to avoid a toxic level. Theophylline, like caffeine, is a central stimulant and may cause insomnia. It also causes nausea, vomiting, diarrhoea, tachycardia, and convulsions. Vomiting, cardiac arrhythmia, and convulsions are especially liable to occur if theophylline is given rapidly through the veins.

3.54 a **False** b **True** c **False** d **False** e **True**
Suxamethonium is a depolarizing agent at the neuromuscular junction. It activates the nicotinic acetylcholine receptor and often causes transient muscular fasciculation before paralysis occurs. It has a short half-life (<10 min), and is used for brief medical procedures such as electroconvulsive therapy or in status epilepticus. It does not cross

the placenta, and can be used for caesarean section. However, in a few individuals with a hereditary low plasma cholinesterase activity, the effect of suxamethonium may persist for a prolonged period of time and the patient needs to be ventilated during this period. Hence, it is important to enquire about any family history of prolonged recovery following anaesthesia.

3.55 a **True** b **False** c **False** d **True** e **True**
Phenytoin is effective against almost all forms of epilepsy except absence seizures. However, it has many side-effects. They include hirsutism, coarsening of facial features, and gingival hyperplasia. Hence, it should be avoided if possible in adolescents. It also has a wide range of neurological side-effects, from headache, tremor, and dizziness to ataxia, peripheral neuropathy, drowsiness, and delirium. It may cause non-specific skin rashes as well as erythema multiforme and toxic epidermal necrolysis. It may also cause folic acid and vitamin D deficiency resulting in megaloblastic anaemia and osteomalacia. Hyperkinesia in children is a characteristic side-effect of barbiturates, and fatal hepatic failure is a characteristic side-effect of sodium valproate.

3.56 a **True** b **True** c **False** d **False** e **True**
Drugs which may cause constipation include opiates (e.g. morphine), antimuscarinic drugs (e.g. orphenadrine, benzhexol), tricyclic antidepressants (e.g. imipramine, amitriptyline), iron preparations, and aluminium-containing antacids. Senna is a stimulant laxative. Lithium usually causes vomiting and diarrhoea.

3.57 a **True** b **True** c **False** d **True** e **True**
Most drugs are safe for mothers who are breast-feeding to take, as the amount present in her milk is usually very small. However, there are some exceptions. They include cytotoxic drugs, some anticonvulsants (e.g. phenobarbitone, phenytoin), some antibiotics (e.g. tetracyline, which discolours the baby's teeth and bones, and chloramphenicol which may rarely cause 'grey baby syndrome'). Tricyclic antidepressants (except doxepin) are safe.

3.58 a **False** b **False** c **True** d **False** e **True**
Tardive dyskinesia is a disorder of involuntary movements of the face, jaw, and limbs usually after prolonged use (>2 years) of a neuroleptic drug. It is due to increased dopamine sensitivity and increase in the number of dopamine receptors following chronic blockade. Tardive dyskinesia is particularly prone to occur in the elderly, and if anticholinergic drugs have been given to alleviate Parkinsonian symptoms. It is less likely to occur for the new 'atypical' neuroleptics such as resperidone and clozapine.

3.59 a **True** b **True** c **False** d **True** e **True**
Anticholinesterases inhibit the enzymes which break down acetylcholine. Hence, they prolong the action of acetylcholine at the neuromuscular junction. The symptoms in myasthenia gravis are due to antibodies to their acetylcholine receptors, and anticholinesterases are effective in improving the symptoms. However, an excessively high dose may exacerbate the symptoms (a cholinergic crisis) by causing an excess accumulation of acetylcholine. Anticholinesterase drugs are less effective in

Eaton-Lambert myasthenic syndrome where there is a deficiency of acetylcholine release from the presynaptic neurone. Some centrally-acting anticholinesterase (e.g. tetrahydroaminoacridine) has been used in Alzheimer's dementia with limited benefits.

3.60 a **False** b **True** c **True** d **False** e **False**
The pharmacological effects of all calcium channel blockers are broadly similar, although the relative strengths of each of these effects differ amongst individual drugs. The pharmacological effects include both arteriole and venodilatation, hypotension, negative inotropic effects, and slowing of the conduction and increasing the refractoriness at the sinoatrial (SA) and atrioventricular (AV) nodes. Hence, they are used in the management of hypertension (via its hypotension effect), angina (via its vasodilatation effect), Raynaud's disease (via its arteriodilatation effect), and in the treatment of supraventricular tachycardia (via its effects on slowing of the conduction at the SA and AV nodes).

4 *Pathology*

Questions

4.1 ***Which of the following are examples of response of tissue by hypertrophy?***

a breast enlargement in puberty
b prostate enlargement in advancing age
c liver nodule formation in cirrhosis of the liver
d enlargement of the left ventricle as a response to hypertension
e adrenal gland enlargement as a response to inappropriate ACTH secretion

4.2 ***Metaplasia***

a is accompanied by a higher proportion of cells undergoing mitosis
b is accompanied by increase in nuclear to cytoplasmic ratio
c is the transformation of one type of differentiated cells to another
d is irreversible
e may progress to dysplasia and neoplasia

4.3 ***Causes of amyloidosis include***

a myeloma
b heart failure
c rheumatoid arthritis
d osteomyelitis
e bronchiectasis

4.4 ***Which of the following disorders are significantly more frequent in bed-rest patients?***

a deep vein thrombosis
b osteoarthritis
c pneumonia
d osteoporosis
e rheumatoid arthritis

4.5 ***According to Virchow, the predisposing factors for thrombus include***

a changes in the muscular layer of the vessel
b changes in the intimal surface of the vessel
c increase in temperature of the blood

d changes in the blood constituents
e changes in the pattern of blood flow

4.6 *Complications resulting from emboli from the left ventricle include*

a transient ischaemic attacks
b dry gangrene of the legs
c pulmonary embolism
d ischaemic bowel
e pulmonary hypertension

4.7 *Causes of acute inflammation include*

a bacterial infection
b infarction
c altered state of immune response
d trauma
e acid burn

4.8 *Which of the following happens in the early stages of an acute inflammatory reaction?*

a the arterioles dilate
b transudate fluid escapes into the extravascular space
c the permeability of small blood vessels decreases
d the blood flow at the site of injury increases
e lymphocytes migrate through the walls of venules

4.9 *The possible roles of neutrophil polymorphs in acute inflammation include*

a opsonization of bacteria
b release of pyrogens
c phagocytosis of bacteria
d intracellular killing of bacteria
e deactivation of the complement system

4.10 *Characteristic pathological features of chronic inflammation include*

a infiltrate containing lymphocytes
b infiltrate containing neutrophils
c infiltrate containing macrophages
d infiltrate containing plasma cells
e formation of fibrous tissue

4.11 *Which of the following statements about the multistep theory of carcinogenesis is/are true?*

a the promotion step precede the initiation step

b the genetic material with neoplastic potential is first introduced in the promotion step
c carcinogenesis requires either the promotion or the initiation step
d the theory explains the long latency period between exposure to carcinogens and clinical malignancy
e the persistence stage may occur without the presence of a promotor

4.12 *Which of the following pathological features of a tumour suggest that it is benign?*

a an epithelial tumour growing away from the surface
b an ulcerative surface
c an well demarcated border
d multiple nuclei in cells
e significant histological difference from parent tissues

4.13 *Teratomas*

a arise from mesoderm cells only
b are almost always malignant
c may contain teeth
d always occur in the gonads
e may contain muscular tissue

4.14 *Which of the following tumour markers is/are correctly matched?*

a choriocarcinoma — alphafetoprotein (AFP)
b colonic adenocarcinoma — carcinoembryonic antigen (CEA)
c hepatocellular carcinoma — β-hCG
d myeloma — Bence Jones protein
e carcinoid tumour — vanillylmandelic acid (VMA)

4.15 *In type I hypersensitivity*

a the immune reaction occurs about 48 h after exposure to an antigen
b rhesus isoimmunization is an example
c igG antibodies are mainly responsible
d degranulation of mast cells occurs
e vasodilatation and increased vascular permeability occurs

4.16 *In type IV hypersensitivity*

a the immune reaction takes more than 12 h to develop
b it is mediated by antibodies
c it occurs in sarcoidosis
d lymphokines are released from sensitized T cells
e intracellular killing may occur inside macrophages

4.17 *Which of the following are risk factors for atherosclerosis?*

a raised high-density lipoprotein (HDL)
b increasing age
c hypertension
d cigarette smoking
e diabetes mellitus

4.18 *Which of the following statements about aneurysms is/are true?*

a they are dilatations throughout the length of blood vessels
b the thoracic aorta is the commonest site for aortic aneurysms
c dissecting aneurysms are commonly associated with degeneration of the aortic media
d berry aneurysms in the circle of Willis predispose to subarachnoid haemorrhage
e microaneurysms in the intracerebral capillaries predispose to subarachnoid haemorrhage

4.19 *Which of the following statements about pathological changes following an acute myocardial infarct is/are true?*

a both microscopic and macroscopic changes can be seen 2 h after an infarct
b fibrous tissue starts to appear 3 months after an infarct
c the infarcted muscle becomes oedematous 1–2 days after the infarct
d granulation tissue follows fibrosis
e neutrophil infiltration occurs within 1–2 days

4.20 *Which of the following complications may occur during the first week of a acute myocardial infarct*

a cardiac failure
b rupture of the papillary muscle causing mitral incompetence
c ventricular aneurysm
d pulmonary embolus
e pericarditis

4.21 *Bronchopneumonia*

a may be caused by staphylococcus
b is commonly unilateral
c commonly affects a single lobe of the lung
d is associated with acute inflammatory exudate in the alveoli
e occurs more frequently in the elderly and in infancy

4.22 *Which of the following statements about lobar pneumonia is/are true?*

a it is commoner in the elderly
b it usually affects an entire lobe of a lung
c the commonest causative organism is streptococcus pneumoniae
d it characteristically undergoes four pathological stages, congestion, red hepatization, grey hepatization, and resolution
e the red hepatization stage is characterized by the accumulation of fibrin

4.23 *Which of the following statements about pulmonary tuberculosis is/are true?*

a the focus of primary TB is usually an unilateral apical lesion
b primary tuberculosis is often associated with hilar lymphanopathy
c secondary tuberculosis usually consist of bilateral mid-zone lesions
d pleural effusion may complicate secondary tuberculosis
e miliary pulmonary tuberculosis is characterized by small granulomas throughout both lungs

4.24 *Bronchiectasis*

a is characterized by permanent dilatation of bronchi and bronchioles
b commonly affects the upper lobes
c is commonly associated with recurrent respiratory tract infection
d may be complicated by amyloidosis
e results from bronchial obstruction

4.25 *Coal-worker's pneumoconiosis may give rise to*

a black pigment in the lung
b extrinsic allergic alveolitis
c progressive massive fibrosis
d lung nodules less than 1 cm in diameter
e mesothelioma

4.26 *Which of the following statements about the histological types of bronchial carcinoma is/are true?*

a small cell carcinoma is the commonest type
b squamous cell carcinoma are usually hilar
c small cell carcinoma typically metastasis early
d ectopic parathyroid hormones are typically secreted by small cell carcinoma
e adenocarcinomas are usually peripheral

4.27 *Barrett's oesophagus*

a usually results from chronic reflux of gastric contents
b is associated with squamous epithelium in the lower oesophagus

c is associated with oesophageal diverticula
d is associated with oesophageal varices
e predisposes to carcinoma of the oesophagus

4.28 *Carcinomas of the stomach*

a are commoner in the United Kingdom than in Japan
b are mostly of the squamous type
c may spread to the ovaries through the peritoneal cavity
d usually present in an early stage before spread through the stomach wall has occurred
e have become more frequent over the last few decades

4.29 *Predisposing factors for carcinoma of the stomach include*

a pernicious anaemia
b chronic gastritis
c blood group O
d excessive vitamin C intake
e excessive salt intake

4.30 *Coeliac disease*

a is due to sensitivity to the gliadin component of gluten
b is caused by metaplasia of the intestinal epithelium
c is autosomal recessive in inheritance
d is caused by exposure of the intestine to fungus
e has a HLA association

4.31 *In coeliac disease*

a crypt atrophy is characteristic
b villous atrophy is characteristic
c the ileum is more commonly affected than the jejunum
d malignant lymphoma is a recognized long term complication
e fat malabsorption is common

4.32 *Which of the following pathological features are characteristic of Crohn's disease?*

a inflammation of the mucosa without involvement of the muscle
b presence of granuloma
c skip lesions
d fistula formation
e macroscopic 'cobblestone' appearance

4.33 *Diverticular disease*

a occurs more frequently in those with high fibre intake

b occurs more frequently in the transverse colon
c is associated with herniations of the bowel mucosa into the bowel wall
d may be complicated by fistula formation
e is a significant risk factor for carcinoma of the colon

4.34 *Carcinoma of the large bowel*

a is of the squamous type in more than 20% of cases
b occurs most frequently in the ascending colon
c may spread to the liver
d causes obstruction more frequently if it occurs in the ascending colon than in the rectum
e is usually staged by the TNM method

4.35 *Viruses which cause liver damage include*

a hepatitis A virus
b Epstein-Barr virus
c rotavirus
d cytomegalovirus
e parainfluenza virus

4.36 *Which of the following abnormalities may be seen in liver disease caused by alcohol?*

a mallory's hyalin in the cytoplasm of hepatocytes
b fat globules in the cytoplasm of hepatocytes
c micronodular cirrhosis
d macronodular cirrhosis
e 'piecemeal' hepatic necrosis

4.37 *Primary haemochromatosis*

a is synonymous with haemosiderosis
b may be due to excessive iron in the diet
c is caused by genetic defect in chromosome 6
d may cause diabetes
e is associated with increased absorption of iron

4.38 *Graves' disease*

a is the commonest cause for hyperthyroidism
b is caused by long-acting thyroid stimulator (LATS) acting on thyroid epithelial cells
c is usually associated with nodules in the thyroid gland
d is associated with infiltration of the orbital tissues by fat and mucopolysaccarides
e may be associated with deposition of mucopolysaccardies in the dermis of the skin in the shins

4.39 *Hashimoto's thyroiditis*

a is associated with a firm bright red thyroid gland macroscopically
b has an HLA association
c is associated with dense lymphocytic infiltration of the thyroid gland microscopically
d may cause transient hyperthyroidism in the early stages of the disease
e is characterized by the presence of thyroglobulin autoantibodies

4.40 *Follicular adenoma of the thyroid*

a is the commonest type of thyroid tumour
b commonly transforms to follicular carcinoma within a year of presentation
c characteristically causes hyperthyroidism
d is usually surrounded by a fibrous capsule
e is usually cystic

4.41 *Which of the following statements about thyroid carcinoma is/are true?*

a follicular carcinoma is the commonest type
b papillary carcinoma typically occurs in the elderly
c anaplastic carcinoma has the worst prognosis
d follicular carcinoma often spread to the bones through the blood stream
e papillary carcinoma is associated with excessive secretion of calcitonin

4.42 *Fibroadenoma of the breast*

a is the commonest benign tumour of the breast
b commonly occurs after menopause
c may grow rapidly during pregnancy
d usually has a smooth outer surface
e often progresses to malignancy

4.43 *Which of the following statements about carcinoma of the breast is/are true?*

a infiltrating ductal type is the commonest
b it never occurs in the male
c the infiltrating ductal type has the best prognosis
d it commonly spread to the lungs via the blood stream
e it commonly spread to the axillary lymph nodes via lymphatics

4.44 *Which of the following statements about squamous carcinoma of the cervix is/are true?*

a it is less common than adenocarcinoma of the cervix
b human papillomaviruses have been implicated as an important predisposing factor
c it is commoner in smokers than non-smokers

d it arises from cells in the cervical transformation zone
e it is often preceded by epithelial changes which can be recognized by cervical smear histology

4.45 *Uterine fibroids*

a usually occur between the ages of 20 and 40
b are associated with high parity
c are leiomyomas
d are the commonest tumours in the female genital tract
e are diffuse ill-circumscribed tumours

4.46 *Compared with seminoma of the testes, teratoma*

a occurs in an older age group
b is commoner
c has a more uniform and homogeneous macroscopic appearance
d is less aggressive
e is more likely to be cystic

4.47 *Causes of focal proliferative glomerulonephritis include*

a Henoch-Schonlein purpura
b poststreptococcal infection
c systemic lupus erythematosus
d hepatitis B
e diabetes mellitus

4.48 *Transitional cell carcinomas of the bladder*

a are less common than squamous cell carcinoma
b are usually solitary
c are commoner in smokers
d may cause secondary hydronephrosis
e are often papillary

4.49 *Which of the following statements about Hodgkin's lymphomas is/are true?*

a they usually occur in the elderly
b the lymphocyte depletion type is associated with the best prognosis
c they are characterized by the presence of Reed-Sternberg cells
d the prognosis is worse if there are systemic symptoms such as weight loss and pyrexia
e the nodular sclerosis type may progress to the lymphocyte predominant type

4.50 *Causes of eosinophil leukocytosis include*

a atopy

b virus infection
c bacterial infection
d parasite infection
e Hodgkin's lymphoma

4.51 *Characteristic haematological features of iron deficiency anaemia include*

a predominance of microcytic red cells
b predominance of hyperchromic red cells
c grossly increased reticulocyte count
d increased serum ferritin
e a high level of mean corpuscular haemoglobin (MCH)

4.52 *Characteristic haematological features vitamin B_{12} deficiency include*

a a slight reduction in platelet count
b a slight increase in white cell count
c neutrophils hypersegmentation
d macrocytes on the blood film
e megaloblasts in the bone marrow

4.53 *Compared with vitamin B_{12} deficiency, anaemia due to folate deficiency*

a develops more gradually
b is more likely to be caused by disease of the terminal ileum
c is more likely to result in neurological disorder
d is more likely to be due to an autoimmune disease
e is more likely to occur in pregnancy

4.54 *Characteristic pathological features of multiple myeloma include*

a presence of monoclonal immunoglobulin (paraproteins)
b polycythaemia
c rouleaux formation
d raised ESR
e increased platelets

Answers

4.1 a **False** b **False** c **False** d **True** e **False**

Growth of tissues may occur in response to either physiological (e.g. puberty, pregnancy) or pathological causes. Growth may be achieved by either hyperplasia or hypertrophy, or a combination of both. In hyperplasia, the number of cells increases although the cell size remains the same. This usually occurs in tissues with a capacity to divide. Examples are breast enlargement as a response to puberty, prostate enlargement in advancing stage, liver nodule formation in cirrhosis of the liver, and endocrine gland enlargement in response to trophic hormones. In hypertrophy, the existing cells become larger but no new cells are formed. This occurs in tissues with little or no capacity to divide. Examples are increase in muscle bulk in athletes, and cardiac hypertrophy in response to hypertension or valvular diseases.

4.2 a **False** b **False** c **True** d **False** e **True**
Metaplasia is the reversible transformation of one type of differentiated cell into another. Common examples are transformation of columnar epithelium of bronchi in smokers to squamous epithelium, and changes from squamous epithelium of the oesophagus to glandular (gastric-like) epithelium in reflux. Dysplasia, but not metaplasia, is associated with increase in the proportion of mitotic cells and presence of atypical morphology such as increase in nuclear to cytoplasmic ratio. Although metaplasia may progress to dysplasia and finally neoplasia, this is not inevitable.

4.3 a **True** b **False** c **True** d **True** e **True**
Amyloidosis can be classified according to either the clinical picture or the amyloid substance. The common causes are myleoma (the amyloid substance being AL amyloid, which consists of immunoglobulin light chains) and reaction to chronic inflammatory disorders (e.g. bronchietasis, osteomyelitis, rheumatoid arthritis). Other rarer causes are haemodialysis, and hereditary disorders. Heart failure may be a complication of amyloidosis.

4.4 a **True** b **False** c **True** d **True** e **False**
Bed rest increases the risk of several disorders. Pressure sores may result from ischaemic necrosis of the skin caused by compression of the capillary network. Osteoporosis and muscle wasting are examples of disuse atrophy. Deep vein thrombosis (and hence pulmonary embolus) may be caused by venous status, as the calf muscles are important in enhancing venous return of blood from the legs. Pneumonia may result from a number of factors, including reduced respiratory movement and gravitational congestion of the posterior parts of the lungs.

4.5 a **False** b **True** c **False** d **True** e **True**
Virchow described three general predisposing factors for thrombosis: changes in the intimal surface of the vessel, changes in the pattern of blood flow, and changes in the blood constituents. These three factors are often closely interrelated. A common example is that of thrombosis due to athermomatous plaque. Atheroma formation may lead to protrusion of the plaque into the vessel lumen, thus altering the pattern of blood flow (factor 2). The resulting turbulence may lead to loss of endothelial cells (factor 1). Patients with atheroma often have high blood cholesterol (factor 3), thus further increasing the risk for thrombus.

4.6 a **True** b **True** c **False** d **True** e **False**
Emboli from the left side of the heart or the major arterial vessels are systemic emboli,

and may be travel to various organs in the body. In the brain, they may cause transient ischaemic attacks or strokes. In the lower limbs, they may cause acute ischaemia of the legs and gangrene. They may be lodged in the mesenteric arteries to cause ischaemic bowel, or in the renal vessels to cause renal infarct. Pulmonary emboli are caused by thrombus from the deep veins of the calf or the pelvis.

4.7 a **True** b **True** c **True** d **True** e **True**
Acute inflammation is the body's initial physiological response to injury. The types of injury include infection (e.g. bacteria, virus, fungal), hypersensitivity reaction (e.g. atopy), chemical burns from acids or alkali, physical agents such as trauma, heat or irradiation, and tissue death (e.g. after myocardial infarct).

4.8 a **True** b **False** c **False** d **False** e **False**
Three processes occur in acute inflammation: the arterioles dilate, the vascular permeability increases, and neutrophil polymorphs accumulate in the extravascular space. Arteriolar dilatation causes increased blood flow through the capillaries. Increased permeability causes relatively more plasma than cells to escape, and hence the blood viscosity increases. This slows the blood flow. Increased permeability causes plasma and plasma proteins to escape into the extravascular space, forming an exudate which has a high protein concentration.

4.9 a **True** b **True** c **True** d **True** e **False**
There are many possible roles for neutrophil polymorphs in acute inflammation. Neutrophils adhere to bacteria to facilitate its phagocytosis either by neutrophils or macrophages. The neutrophils have both oxygen dependent and oxygen independent mechanisms for intracellular killing of microorganisms. Both neutrophils and macrophages may discharge their lysosomal products. These include pyrogens which may induce fever, and other products which may help to activate the complement system or increase the vascular permeability still further.

4.10 a **True** b **False** c **True** d **True** e **True**
Infiltrate containing lymphocytes, plasma cells, and macrophages predominate in chronic inflammation. The B lymphocytes are transformed into plasma cells which produce antibodies when they encounter antigens. The T lymphocytes produce macrophage inhibition factor (which traps macrophages) and macrophage activation factor (which causes macrophages to phagocytose and kill bacteria) when they encounter antigens. There is often evidence of tissue destruction as well as tissue repair and regeneration. Fibrous tissue formation is the characteristic feature in the late stages of chronic inflammation.

4.11 a **False** b **False** c **False** d **True** e **True**
There are three steps in the multistep theory of carcinogenesis. In the initiation step, the abnormal genetic material is introduced into the cell. In the promotion step, the presence of promotors stimulate proliferation of cells containing the abnormal transformed cells. Both the initiation and the promotion steps are required for carcinogenesis to occur. In the last step, persistence, proliferation of the transformed cells

occurs without the presence of promotors. These steps explain the long latency period between the initial exposure to carcinogens and the clinical development of malignancy.

4.12 a **True** b **False** c **True** d **False** e **False**
Macroscopic features of a benign tumour are characteristically exophytic (grows away from the mucosal surface for an epithelial tumour) with intact surface, well circumscribed, and without evidence of infiltration and metastasis. Histologically, they are similar to the parent tissues. Necrosis and ulceration suggest malignancy.

4.13 a **False** b **False** c **True** d **False** e **True**
Teratomas are tumours of germ-cell origin. They contain cells representing all three germ layers: ectoderm, mesoderm, and endoderm. Hence, they may contain ectodermal tissues such as teeth and hair, and mesodermal tissues such as muscles and cartilage. They are almost always cystic and benign in the ovaries, but almost always solid and malignant in the testis. They may occasionally occur outside the gonads, such as the sacrococcygeal region.

4.14 a **False** b **True** c **False** d **True** e **False**
The following tumour markers are correctly matched:

choriocarcinoma	-	β-hCG
colonic adenocarcinoma	-	raised carcinoembryonic antigen (CEA)
hepatocellular carcinoma	-	AFP
myeloma	-	Bence Jones protein in urine and monoclonal serum immunoglobulin
carcinoid tumour	-	5-HIAA
phaeochromocytoma	-	VMA

4.15 a **False** b **False** c **False** d **True** e **True**
Type I hypersensitivity is of the anaphylactoid type, and occurs within minutes of exposure to the antigen. It is responsible for atopy such as hayfever, childhood asthma, and systemic anaphylaxis. Type I hypersensitivy is mediated by IgE antibodies which bind to mast cells and basophils with their Fc component. This leads to degranulation and release of mast cell contents such as histamine, eosinophil chemotactic factors, and slow releasing substances of anaphylaxis. These products cause vasodilatation, increased vascular permeability, recruitment of eosinophils and oedema.

4.16 a **True** b **False** c **True** d **True** e **True**
Type IV hypersensitivity is also known as delayed type hypersensitivity, and the immune reaction takes longer than 12 h to develop. Examples are response to virus, fungus, and tuberculosis. It also occurs in sarcoidosis and in transplant graft rejection. It is mediated by T lymphocytes which are sensitized by the antigen release lymphokines, which activate cytotoxic T cells and recruit macrophages. Intracellular killing occurs inside macrophages.

4.17 a **False** b **True** c **True** d **True** e **True**
Risk factors for atherosclerosis include increasing age, cigarette smoking, hypertension, raised low density lipoprotein-cholesterol levels, diabetes mellitus, obesity, and reduced physical activity. A high level of high density lipoprotein protects against atherosclerosis. Atherosclerosis is more common in male than female before menopause.

4.18 a **False** b **False** c **False** d **True** e **False**
Aneurysms are localized abnormal dilatations of a blood vessel. The commonest type is due to atherosclerosis and occur in the lower abdominal aorta. Dissecting aneurysms are associated with cystic medial necrosis associated with mucinous degeneration, and occur in the thoracic aorta. They usually occur in elderly subjects, but are also characteristically seen in Marfan's syndrome. They are liable to rupture and cause haemopericardium or retroperitoneal haemorrhage. Berry aneurysms occur at the branching points in the circle of Willis, and predispose to subarachnoid haemorrhage. Intracerebral capillary aneurysms predispose to intracerebral haemorrhage.

4.19 a **False** b **False** c **True** d **False** e **True**
The macroscopic and microscopic changes after an acute myocardial infarct follow a predictable sequence. Usually no changes can be seen in the first day. Within 1–2 days, the infarcted muscle becomes oedematous, and an acute inflammatory picture can be detected microscopically. Necrosis occurs about 4 days, and granulation tissue appears about 1 week after the event. The infarcted areas are replaced by fibrous tissues 1–2 months after the event.

4.20 a **True** b **True** c **False** d **False** e **True**
The immediate complications after a myocardial infarct include arrhythmia and sudden death from ventricular fibrillation. In the first few days, cardiac failure may occur as a result of ventricular dysfunction. Pericarditis may occur if the infarct involves the whole thickness of the myocardium. Rupture of the ventricular septum or the papillary muscles may occur due to necrosis and subsequent weakening of the muscles. Ventricular aneurysm usually occur after the first month of the infarct, as it represents stretching of the newly formed fibrous tissues. Pulmonary emboli usually occur after the first week resulting from deep vein thrombosis which develops as a result of bed rest.

4.21 a **True** b **False** c **False** d **True** e **True**
Bronchopneumonia causes patchy consolidation of the lungs, and usually occurs in the elderly, in infancy, in the immunocompromised, and in those with chronic illnesses. They may be caused by a number of organisms including haemophilus influenzae, streptococci, staphylococci, or coliforms. The lesions are usually bilateral and in the bases of the lungs.

4.22 a **False** b **True** c **True** d **True** e **False**
Lobar pneumonia, in contrast to bronchopneumonia, commonly affects healthy

middle-aged subjects. An entire lobe of a lung is typically affected. ***Streptococcus pneumoniae*** (pneumococcus) is the causative organism in the vast majority of the cases. The pathology is typically of acute inflammation and its resolution, and consists of four stages. The first congestion stage is characterized by accumulation of exudate in the alveoli. The second red hepatization stage is characterized by accumulation of polymorphs, together with some lymphocytes and macrophages. The lung is red and solid like the liver. The third grey hepatization stage is characterized by accumulation of fibrin and destruction of the white and red cells. The last resolution stage is characterized by removal of the exudate and debris.

4.23 a **False** b **True** c **False** d **True** e **True**
Primary pulmonary tuberculosis usually consists of a small mid-zone lesion (a Ghon complex) associated with hilar lymph nodes involvement. This usually become calcified. This may be reactivated and the lesions are usually bilateral in the apices of the lungs. This may be complicated by pleural effusion, pneumonia, and intestinal tuberculosis. If the subject is immunocompromised, the disease may become disseminated throughout the lungs, as well as other organs such as bone marrow, kidneys, and meninges. Pulmonary miliary tuberculosis is characterized by numerous small granulomata scattered throughout both lungs.

4.24 a **True** b **False** c **True** d **True** e **True**
Bronchiectasis results from bronchial obstruction, leading to distal inflammation and fibrosis, and dilatation of bronchi and bronchioles. The lower lobes are preferentially affected, and recurrent respiratory infections result from inability to clear the secretions. Complications include septicaemia, meningitis, and amyloid formation.

4.25 a **True** b **False** c **True** d **True** e **False**
The coal dust is ingested by alveolar macrophages which may then gather around bronchioles. The black pigment in the lung is called anthracosis and reflects the amount of exposure to carbon. This has no clinical significance. However, this may progress to macular coal-worker pneumoconiosis with mild centrilobular emphysema and to nodular coal-worker pneumoconiosis with the formation of nodules less than 1 cm. In some cases, it may progress to massive pulmonary fibrosis with large irregular nodules in mid or upper zones, associated with scarring. Extrinsic allergic alveolitis is caused by organic dusts, and mesothelioma is usually caused by asbestos exposure.

4.26 a **False** b **True** c **True** d **False** e **True**
There are four main types of bronchial carcinomas: squamous cell carcinoma, small cell carcinoma, adenocarinoma, and large cell undifferentiated carcinoma. Squamous cell carcinoma accounts for just over half of all bronchial carcinomas. They are usually hilar, and results from squamous metaplasia, and are most closely related to cigarette smoking. They typically secrete ectopic parathyroid hormones. Small cell carcinoma is also known as 'oat-cell' carcinoma. They usually metastasize early. Adenocarcinomas arise from glandular (e.g. globlet) cells, are usually peripheral. Large cell undifferentiated carcinomas are usually central and highly invasive.

4.27 a **True** b **False** c **False** d **False** e **True**
Barrett's oesophagus usually results from long-standing reflux of gastric contents, and the lining of the lower oesophagus changes from the normal squamous epithelium to columnar epithelium. This predisposes to adenocarcinoma, and must be observed closely by regular endoscopy.

4.28 a **False** b **False** c **True** d **False** e **False**
Carcinomas of the stomach are commoner in Japan and China than in the United Kingdom. The incidence has been decreasing in the last few decades. They are adenocarcinomas arising from mucus-secreting epithelial cells. As they have few symptoms in the early stages, most carcinomas of the stomach present at an advanced stage. Carcinoma of the stomach may spread directly to the pancreas, liver, and spleen, through the peritoneal cavity to the ovaries (Krukenberg tumours), through the lymphatics, or through the portal vein to the liver.

4.29 a **True** b **True** c **False** d **False** e **True**
Excessive salt intake predisposes to carcinoma of the stomach, but vitamin C has protective effect. Chronic gastritis, pernicious anaemia, and achlorhydria are predisposing conditions for carcinoma of the stomach.

4.30 a **True** b **False** c **False** d **False** e **True**
Coeliac disease is due to sensitivity of the intestine to gliadin, a component of gluten, which is present in wheat flour. It has a strong HLA–B8 association, and there is often a family history. However, the inheritance appears not to be Mendelian. It appears that the condition is immune mediated and T lymphocytes are involved, but the exact mechanism is uncertain.

4.31 a **False** b **True** c **False** d **True** e **True**
In coeliac disease, there is accelerated loss of cells from the villi compared with normal, and there is increased proliferation and mitotic activities in the crypts in an attempt to replace them. Hence, there is total villous atrophy and crypt hyperplasia. There is malabsorption of carbohydrates, proteins, and fats as a result. The proximal small intestine is affected more than the distal small intestine, presumably because there is higher exposure of the proximal small intestine to gluten. The development of malignant lymphomas is a recognized complication.

4.32 a **False** b **True** c **True** d **True** e **True**
In Crohn's disease, all parts of the gastrointestinal tract may be affected. The lesions are usually segmental in distribution (i.e. skipped lesions). There are deep fissured ulcers, with patchy inflammatory changes affecting the full thickness of the bowel. Where the fissures cross mucosal folds, a 'cobblestone' appearance results. Fistula formation may occur where deep ulcers occur. Inflammation of the mucosa without involvement of the muscle is characteristic of ulcerative colitis.

4.33 a **False** b **False** c **True** d **True** e **False**
Diverticula are herniations of the bowel mucosa into the bowel wall. They occur most

frequently in the sigmoid colon. It is thought that the aetiology for diverticular disease is high intraluminal pressure resulting from a low fibre diet. Clinically, the patient may have abdominal pain and change of bowel habits. The herniated mucosa may become infected with faecal organisms, and diverticulitis results. Abscesses and fistulas are complications of diverticular disease. Unlike inflammatory bowel disease, diverticular disease does not significantly predispose to carcinoma of the colon.

4.34 a **False** b **False** c **True** d **False** e **False**
About half of the carcinomas of the large bowel occur in the rectum, and about a quarter occur in the sigmoid colon. Hence, the majority of these carcinomas can be detected by sigmoidoscopy. All carcinomas of the large bowel are adenocarcinomas. Since the bowel content is more fluid in the right side of the colon than in the left, carcinoma of the rectum is more likely to cause obstruction. Carcinomas of the large bowel may spread through the peritoneal cavity, and to the liver through the blood stream. The Duke's staging method is used, depending on whether the carcinoma has spread through the submucosa, muscle layer, or lymph nodes.

4.35 a **True** b **True** c **False** d **True** e **False**
Viruses which cause liver damage include all hepatitis viruses (A, B, C, and other non-A non-B viruses), cytomegalovirus, herpes simplex virus, and yellow fever virus.

4.36 a **True** b **True** c **True** d **True** e **False**
Alcohol may cause both acute and chronic liver damage. The appearance of fat globules within the cytoplasm of the liver cells is often an early abnormality. Mallory hyalin, an aggregate of filaments in the cytoplasm of liver cells, may be seen in acute alcoholic hepatitis, and is associated with risk of progression to micronodular and macronodular cirrhosis. 'Piecemeal' hepatic necrosis is necrosis of liver cells at the margin of the portal tract, and is associated with chronic active (autoimmune) hepatitis.

4.37 a **False** b **False** c **True** d **True** e **True**
Haemosiderosis describes excessive iron deposition in the liver in the form of haemosiderin without cirrhosis. Haemochromatosis describes excessive iron deposition with consequent cirrhosis of the liver. It is classified into primary and secondary haemochromatosis. Primary haemochromatosis is due to a gene defect in chromosome 6. Heterozygotes have slightly increased absorption of iron, but they do not usually manifest clinically. Clinical manifestation is commoner in men than women in homozygotes, as women partially compensate for the excessive iron by menstruation. Excessive iron may also deposit in the pancreas to cause diabetes, the heart to cause heart failure, and melanotrophin levels in the skin may be increased resulting in bronze coloration.

4.38 a **True** b **True** c **False** d **True** e **True**
Graves' disease is the commonest cause for hyperthyroidism. This is an organ-specific autoimmune disease caused by the stimulatory action of an autoantibody (LATS) on the thyroid epithelium. Graves' disease usually causes a diffusely enlarged goitre. It is often associated with infiltration of the orbital tissues by fat and mucopolysaccarides

(resulting in exophthalmos), and deposition of mucopolysaccharide in the dermis in the shins (resulting in pretibial myxoedema).

4.39 a **False** b **True** c **True** d **True** e **True**
Hashimoto's thyroiditis is the commonest cause of hypothyrodism. It is an autoimmune disease, and has an association with HLA–B8. Autoantibodies to the endoplasmic reticulum of the thyroid epithelial cells and to thyroglobulin are often present. Macroscopically, it appears firm and pale. This contrasts with the bright red appearance in Graves' disease. Microscopically, there is dense lymphocytic and plasma cells infiltration of the thyroid gland.

4.40 a **True** b **False** c **False** d **True** e **False**
Folliclar adenoma is the commonest type of tumour of the thyroid gland. It is a solid benign tumour usually surrounded by a fibrous capsule. Only about 1% of adenomas are functional and cause hyperthyroidism.

4.41 a **False** b **False** c **True** d **True** e **False**
About two-thirds of all thyroid carcinoma is of the papillary type. Papillary carcinoma typically occurs in young adults. It may spread via lymphatics to other parts of the thyroid gland or to cervical lymph nodes. However, it grows very slowly, and the prognosis is very good. Follicular carcinoma is the next commonest, and typically occurs in the young adult or the middle aged. It may spread to the bones or lungs via the blood stream. Anaplastic carcinoma is an undifferentiated adenocarcinoma which typically occurs in the elderly. The prognosis is very poor. Medullary carcinoma typically produces excessive calcitonin.

4.42 a **True** b **False** c **True** d **True** e **False**
Benign tumours of the breast include fibroadenoma, duct papilloma, and adenoma. Fibroadenoma is the commonest. It commonly occur in young women and presents clinically as a mobile breast lump or 'breast mouse'. It may enlarge rapidly during pregnancy due to hormonal influences, but it does not progress to malignancy. Macroscopically, it has a smooth surface, and is well circumscribed.

4.43 a **True** b **False** c **False** d **True** e **True**
About 1% of carcinoma of the breast occur in men, and patients with Klinefelter's syndrome have an increased risk. The infiltrating ductal type constitutes more than 80%. The other types are infiltrating lobular, mucinous, and tubular. These generally have a better prognosis. Breast carcinoma may spread directly into skin and muscle, via lymphatics to local and axillary lymph nodes, and via the blood stream to the other breast, bones, lungs, or the brain.

4.44 a **False** b **True** c **True** d **True** e **True**
Squamous cervical carcinoma is commoner than cervical adenocarcinoma, although the proportion of cervical adenocarcinoma is increasing now that the incidence of squamous carcinoma is decreasing due to the cervical screening programme. Squamous cervical carcinoma is most likely to be mediated by human papillomaviruses.

A large number of sexual partners, early age of first intercourse, and smoking are important risk factors. Cervical squamous carcinoma arises from cells in the cervical transformation zone where endocervical epithelium undergoes eversion at puberty and continuous squamous metaplasia on exposure to the low pH of vaginal mucus. Cervical intraepithelial neoplasia is epithelial changes such as mitotic figures and abnormal nuclei which can be recognized on histological examination of cervical smears.

4.45 a **False** b **False** c **True** d **True** e **False**
Uterine fibroids are the commonest tumours in the female genital tract. They are leiomyomas, and are usually multiple round well-circumscribed tumours. They commonly occur between the ages of 40 and 60. They are associated with low parity.

4.46 a **False** b **False** c **False** d **False** e **True**
Seminomas are the commonest type of testicular tumour, followed by teratomas. Seminomas typically occur in the middle aged, whereas teratomas occur before the age of 30. Seminomas are usually solid and homogeneous on macroscopic appearance. Differentiated teratomas are usually cystic. Teratomas are more aggressive than seminomas.

4.47 a **True** b **False** c **True** d **False** e **False**
In focal proliferative glomerulonephritis, some glomeruli are affected whilst others are spared. This can be caused by a number of systemic diseases including Henoch-Schonlein purpura, systemic lupus erythematosus, subacute bacterial endocarditis, and polyarteritis. They may be immune-mediated. Poststreptococcal infection usually causes diffuse proliferative glomerulonephritis. Hepatitis B causes membranous glomerulonephritis. Diabetes mellitus typically causes nodular glomerulosclerosis.

4.48 a **False** b **False** c **True** d **True** e **True**
Transitional cell carcinomas are the commonest bladder tumours. Predisposing factors include smoking and industrial exposure to dyes. Schistosomiasis predisposes to squamous bladder carcinoma. The low grade tumours are usually multiple papillary tumours. They usually present with painless haematuria. However, they may cause secondary hydronephrosis or pyelonephritis if they occur near a ureteric orifice.

4.49 a **False** b **False** c **True** d **True** e **False**
Hodgkin's lymphoma typically occurs between the age of 25 and 45. It is characterized by the presence of Reed-Sternberg cells with binucleate appearance and prominent nucleoli. According to the Rye classification system, there are four subgroups: nodular sclerosis, lymphocyte-predominant, mixed cellularity, and lymphocyte-depleted. The lymphocyte-predominant type has the best prognosis, and the lymphocyte-depleted type the worst. The nodular sclerosis type is a distinct type and does not progress to the other types. Poor prognostic factors include old age, systemic symptoms such as weight loss, fever and night sweats, advanced TMN stage, lymphocyte-depleted type, and haematological abnormalities at presentation such as anaemia or increased ESR.

4.50 a **True** b **False** c **False** d **True** e **True**
Causes of eosinophil leukocytosis include atopy (e.g. hayfever, asthma), parasite infections, Hodgkin's lymphoma, and polyarteritis nodosa. There is neutrophilia in bacterial infection, and lymphcytosis in viral infection.

4.51 a **True** b **False** c **False** d **False** e **False**
The characteristic haematological features of iron deficiency anaemia are microcytic (small) and hypochromic (low haemoglobin content) red cells. Hence, both the mean corpuscular volume (MCV) and MCH are low. As the bone marrow is unable to manufacture sufficient haemoglobin through the lack of iron, the reticulocyte count is low in relation to the degree of anaemia. The serum iron level is low, and the total iron binding capacity is high. The ferritin level reflects the total body iron content, and is low.

4.52 a **True** b **False** c **True** d **True** e **True**
Vitamin B_{12} is essential for DNA synthesis. Hence, vitamin B_{12} deficiency affects the production of red blood cells, white cells, and platelets. The white cells and platelet levels are often slightly low. The defect in DNA synthesis is associated with a reduction of mitosis. As RNA and protein synthesis are normal, large red cells are seen in the bone marrow (megaloblasts) and in the peripheral film (macrocytes). Some neutrophil shows neutrophil hypersegmentation (large with excessive lobulation of the nucleus).

4.53 a **False** b **False** c **False** d **False** e **True**
Vitamin B_{12} is absorbed in the terminal ileum whereas folate is absorbed in the jejunum. The commonest cause for vitamin B_{12} deficiency is pernicious anaemia, which is an autoimmune disease. Folate deficiency often occurs in pregnancy when the demand increases. However, vitamin B_{12} deficiency is rare. This is because fertility is impaired in vitamin B_{12} deficiency, and that the body store for vitamin B_{12} is sufficient to last for several years. Subacute degeneration of the spinal cord and peripheral neuropathy may result from vitamin B_{12} deficiency, but neurological complications do not occur with folate deficiency.

4.54 a **True** b **False** c **True** d **True** e **False**
Multiple myeloma is a disease with multiple plasma cell tumours which produce monoclonal immunoglobulin or light chains. Light chains may be detected in the urine as Bence Jones protein. Anaemia is common, and the ESR is often over 100 mm/h. In the late stages, pancytopenia may occur. The high concentration of immunoglobulin causes the red cells to adhere to each other, which gives rise to rouleaux formation.

5 *Obstetrics and gynaecology*

Questions

5.1 ***The following parameters are recorded in the Bishop score in the assessment of readiness for induction of labour***

a dilatation of the cervix
b viscosity of the cervical mucus
c consistency of the cervix
d position of the cervix
e fundal height

5.2 ***Which of the following statements about ultrasound in early pregnancy is/are true?***

a the gestation sac may be visualized earlier with transvaginal ultrasound than with transabdominal ultrasound
b no gestation sac can be seen in missed abortion
c ectopic pregnancy can be visualized with transabdominal ultrasound in over 50% of cases
d ectopic pregnancy can be visualized with transvaginal ultrasound in over 50% of cases
e no fetal heart activity can be detected in missed abortion

5.3 ***An ultrasound examination at 18 weeks of pregnancy may be used to***

a establish the gestational age
b localize the placenta
c exclude cystic fibrosis
d confirm or exclude multiple pregnancy
e exclude Down's syndrome

5.4 ***Causes for asymmetrical intrauterine growth retardation (i.e. abdominal growth more affected than head growth) include***

a placental insufficiency
b congenital rubella infection
c chromosomal abnormalities

d pregnancy induced hypertension
e multiple pregnancy

5.5 *Current acceptable methods for assessing fetal well-being antenatally include*

a the kick chart
b antenatal cardiotocography (CTG)
c AFP level
d Doppler waveform of the fetal descending aorta and middle cerebral artery
e ultrasound assessment of amniotic fluid volume

5.6 *Causes for antepartum haemorrhage include*

a placenta praevia
b cervical polyp
c hydatiform mole
d cervical carcinoma
e placental abruption

5.7 *Signs of severe placental abruption with concealed haemorrhage include*

a hypotension
b uterus resonant on percussion
c extreme tenderness over uterus
d absence fetal heart sound
e prominence of fetal parts on palpation

5.8 *Which of the following are appropriate immediate assessment for moderately severe antepartum haemorrhage of uncertain cause at 34 weeks gestation*

a immediate vaginal examination to assess cervical dilatation
b cross-match blood
c put up an intravenous infusion
d arrange an ultrasound scan
e CTG

5.9 *Causes of polyhydramnios include*

a Potter's syndrome
b duodenal atresia
c multiple pregnancy
d maternal diabetes
e fetoplacental insufficiency

5.10 *Significant risk factors for pregnancy induced hypertension include*

a multiparity

b maternal age over 35
c maternal diabetes mellitus
d multiple pregnancy
e past history of placenta praevia

5.11 *Signs and symptoms for imminent eclampsia include*

a severe headache
b hyporeflexia
c visual disturbance
d epigastric pain
e rapidly rising blood pressure

5.12 *Significant risk factors for developing diabetes in pregnancy include*

a previous babies over 4.5 kg birth weight
b previous unexplained stillbirth
c previous forceps delivery
d abnormal glucose tolerance tests during previous pregnancies
e family history of diabetes in a first degree relative

5.13 *Complications significantly associated with maternal diabetes in pregnancy include*

a premature labour
b shoulder dystocia
c oligohydramnios
d neonatal hyperglycaemia
e neonatal idiopathic respiratory distress syndrome

5.14 *Which of the following statements about postnatal depression is/are true?*

a the incidence is about 1 in every 500 live births
b it usually occurs 4 weeks after the birth of the baby
c treatment with antidepressants and psychotherapy is usually effective
d it usually lasts less than a week
e excessive anxiety about the baby's health may be a feature

5.15 *Complications seen more commonly in twin pregnancies than in singleton pregnancies include*

a postmaturity
b pregnancy-induced hypertension
c postpartum haemorrhage
d maternal anaemia
e cord prolapse

5.16 *Which of the following statements regarding management of twin pregnancies is/are true?*

a home deliveries should be encouraged if there are no other risk factors
b epidural analgesia is contraindicated
c intravenous oxytocin is contraindicated
d CTG monitoring of one of the two twins is sufficient
e caesarean section is indicated if the first twin presents by vertex and the second twin by breech

5.17 *Risk factors for ectopic pregnancy include*

a combined oral contraceptives
b intrauterine contraceptive device
c history of pelvic infections
d in vitro fertilization
e a history of tubal surgery

5.18 *Which of the following statements about the stages of normal labour is/are true?*

a the first stage of labour begins when there is significant descent of the fetus
b dilatation of the cervix is more rapid in the active phase than the latent phase of the first stage of labour
c the second stage begins when the contractions become very strong
d the second stage ends when the anterior shoulder of the baby is delivered
e the third stage usually lasts for about 2 hours

5.19 *Which of the following fetal monitoring findings (CTG) are normal?*

a the basal heart rate is 100 beats/min
b the basal heart rate is 150 beats/min
c the beat-to-beat variation is 10 beats/min
d there is slowing of about 10 beats/min with each contraction with rapid recovery
e there is slowing of about 40 beats/min half a minute after each uterine contraction

5.20 *Which of the following statements about the use of analgesia during labour is/are true?*

a oral morphine is a good analgesic agent
b intramuscular pethidine given 30 min before birth may result in respiratory depression of the newborn
c epidural block should be commenced during the second stage of labour
d hypotension is a recognized complication of epidural block
e Entenox is a mixture of nitrous oxide and oxygen

5.21 *Causes for prolonged labour include*

a fetal hydrocephaly
b brow presentation
c primary uterine dysfunction
d intrauterine growth retardation
e polyhydramnios

5.22 *Which of the following statements about breech presentation is/are true?*

a it is commoner in premature births
b flexed breech (with flexion of both knees and hips) is the commonest type
c extended breech is often complicated by prolapse of the cord
d it occurs in about 3% of all term pregnancies
e external cephalic version may be attempted at 30 weeks

5.23 *Which of the following statements about unstable lie is/are true?*

a it can be diagnosed if the presentation is cephalic in one week and breech in the next
b it is associated with oligohydramnios
c it occurs more commonly in primigravida
d the patient should be admitted routinely at 38 weeks for induction by amniotomy
e it is never possible to deliver the baby vaginally

5.24 *Effective tocolytic drugs (drugs delaying progress of labour) include*

a salbutamol
b atenolol
c ritrodrine
d prostaglandin E2
e indomethacin

5.25 *Predisposing factors for rupture of the uterus during pregnancy or labour include*

a previous classical caesarean section scar
b attempts of internal cephalic version
c primigravida
d excess syntocinon infusion
e previous pelvic infection

5.26 *Causes of primary postpartum haemorrhage include*

a atonic uterus
b multiple pregnancy

c retained placenta
d attempt to deliver the placenta before separation
e intrauterine infection

5.27 *Indications for the use of forceps include*

a fetal distress in the first stage of labour
b fetal distress in the second stage of labour
c delay in the second stage of labour
d delivery of the head in breech presentation
e delivery of the head in brow presentation

5.28 *Which of the following conditions must be satisfied before forceps are applied?*

a the bladder must be empty
b the membranes must be intact
c the uterus must be relaxed
d the cervix must be fully dilated
e the head must be engaged (in cephalic presentation)

5.29 *Situations in which a caesarean section is mandatory include*

a conjoined twins
b prolapse of the cord in the first stage of labour
c pregnancy-induced hypertension
d severe fetal distress in the first stage of labour
e breech presentation

5.30 *Which of the following statements about chorionic villous biopsy is/are true?*

a it cannot be performed transabdominally
b it may be performed at 9 weeks of pregnancy
c the risk of miscarriage is less than after amniocentesis
d biopsy samples may be examined for rubella infection
e Down's syndrome may be diagnosed from biopsy samples

5.31 *Which of the following statements about hormone replacement therapy is/are true?*

a all patients with menopausal symptoms may be given oestrogen without progesterone
b it is effective in abolishing hot flushes
c it may significantly increase the risk of cardiovascular disease
d it protects the woman against osteoporosis
e admission to hospital is required for oestrogen implantation

5.32 *In testicular feminization syndrome*

a the patient has a male external appearance

b the sex chromosome is XX
c the testosterone level is similar to that in a normal male
d testes may be present in the inguinal canal
e the patient should be reared as female

5.33 *Factors which contribute to genital prolapse include*

a past history of difficult forceps delivery
b postmenopausal atrophy of uterine supports
c chronic constipation
d menorrhagia
e nulliparity

5.34 *Symptoms of genital prolapse may include*

a frequency of micturition
b backache exacerbated by lying down
c vaginal discomfort exacerbated by lying down
d dyspareunia
e stress incontinence

5.35 *Which of the following statements about retroversion of the uterus is/are true?*

a it refers to the uterus bending backwards on itself
b the fundus is directed backwards with the opening of the cervix in the anterior fornix
c all retroverted uteri are indications for urgent referral to the gynaecologist
d it occurs in about 0.5% of all women
e mobile retroversion of the uterus is a common cause for infertility

5.36 *Viral vulva warts*

a are also known as condylomata lata
b are caused by human papillomaviruses
c are sexually transmitted
d are an indication for following up male contacts
e are best treated by application of phenol

5.37 *Monilial vaginitis*

a is caused by a bacterial infection
b is commoner in those with glycosuria
c is less common in those being treated with broad spectrum antibiotics
d is characteristically associated with thick white discharge
e is seldom associated with vulval irritation

5.38 *Trichomonas vaginalis*

a is always sexually transmitted
b is characteristically associated with a scanty white discharge

c is characteristically associated with a odorous discharge
d may be treated with vaginal pessaries
e is an indication for treating the patient's male partner

5.39 *Characteristic features of pelvic inflammatory disease include*

a missed menstrual period
b dyspareunia
c cervical excitation
d unilateral abdominal tenderness
e obvious vaginal discharge

5.40 *Which of the following statements about fibroids is/are true?*

a they are often multiple
b they are commoner in multiparous women
c they frequently become malignant
d the are commoner in white women than black women
e the peak incidence is after menopause

5.41 *Symptoms and signs due to uncomplicated fibroids include*

a oligomenorrhoea
b tenderness on abdominal palpation
c nodular abdominal masses
d frequency of micturition
e early menopause

5.42 *Complications following a cone biopsy include*

a secondary haemorrhage
b cervical stenosis
c future midtrimester abortions
d future pregnancies complicated by intra-uterine growth retardation
e future first trimester abortions

5.43 *Colposcopy*

a is an examination of the cervix with a high-powered binocular microscope
b can be used to examine the inside surface of the uterus
c should be performed for every women with severe cervical intraepithelial neoplasia
d allows the epithelial vascular pattern of the transformation zone to be visualized after the application of acetic acid
e cannot yield further information if the cervical cytology shows inflammatory changes

5.44 *Which of the following statements about management of carcinoma of the cervix is/are true?*

a the majority of the early tumours may be treated by chemotherapy alone
b most tumours respond to radiotherapy
c external radiation alone is more effective than radiation via intrauterine and vaginal applicators
d young women with early carcinoma of the cervix should be treated by radiotherapy alone
e Wartheim hysterectomy is most suitable for cancer of the cervix with distant metastasis

5.45 *Risk factors associated with carcinoma of the uterus include*

a low social class
b obesity
c early menopause
d polycystic ovarian syndrome
e multiple sexual partners

5.46 *Which of the following statements about post-menopausal bleeding is/are true?*

a the cause is malignancy of the genital tract in about 60% of cases
b it may be caused by hormone replacement therapy
c if no abnormalities apart from atrophic vaginitis are found on examination, further investigations are unnecessary
d if fibroids are found on examination, further investigations are unnecessary
e a negative physical examination and a negative histology report on endometrial curettage excludes the diagnosis of malignancy of the genital tract

5.47 *Gestational trophoblastic disease (choriocarcinoma)*

a only occurs when there is a previous history of a hydatiform mole
b has β-hCG as a tumour marker
c often responds to radiotherapy treatment
d often responds to treatment by methotrexate or a combination chemotherapy
e has a 5 year survival rate of about 50% for non-metastatic disease given optimal treatment

5.48 *In the assessment of a case of ovarian tumour, which of the following features suggest the tumour is malignant?*

a unilateral mass

b irregular surface
c presence of shifting dullness
d large size
e elevated CEA level

5.49 *Symptoms due to endometriosis include*

a deep dyspareunia
b pelvic pain a few days after menstruation
c oligomenorrhoea
d infertility
e offensive vaginal discharge

5.50 *Endometriosis is commoner in*

a Africans
b multiparous women
c postmenopausal women
d women taking combined oral contraceptives
e during pregnancy

5.51 *Polycystic ovarian syndrome*

a is a cause of secondary amenorrhoea
b is associated with obesity
c is associated with alopecia
d is associated with an abnormally high FSH to LH ratio
e may be treated with clomiphene if fertility is desired

5.52 *Causes of secondary amenorrhoea include*

a pregnancy
b premature ovarian failure
c prolactinoma
d anorexia nervosa
e emotional stress

5.53 *Treatments which may be effective for dysfunctional uterine bleeding in a 35 year old women include*

a mefanamic acid
b danazol
c endometrial ablation
d GnRH analogues
e dilatation and curettage

5.54 *In the investigation of infertility, tests for ovulation include*

a progesterone level 7 days after menstruation
b urinary LH test at mid-cycle

c monitoring of the size of the dominant follicle by vaginal ultrasound
d assessment of cervical mucus in the postcoital test
e oestradiol level 7 days before menstruation

5.55 *Causes of infertility include*

a mumps in the male partner
b pelvic inflammatory disease in the female partner
c presence of anti-sperm antibodies in the cervical mucus
d retroversion of the uterus
e poorly controlled diabetes mellitus in the female partner

5.56 *Detrusor instability*

a can be diagnosed from the history alone
b may be treated by anticholinergic drugs
c may be treated by bladder retraining
d may be treated by bladder neck suspension
e is associated with urgency

5.57 *Laparoscopy may be used to*

a diagnose suspected ectopic pregnancy
b investigate infertility
c perform sterilization
d puncture a suspected malignant ovarian cyst
e divide the uterosacral and cardinal ligaments in a vaginal hysterectomy

5.58 *Of which of the following must a woman be advised before sterilization?*

a there is a small risk that she may still become pregnant in spite of the operation
b the operation must be regarded as irreversible
c if the patient is already pregnant, the sterilization operation should be performed immediately after delivery
d there is a small risk that a mini-laparotomy may be needed if the attempt by laparoscopy is unsuccessful
e she may enter menopause earlier as a result of this operation

5.59 *Complications of an intrauterine contraceptive device include*

a menorrhagia
b dysmenorrhoea
c perforation of the uterus
d expulsion of the device from the uterus
e pelvic inflammatory disease

5.60 *Compared with the combined oral contraceptives, progesterone-only pills are more*

a suitable for breast-feeding women
b effective
c likely to cause deep vein thrombosis
d likely to be associated with irregular vaginal bleeding
e suitable for younger women

Answers

5.1 a **True** b **False** c **True** d **True** e **False**
The Bishop score is used to assess whether labour is ready to be induced. The five parameters to be recorded are dilatation of the cervix, consistency of the cervix, length of the cervical canal, position of the cervix, and station of the presenting part above ischial spines. In the modified Bishop score, each of these parameters is scored out of a maximum of 3. A dilated, short, soft, anterior cervix at below the ischial spine indicates that labour should commence easily. A total score of less than 5 indicates that ripening of the cervix with vaginal prostaglandin is necessary before induction.

5.2 a **True** b **False** c **False** d **True** e **True**
Transvaginal ultrasound has a better resolution than transabdominal ultrasound, as the transducers may be placed closer to the uterus. Transvaginal ultrasound may detect the gestation sac a week at 4 weeks, a week earlier than if transabdominal ultrasound is used. In missed abortion, the gestation sac can be seen, but fetal heart activity is absent. Ectopic pregnancy can very rarely be visualized with transabdominal ultrasound, and its main use is to exclude intrauterine pregnancy. However, ectopic pregnancy can be diagnosed positively by transvaginal ultrasound in over 80% of cases.

5.3 a **True** b **True** c **False** d **True** e **False**
The purposes of a routine ultrasound between 16 and 20 weeks are to establish gestational age, to exclude structural abnormalities (e.g. neural tube defect), to localize the placenta (to detect low lying placenta), and to diagnose whether the pregnancy is single or multiple. While there are often non-specific ultrasound markers for chromosomal abnormalities (e.g. duodenal atresia, cardiac abnormalities, nuchal fat pads, etc.), Down's syndrome cannot be diagnosed or excluded by ultrasound appearance alone. Amniocentesis is needed. Cystic fibrosis may be diagnosed antenatally be screening for carrier status in the parents, and to perform amniocentesis if both parents are carriers.

5.4 a **True** b **False** c **False** d **True** e **True**
Intrauterine growth retardation may be broadly divided into symmetrical and asymmetrical types. The symmetrical type is generally caused by external factors which

affect all the tissues of the fetus, such as congenital infections (e.g. TORCHS infection), fetal alcohol syndrome, maternal drug addiction, maternal smoking, and chromosomal abnormalities. Asymmetrical intrauterine growth retardation is generally caused directly or indirectly through placental insufficiency, such as pregnancy-induced hypertension and multiple pregnancy. In this case, the growth of the fetal head is protected at the expense of the rest of the body. This distinction is important, as babies with asymmetrical intrauterine growth retardation are most at risk of asphyxia or intrauterine death, and regular frequent assessments must be made to deliver at the appropriate time.

5.5 a **True** b **True** c **False** d **True** e **True**
In the past, biochemical methods such as oestriol level were used to assess fetal well-being antenatally. The current acceptable methods for assessing fetal well-being, in descending order of simplicity and widespread use, include the kick chart, antenatal CTG, ultrasound assessment of amniotic volume, and Doppler waveforms of the descending aorta and middle cerebral artery of the fetus. Ultrasound assessment of the whole biophysical profile (by recording movements, breathing movements, tone, amniotic volume) may also be used, but this examination may take more than an hour to perform.

5.6 a **True** b **True** c **False** d **True** e **True**
Antepartum haemorrhage is bleeding from the vagina occurring after 24 weeks of pregnancy and before the birth of the child. The main causes for antepartum haemorrhage are placenta praevia (usually presents with painless bleeding), placental abruption (usually presents with painful bleeding), and local lesions such as cervical polyp and cervical carcinoma. Vasa praevia, bleeding from the fetus due to velamentous insertion of the cord, is a rare cause. Hydatidiform moles present before 24 weeks of pregnancy.

5.7 a **True** b **False** c **True** d **True** e **False**
In severe placental abruption with concealed haemorrhage, there is separation of a portion of the placenta from its uterine attachment. There is bleeding from the placenta, but the blood remains inside the uterus. Hence, the degree of shock if more marked than expected from the degree of external blood loss. The blood pressure is low. The uterus may be larger than expected due to overdistension, and assume a globular shape. It is hard and extremely tender. It is often difficult to feel the fetal parts due to the tenderness and distension of the uterus. The fetal heart may not be heard, which may either be due to the collection of blood makes fetal heart more difficult to detect, or due to fetal intrauterine death.

5.8 a **False** b **True** c **True** d **True** e **True**
Moderately severe antepartum haemorrhage should be managed by immediate admission to hospital. Pulse and blood pressure should be taken. Blood should be taken for full blood count, clotting studies, and crossmatch. An intravenous infusion should be set up to replace blood loss. CTG should be performed to assess fetal well-being. Vaginal examination must not be performed until an ultrasound has been

performed to exclude placenta praevia. An ultrasound should be arranged to localize the placenta, to look for retroplacental clot, and to assess fetal growth and wellbeing.

5.9 a **False** b **True** c **True** d **True** e **False**
Polydramnios is an excess of amniotic fluid. Often no causes can be found. The known causes can be divided into fetal and maternal causes. Fetal causes include multiple pregnancy, and conditions associated with reduction of fetal swallowing. This may be due to neurological abnormality (e.g. anencephaly), mechanical abnormality (e.g. oesophageal or duodenal atresia), and severe rhesus isoimmunization. Maternal causes include maternal diabetes, as this causes glucose-induced osmotic diuresis in the fetus. Potter's syndrome and fetoplacental insufficiency are causes of oligohydramnios.

5.10 a **False** b **True** c **True** d **True** e **False**
Significant risk factors for pregnancy-induced hypertension include primigravida, maternal age over 35, maternal diabetes mellitus, previous history of hypertension or renal disease, and multiple pregnancy. Although pregnancy induced hypertension may recur, its severity tends to decrease with subsequent pregnancies.

5.11 a **True** b **False** c **True** d **True** e **True**
Symptoms for imminent eclampsia include increasing oedema, oliguria, headache, visual disturbance, vomiting, and epigastric pain. Epigastric pain may indicate hepatic haemorrhage. Signs may include rapidly increasing blood pressure, heavy proteinuria, brisk reflex, tenderness over the liver, and retinal haemorrhages.

5.12 a **True** b **True** c **False** d **True** e **True**
Significant risk factors for developing diabetes in pregnancy include a family history of diabetes in first degree relatives, previous large babies (especially if there had been a trend of increasing birth weight in past pregnancies), previous unexplained stillbirth, abnormal glucose tolerance during previous pregnancies, persistent glycosuria, and polyhydramnios.

5.13 a **True** b **True** c **False** d **False** e **True**
Antenatal complications of diabetes in pregnancy include pre-eclampsia, polyhydramnios, premature labour, and sudden intrauterine death. Perinatal complications include obstructed labour and shoulder dystocia due to large baby size. The incidence of idiopathic respiratory syndrome is increased by a factor of 9. Polycythaemia and physiological jaundice are significantly commoner, and neonates of diabetic mothers often have hypoglycaemia after delivery owing to increased insulin production by the fetus in response to high maternal glucose level antenatally.

5.14 a **False** b **False** c **True** d **False** e **True**
Postnatal depression must be distinguished from postnatal blues and puerperal psychosis. Postnatal blues occurs after about half of all pregnancies. It usually occurs about 4–6 days postpartum, and may last for 2–3 days. The commonest symptoms are weeping episodes, irritability, depersonalization, and forgetfulness. Postnatal depression occurs after about 10% of all pregnancies. Clinical features may include excessive

anxiety about the baby's health, and irrational doubts about her ability as a mother leading to reluctance to feed and handle the baby. Depressive symptoms such as tearfulness, irritability, sleep, and appetite disturbance may be present. In severe cases, there may be suicidal thoughts or thoughts of harming the baby. It is important to diagnose postnatal depression early, as treatment with antidepressants and psychotherapy is usually effective. Puerperal psychosis occurs in 1 every 500 livebirths. It usually starts 2–4 weeks after delivery. There are often psychotic features such as delusions, hallucinations, and thoughts of harming the baby in the belief that this would be the best option for the baby. Admission to a mother and baby psychiatric unit is required.

5.15 a **False** b **True** c **True** d **True** e **True**
Antenatal complications of twin pregnancies include maternal anaemia, polyhydramnios, pregnancy-induced hypertension, and premature labour. Perinatal complications include malpresentations (breech presentation or transverse lie), cord prolapse associated with malpresentation, and postpartum haemorrhage. Locked twins are rare and occurs in less than 0.1% of all twin pregnancies. Fetal complications include congenital malformation and twin-to-twin transfusion.

5.16 a **False** b **False** c **False** d **False** e **False**
As both maternal and neonatal complications are commoner in twin labour, delivery must be performed in a well-equipped maternity unit with resuscitative equipment and a special care unit for neonates. Epidural analgesia is particularly suitable, as it allows rapid intervention by forceps, vacuum extraction, or caesarean section. Syntocinon may be used both in the first stage of labour, and a few minutes after the delivery of the first twin if uterine contractions do not return. Attempts should be made to monitor both fetuses. Caesarean section may be indicated for prolonged first stage of labour, if both twins present by breech, in the rare cases of conjoint or locked twins, or if there are signs of fetal distress.

5.17 a **False** b **True** c **True** d **True** e **True**
Ectopic pregnancy occurs when the fertilized egg is implanted in sites other than the uterine cavity. Most ectopic pregnancies occur in the fallopian tubes. This is caused by delay in the transit of the fertilized egg from the ampula of the fallopian tube to the uterus. Hence, previous pelvic infections and adhesions, previous tubal surgery, and conception by assisted reproductive techniques are all predisposing factors for ectopic pregnancies. An intrauterine contraceptive device also increases the risk for ectopic pregnancy.

5.18 a **False** b **True** c **False** d **True** e **False**
The first stage of labour begins from the onset of labour to full dilatation of the cervix. It is divided into the latent phase and the active phase. In the latent phase, which may take more than 6 h, the cervix dilates from 0 cm to 3 cm. It is often pain free. In the active phase, the cervix typically dilates at a rate of 1 cm/h, and this is often associated with pain. The second stage of labour begins with full dilatation of the cervix, and

ends with the birth of the baby. The third stage of labour ends when the placenta and membranes are delivered and the uterus is firmly contracted. This usually lasts less than 15 min.

5.19 a **False** b **True** c **True** d **True** e **False**
The normal basal heart rate is 120–160 beats/min. There should be beat-to-beat variations of more than 5 beats per minute. Occasional accelerations (increase from the basal heart rate) are signs of fetal wellbeing. Fetal bradycardia is more ominous than tachycardia. Slight transient slowing of fetal heart rate with each uterine contraction is normal, but prolonged decelerations which occurs some time after uterine contraction, or which last a significant period of time, are abnormal.

5.20 a **False** b **True** c **False** d **True** e **True**
Analgesia during labour include inhalation agents, intramuscular injections, and epidural block. Transcutaneous electrical nerve stimulation (TENS) may be used to postpone the use of stronger analgesia. The usual inhalation agent, Entenox, is a 50 : 50 mixture of nitrous oxide and oxygen. It is most useful in the second stage of labour. Pethidine is the most widely used intramuscular analgesia given during labour. Oral analgesia is not used owing to unreliable absorption. Intramuscular pethidine given within a short time before delivery may result in neonatal respiratory depression, but this may be reversed by administering naloxone to the neonate. Epidural block should be commenced in the first stage of labour. The commonest complication is hypotension. Headache may occur if a spinal block is accidentally given. Other rarer complications include respiratory paralysis or neurological sequele of the legs.

5.21 a **True** b **True** c **True** d **False** e **False**
The main causes for prolonged labour are primary uterine dysfunction, cephalopelvic disproportion, and obstructive lesions in the birth canal. In primary uterine dysfunction, there are either inert or uncoordinated uterine contractions. Cephalopelvic disproportion may be due to fetal or maternal causes. Fetal causes include malposition, malpresentation, malformation such as hydrocephaly, and a large baby. Maternal causes include a contracted pelvis, such as that associated with short stature. Obstructive lesions in the birth canal include pelvic tumour or stenosis of the cervix.

5.22 a **True** b **False** c **False** d **True** e **False**
About a quarter of all pregnancies are breech at 30 weeks, but this decreases to 3% at term. Hence, it is commoner in premature deliveries than in full-term deliveries. External cephalic version should be performed between 32 and 38 weeks, as there is significant chance of spontaneous version after 32 weeks, and that external cephalic version becomes difficult after 38 weeks. There are three types of breech. The commonest type is the extended breech, where the hips are flexed while the knees are extended. The next commonest type is the flexed breech, where knees and hips are flexed. In the half breech, one leg is extended both at the hip and the knee while the other is flexed at the hip and extended at the knee.

5.23 a **False** b **False** c **False** d **False** e **False**

Unstable lie is said to occur if the axis of the fetus frequently changes from longitudinal to oblique or transverse. Both cephalic and breech presentations are of longitudinal lie. Hence, changes from cephalic to breech presentation or vice versa are not indicative of unstable lie. It commonly occurs in the multiparous with lax uterus. It can also occur in polyhydramnios, pelvic tumour, or placenta praevia. The most dangerous complication of unstable lie is cord prolapse. Hence, patients should be admitted if there are any suggestion of onset of labour. Routine amniotomy should be avoided as far as possible due to the risk of cord prolapse. High rupture of membranes is preferable, and one should be ready for caesarean section should cord prolapse occurs. However, it is sometimes possible to deliver the baby vaginally.

5.24 a **True** b **False** c **True** d **False** e **True**

Effective tocolytic agents include β-agonists (e.g. salbutamol, ritrodrine), cyclo-oxygenase inhibitors (e.g. indomethacin), and calcium channel blockers (e.g. nifedipine). Prostaglandin pessaries are often used to ripen the cervix for induction of labour.

5.25 a **True** b **True** c **False** d **True** e **False**

Rupture of the uterus during pregnancy is now rare. The commonest cause is previous surgery, especially the classical caesarean section or hysterostomy. Rupture of the uterus during labour may be caused by obstructed labour, interventions by instruments, internal cephalic version, or grand multiparity.

5.26 a **True** b **True** c **True** d **True** e **False**

Primary postpartum haemorrhage is defined as loss of more than 500 ml of blood from the genital tract within 24 h after the birth of the child. Secondary postpartum haemorrhage occurs within 6 weeks after the birth of the child. The two major causes for primary postpartum haemorrhage are retained placenta and ineffective uterine contraction. Retained placenta may be due to abnormally adherent placenta. Attempts to deliver the placenta before it separates will also result in bleeding. Ineffective uterine contraction may be due to atonic uterus in mulipara, or after prolonged labour. Other causes are multiple pregnancies (due to increased placental area) and disseminated intravascular coagulation. Uterine infection is a predisposing factor for secondary postpartum haemorrhage.

5.27 a **False** b **True** c **True** d **True** e **False**

Forceps cannot be used in the first stage of labour, as the cervix is not fully dilated. They may be used for delay in the second stage of labour, fetal distress in the second stage of labour, maternal exhaustion, and maternal conditions in which excess maternal effort is undesirable (e.g. heart disease). Besides cephalic presentation with occipital anterior position, forceps may be used to deliver the head in breech presentation and face presentation with chin anterior. Rotation with Kjelland forceps may be required for occipital transverse or occipital posterior presentations. Brow presentation cannot be delivered by forceps. The mentovertical diameter is 13 cm, which is too large to be delivered vaginally without correction.

5.28 a **True** b **False** c **False** d **True** e **True**
Before applying the forceps, the cervix must be fully dilated. Otherwise, the cervix may be torn. The head must be engaged and the pelvic outlet must be of the adequate size, as cephalopelvic disproportion must be excluded. The membranes should have been ruptured. Spontaneous delivery may follow after rupture, and forceps delivery may be unnecessary. The bladder must be empty to avoid injury by the application of forceps. The uterus must be contracting to maximize the chance of success in delivering the baby with forceps.

5.29 a **True** b **True** c **False** d **True** e **False**
Most indications for caesarean section are relative, and all the maternal and fetal factors should be taken into account in reaching a decision. Conditions in which a caesarean section is *mandatory* include gross cephalopelvic disproportion, placenta praevia major, conjoined twins, severe fetal distress in the first stage of labour, and prolapse of the cord in the first stage of labour. Breech presentation and pregnancy-induced hypertension are relative contraindications.

5.30 a **False** b **True** c **False** d **True** e **True**
Chorionic villous biopsy can be performed either transabdominally or transcervically. A sample is taken from the edge of the placenta via a hollow needle. The miscarriage rate is 2% above the natural rate. In amniocentesis, the miscarriage rate is about 1% above the natural rate. Chorionic biopsy samples may be examined for karoytypes, enzyme levels to detect inborn errors of metabolism, and DNA analysis to detect single gene disorders. Virus particles may be detected by electron microscopy.

5.31 a **False** b **True** c **False** d **True** e **False**
Hormone replacement therapy may be given orally, by dermal patches, and by implantation. Implantation of oestrogen is relatively simple, and can be done as an outpatient procedure. Continuous administration of unopposed oestrogen without progesterone carries an increased risk of endometrial hyperplasia and endometrial carcinoma. Hence, only those without a uterus (i.e. those who have had a hysterectomy) should be given unopposed oestrogen without progesterone. Hormone replacement therapy is effective in reversing the tissue atrophy (e.g. vaginal dryness, dyspareunia) and vasomotor symptoms (e.g. hot flushes). It protects the woman against coronary heart disease and osteoporosis.

5.32 **False** b **False** c **True** d **True** e **True**
In testicular feminization syndrome, the sex chromosome is XY (genetic male). Testes are present, but they are often in the abdomen or in the inguinal canal. The testosterone level is similar to that of a normal male. However, due to either end-organ insensitivity to testosterone or to the deficiency of the enzyme converting testosterone to the more potent androgen dihydrotestosterone, virilization of the fetus does not occur, and the patient appears to be female externally. As the risk of malignancy of the intra-abdominal or inguinal testes is high, they should be surgically removed. The patient should be reared as female, and oestrogen replacement therapy should be given.

5.33 a **True** b **True** c **True** d **False** e **False**
The most important factors which contribute to genital prolapse are childbirth (especially when associated with obstetric injury) and postmenopausal atrophy. Hence, it is commonly seen in elderly women who have undergone several deliveries. Conditions associated with increased intra-abdominal pressure such as chronic constipation, chronic cough, and heavy lifting also predispose to genital prolapse.

5.34 a **True** b **False** c **False** d **True** e **True**
The main symptoms of genital prolapse are dragging sensation and feeling 'a lump coming down'. Backache may occur which is worse on standing up and relieved by lying down. Dyspareunia may also occur. Other symptoms of genital prolapse depend on the structures sagging. When a cystocele (prolapse of bladder and anterior vaginal wall) is present, urinary symptoms such as frequency of micturition and stress incontinence occur. There may be difficulty in emptying the bowel and straining if a rectocele is present.

5.35 a **False** b **True** c **False** d **False** e **False**
Most uteri lie at an angle to the vagina with the fundus directed forwards and the cervix opening into the posterior fornix. They are said to be anteverted. If the fundus is directed backwards with the cervix opening into the anterior fornix, the uterus is said to be retroverted. A anteverted uterus that bends forwards on itself is said to be anteflexed, and a retroverted uterus that bends backwards on itself is said to be retroflexed. About 20% of all women have retroverted uterus. If the retroverted uterus is mobile and can be manually pushed back into anteversion, this is of little clinical significance except that it occasionally causes intermittent dyspareunia. An immobile retroverted uterus may be caused by pathology such as pelvic inflammatory disease and endometriosis.

5.36 a **False** b **True** c **True** d **True** e **False**
Viral vulva warts are also known as condylomata acuminata. Condylomata lata are second stage syphilitic lesions. Viral vulval warts are caused by human papillomaviruses, and are sexually transmitted. Penile warts may appear in male partners, who should be traced. The most effective treatment is diathermy under general anaesthetic. Alternative treatments include cryosurgery, laser treatment, and application of 20% podophyllin.

5.37 a **False** b **True** c **False** d **True** e **False**
Monilial vaginitis is caused by infection with candida albicans. It is commoner in those with glycosuria, those using oral contraceptives, and those taking broad spectrum antibiotics such as amoxycillin. The characteristic symptoms are intense vulval irritation and thick white vaginal discharge. Treatments include either vaginal pessaries of the imidazole group of drugs (e.g. clotrimazole), or oral fluconazole or itraconazole. However, liver damage may rarely occur with these oral drugs.

5.38 a **False** b **False** c **True** d **False** e **True**
Trichomonas vaginalis is a protozoal infection. Although it is often transmitted by

sexual intercourse, it may also be transmitted via toilet articles or instruments in the gynaecology clinic. It characteristically presents with a profuse yellow odorous discharge. The treatment is oral metronidazole. Male partners should also be treated to avoid cross infection.

5.39 a **False** b **True** c **True** d **False** e **True**
Characteristic symptoms of pelvic inflammatory disease are bilateral abdominal pain and dyspareunia, fever, and profuse vaginal discharge. There may be associated symptoms of irregular vaginal bleeding, nausea, and vomiting. Characteristic signs include tenderness and mass on bimanual examination, and cervical excitation (tenderness when the cervix is moved).

5.40 a **True** b **False** c **False** d **False** e **False**
Fibromyoma (fibroids) are the commonest benign tumour in the female genital tract. They frequently occur in multiples rather than singly. The development of fibroids appears to be related to oestrogen effects. They are commoner in nulliparous women and in black women. They usually start to develop in young adulthood, although they may not have symptoms until later. They tend to decrease in size after menopause. They very rarely become malignant.

5.41 a **False** b **False** c **True** d **True** e **False**
Uncomplicated fibroids may not be symptomatic. The symptoms and signs depend on the numbers, size, and position of the fibroids. The commonest symptoms are abdominal masses which may be nodular and asymmetrical, and menorrhagia. Anaemia may result from menorrhagia. Large fibroids may exert pressure on the bladder and cause urinary symptoms such as frequency of urine. Fibroids are usually associated with late menopause.

5.42 a **True** b **True** c **True** d **False** e **False**
Immediate complications following a cone biopsy include bleeding and infection. Secondary haemorrhage occasionally occurs a week or more after the operation. Long term complications include cervical stenosis and cervical incompetence. Cervical incompetence may cause midtrimester abortions.

5.43 a **False** b **False** c **True** d **True** e **False**
The colposcope is a low-powered binocular microscope. It is mainly used to localize the abnormal epithelium in the transformation zone. After acetic acid is applied, the abnormal epithelium can be visualized its their white colour and an abnormal capillary pattern. It allows accurate diagnosis to be made even if cervical cytology shows inflammatory changes. It should be ideally performed for every women with cervical intraepithelial neoplasia.

5.44 a **False** b **True** c **False** d **False** e **False**
The options for the treatment of carcinoma of the cervix include surgical treatment, radiotherapy, combination of surgery and radiotherapy, chemotherapy and palliative treatment. Surgical treatments (e.g. the Wertheim operation which involves removal

of the uterus, cervix, upper third of the vagina, and the cardinal and uteroscacral ligaments) are most suitable for young fit women with early disease. Most cervical carcinomas are radiosensitive. Radiotherapy is usually given via intrauterine and vaginal applicators, although they are sometimes augmented by external radiation to affected lymph nodes in the pelvic wall. Chemotherapy has not been conclusively shown to be effective, but may be preferred if the carcinoma has metastasized and recurred.

5.45 a **False** b **True** c **False** d **True** e **False**
Risk factors associated with carcinoma of the uterus are those associated with excessive exposure to oestrogen, such as unopposed hormone replacement therapy (i.e. oestrogen replacement without progesterone), oestrogen-secreting tumour, late menopause, polycystic ovarian syndrome, and obesity. Diabetes is also associated with increased risk. Low social class and multiple sexual partners are not significant risk factors for carcinoma of the uterus, unlike carcinoma of the cervix.

5.46 a **False** b **True** c **False** d **False** e **False**
Malignancy of the genital tract is the cause for about a fifth of all cases of post-menopausal bleeding. Other causes include atrophic vaginitis or endometritis, hormone replacement therapy, uterine or cervical polyps and fibroids. However, all cases should be investigated with either a curettage or an endometrial biopsy, as carcinoma of the uterus may coexist with these less serious causes. A negative physical examination and curettage is reassuring, but does not exclude carcinoma of the fallopian tubes or ovaries, or an early endometrial carcinoma.

5.47 a **False** b **True** c **False** d **True** e **False**
Gestational trophoblastic disease (choriocarcinoma) is a highly malignant tumour of the syncitio- and cytotrophoblast tissues. It is much commoner in the Far East. About a half of all tumours occur in those with a previous history of hydatidiform mole, a quarter in those with a previous history of abortion or ectopic pregnancy, and a quarter in those with a normal pregnancy. The tumour produces a large quantity of beta human chorionic gonadotrophin (β-HCG), which can be used both for diagnosis and for monitoring treatment progress. Fortunately, the tumour is highly chemosensitive. Non-metastatic tumour can be effectively treated by methotrexate, whilst metastatic tumour can often be treated by a combination chemotherapy with or without hysterectomy. The 5 year survival rate for non-metastatic tumour is over 95% if the optimal treatment is given.

5.48 a **False** b **True** c **True** d **False** e **True**
It is often not possible to determine preoperatively whether an ovarian tumour is benign or malignant. However, bilateral masses, irregular mobile masses, with the presence of ascites, are more likely to be malignant. Solid elements within the tumour seen on ultrasound also suggest malignancy. Tumour markers such as carcinoembryonic antigen (for mucinous cystadenocarcinoma), alfafetoprotein or β-HCG (for germ cell tumours) may be raised for malignant tumours.

5.49 a **True** b **False** c **False** d **True** e **False**
Endometriosis may often be asymptomatic. The commonest symptoms are pelvic pain occurring before or during menstruation, deep dyspareunia, and menorrhagia. Infertility may occur.

5.50 a **False** b **False** c **False** d **False** e **False**
Endometriosis occurs more frequently in white women than in black women. It occurs in the child-bearing years, and usually regress in the absence of cyclical ovarian function (e.g. pregnancy, after menopause, premature ovarian failure, on combined oral contraceptive). It occurs more often in those who either have no children or who have their first child late.

5.51 a **True** b **True** c **False** d **False** e **True**
In polycystic ovarian syndrome, there is bilateral enlargement of ovaries with multiple follicular cysts. The cause is uncertain. The patient may present with absent or irregular menstruation, and signs of virilism (e.g. acne, hoarse voice, hirsuitism). Investigations may show a normal level of FH, raised level of LH, and increased level of testosterone. In the past, the treatment was bilateral wedge resection of the ovaries. Nowadays, the treatment of choice is a combined oral contraceptive if fertility is not desired, or clomiphene if fertility is desired.

5.52 a **True** b **True** c **True** d **True** e **True**
Secondary amenorrhoea may be physiological or pathological. Physiological causes include pregnancy and lactation. Pathological causes include hypothalmaic disorders (e.g. psychological stress, severe weight loss), pituitary disorders (e.g. prolactinoma, ischaemic necrosis of pituitary gland after postpartum haemorrhage), ovarian disorders (e.g. premature ovarian failure, polycystic ovarian syndrome), and other endocrine abnormalities (e.g. Cushing's syndrome).

5.53 a **True** b **True** c **True** d **True** e **False**
Dysfunctional uterine bleeding may be caused by imbalance of gonadotrophic hormones, ovarian hormones, and prostaglandin in the endometrium. Treatments which are commonly used include non-steroidal inflammatory drugs (e.g. mefanamic acid), combined oral contraceptives, and danazol. If these are ineffective, the new GnRH analogues may be used to induce menopause artificially. However, there are serious menopausal side-effects, including osteoporosis. Hence, this should be used only temporarily. Endometrial ablation is a relatively new technique. Hysterectomy is generally reserved for those after child-bearing age. Dilatation and curettage is an investigation to exclude local cause for bleeding, and is not a treatment.

5.54 a **False** b **True** c **True** d **True** e **False**
In the investigation of infertility, traditional tests for ovulation include body temperature charts and assessment of cervical mucus. More accurate tests indicating ovulation include a raised progesterone level at the luteal phase (usually 7 days before the next period), a surge in LH at mid-cycle indicated by urine dipstick, demonstration of a sudden reduction in size of the dominant follicle by vaginal ultrasound, and

changes in cervical mucus seen on microscopy in the post-coital test. When ovulation occurs, the LH level surges at mid-cycle, and the progesterone level rises in the luteal phase. This causes a rise in basal body temperature and the cervical mucus to become more abundant and stringy, and less viscous, which are important for sperm survival.

5.55 a **True** b **True** c **True** d **False** e **True**
Causes of infertility include psychological and physical factors. Physical factors may be divided into male factors, female factors, and an interaction between the two. Male factors are due to inadequate production of healthy spermatozoa or ineffective delivery into the upper vagina. Causes for inadequate production may be idiopathic oliogozoospermia, or may be testicular atrophy, previous mumps infection, undescended testes or varicocoeles. Female factors include failure of ovulation and blockage of the fallopian tubes. Causes of failure of ovulation include hypothalamic causes (e.g. psychological stress, severe weight loss), pituitary causes (e.g. prolactinoma), ovarian causes (e.g. resistant ovary syndrome, premature ovarian failure), other endocrine causes (e.g. hypothyroidism, diabetes mellitus). Causes for fallopian tube blockage include severe endometriosis and pelvic inflammatory disease. Combined causes include presence of anti-sperm antibodies in the cervical mucus.

5.56 a **False** b **True** c **True** d **False** e **True**
Two major causes for incontinence in women are urethral sphincter incompetence and detrusor instability. Although stress incontinence is commoner in urethral sphincter incompetence and urge incontinence is commoner in detrusor instability, both types of incontinence may occur in either conditions in practice. Hence, urodynamic study (cystometry) must be performed. Detrusor instability can be treated by bladder training or anticholinergic drugs, whereas urethral sphincter incompetence is treated by bladder neck suspension.

5.57 a **True** b **True** c **True** d **False** e **True**
Laparoscopy may be used for both diagnostic and therapeutic purposes. It may be used to diagnose the cause for unexplained abdominal or pelvic pain and the cause for infertility (e.g. by inspecting the ovaries, uterus, and fallopian tubes, and the patency of the tubes by introducing a dye via the cervix). Therapeutic uses include sterilization, rupture of a benign ovarian cyst, ablation of endometriosis, and laparoscopic-assisted vaginal hysterectomy. This is a relatively new technique for removing the uterus, which may otherwise require an abdominal approach. The various ligaments are identified and divided through the laparoscope, and the uterus and cervix are removed vaginally.

5.58 a **True** b **True** c **False** d **True** e **False**
Before performing a sterilization operation, informed consent must be obtained from the patient. She must be informed that the operation has a small failure rate, and that it must be regarded as irreversible. Although most operations are successfully performed by laparoscopy, there is a small chance that an attempt by this method will fails and a mini-laparotomy will be needed. This is especially true if the patient is obese. Sterilization should not be performed immediately after delivery, as the uterus

is still large; the operation is technically more difficult and carries a higher failure rate. The ovarian function is unaffected by tubal ligation.

5.59 a **True** b **True** c **True** d **True** e **True**
The commonest complications of an intrauterine contraceptive device are menorrhagia and dysmenorrhoea. Pelvic infection and ectopic pregnancy are commoner with an intrauterine contraceptive device *in situ*. Occasionally, perforation of the uterus may occur during insertion, and the device may be expelled after insertion.

5.60 a **True** b **False** c **False** d **True** e **False**
Progesterone-only pills are taken continuously, and must be taken at the same time each day. They are less effective than combined oral contraceptives. However, they are more suitable for breast-feeding women, as oestrogen but not progesterone suppresses lactation. Progesterone-only pills are probably more suitable for older women when the natural fertility rate is lower. There is no increased risk in thromboembolism for progesterone-only pills. Menstrual irregularities, ranging from amenorrhoea to irregular menstrual bleeding, are commoner with these pills.

6 *Paediatrics*

Questions

6.1 The average 9 month old baby can

a walk alone unaided
b pass an object from one hand to the other
c put two words together
d sit without support
e scribble

6.2 The average 18 month old child can

a walk alone steadily
b say four recognizable words
c scribble with a pencil
d walk upstairs, two feet per step
e copy a circle

6.3 The average 3 year old child can

a give his or her own full name
b copy a triangle
c drink from a cup
d walk downstairs, two feet per step
e build a tower of six cubes

6.4 Which of the following conditions are autosomal recessive in inheritance?

a tuberose sclerosis
b galactosaemia
c phenylketonuria
d neurofibromatosis
e Hunter's syndrome

6.5 Which of the following statements about Down's syndrome is/are true?

a it affects about 1 in every 6000 live births
b it occurs more frequently with increasing maternal age
c adults with Down's syndrome have increasing risk for Alzheimer's dementia

d it may be diagnosed antenatally by amniocentesis
e it occurs more than twice as frequently in females compared to males

6.6 *Characteristic features of Down's syndrome include*

a short stature
b single palmar crease
c fusion of first and second toes
d congenital heart disease
e duodenal atresia

6.7 *Clinical features of Turner's syndrome include*

a rocker-bottom feet
b coarctation of the aorta
c long neck
d increased carrying angle
e primary amenorrhoea

6.8 *Organisms which may pass from the mother to the fetus through the placenta include*

a rubella virus
b chickenpox virus
c streptococcus
d parvovirus
e toxoplasmosis

6.9 *Which of the following conditions occur significantly more often in the preterm than in term infants?*

a idiopathic respiratory distress syndrome
b jaundice
c intraventricular haemorrhage
d rhesus incompatibility
e hypothyroidism

6.10 *Causes of jaundice within the first 24 h of life include*

a biliary atresia
b physiological jaundice
c breast milk jaundice
d ABO incompatibility
e congenital spherocytosis

6.11 *Compared to bottle-fed infants, breast-fed infants are significantly less likely to suffer from*

a febrile convulsion
b gastrointestinal infection
c atopic eczema

d viral laryngotracheobronchitis (croup)
e sudden infant death syndrome

6.12 *Gastro-oesophageal reflux in the first year of life*

a is extremely rare
b usually requires elective surgical treatment
c may cause aspiration pneumonia
d may cause iron deficiency anaemia
e may be alleviated by thickening the feeds

6.13 *Which of the following statements about congenital hypertrophic pyloric stenosis is/are true?*

a it usually presents within the first week after birth
b it occurs more frequently in females than males
c regurgitation of feed is the characteristic symptom
d the infant usually refuses feeds
e the diagnosis may be confirmed by ultrasound

6.14 *Recognized causes of rickets in children include*

a lack of sunshine
b dietary deficiency
c chronic liver disease
d diabetes mellitus
e chronic renal failure

6.15 *Which of the following vaccines are usually given below 6 months of age?*

a polio vaccine
b pertussis vaccine
c measles vaccine
d meningococcus type B vaccine
e rubella vaccine

6.16 *Clinical features of mumps include*

a enlargement of parotid glands
b aseptic meningitis
c pneumonia
d orchitis
e sensori-neural deafness

6.17 *Which of the following statements about acute laryngotracheobronchitis (croup) is/are true?*

a it is caused by Haemophilus influenzae type B
b it occurs most frequently in summer
c drooling of saliva is a characteristic symptom

d hoarseness is a frequent symptom in older children
e a 'cherry red' epiglottis is often seen

6.18 Clinical features of cystic fibrosis in the late teens include

a bronchiectasis
b subacute intestinal obstruction
c diabetes mellitus
d delayed puberty
e biliary cirrhosis

6.19 Common signs of heart failure in infancy include

a tachypnoea
b gallop rhythm
c oedema of the ankles
d raised jugular venous pressure
e hepatomegaly

6.20 Acyanotic congenital heart diseases include

a atrial septal defect
b transposition of the great vessels
c coarctation of the aorta
d Fallot's tetralogy
e patent ductus arteriosus

6.21 Which of the following statements about ventricular septal defects is/are true?

a they are the commonest congenital heart lesions
b they always require surgical closure
c the onset of symptoms is earlier the larger the defects
d the risk of bacterial endocarditis is higher than in atrial septal defects
e the characteristic sign is an ejection systolic murmur at the lower left sternal edge

6.22 Which of the following statements about coarctation of the aorta is/are true?

a the lesion is in the ascending aorta
b the systolic blood pressure in the upper limb is often elevated
c the brachial pulses are often weak
d radiofemoral delay is a characteristic sign
e chest radiography may show notching of the ribs in older untreated children

6.23 Signs of dehydration in infancy and childhood include

a bulging fontanelle

b loss of skin turgor
c tachycardia
d sunken eye
e dry tongue

6.24 *Which of the following statements about Hirschprung disease is/are true?*

a it characteristically presents with diarrhoea
b it almost always presents in the neonatal period
c it may present with intestinal obstruction in the neonatal period
d the rectum is characteristically full of faeces on rectal examination
e the diagnosis may be confirmed by rectal biopsy

6.25 *Which of the following statements about viral gastroenteritis in infancy is/are true?*

a adenovirus is the commonest causative organism
b it occurs most frequently in winter
c almost all infants should be admitted to hospital for observation
d anti-diarrhoeal agents should be given in the majority of the cases
e prophylactic antibiotics should be given

6.26 *Potter's syndrome is associated with*

a renal agenesis
b polydramnios
c pulmonary hypoplasia
d characteristic facies
e talipes

6.27 *Posterior urethral valves*

a have an equal sex incidence
b may be diagnosed antenatally
c may present with a distended bladder in the first month of life
d may cause bilateral hydronephrosis
e require ureteric diversion in more than half of the cases

6.28 *Which of the following statements about urinary tract infection in infancy is/are true?*

a the diagnosis is confirmed if more than 10^5/ml of urine is grown from a sample of bag urine
b most infants present with urinary symptoms
c it is a cause of prolonged jaundice in the neonatal period
d infants with a characteristic history may be given antibiotics without urinary culture
e all infants with a confirmed urinary tract infection should undergo further radiological examination of the urinary tract

6.29 *Nephrotic syndrome in children*

a is commoner in white than in Asian children
b occurs more frequently in males than in females
c predisposes to pneumococcal infection
d is usually associated with focal sclerosing glomerulonephritis
e usually responds to corticosteroid treatment

6.30 *Clinical features of Henoch-Schönlein purpura may include*

a hypertension
b urticaria
c abdominal pain
d bronchospasm
e a low platelet count

6.31 *Which of the following statements about homozygous β-thalassaemia is/are true?*

a the level of HbA is increased
b the level of HbA_2 is reduced
c macrocytic anaemia is characteristic
d children should be given regular oral iron supplements
e antenatal diagnosis is available

6.32 *Conditions associated with an increased bleeding time include*

a Christmas disease (factor IX deficiency)
b Von Willebrand disease
c idiopathic thrombocytopenic purpura
d vitamin K deficiency
e haemophilia A (factor VIII deficiency)

6.33 *Which of the following statements about idiopathic thrombocytopenic purpura is/are true?*

a the white cell count is characteristically reduced
b the haemoglobin level is characteristically reduced
c reduced numbers of megakaryocytes are characteristically seen on bone marrow examination
d more than 50% of the children require splenectomy
e corticosteroids may temporarily increase the platelet level

6.34 *Which of the following are characteristic features of physical child abuse?*

a multiple fractures of different ages
b torn frenulum

c generalised petechiae
d Mongolian blue spot
e spiral fracture of the humerus

6.35 *Which of the following conditions are significantly associated with microcephaly*

a fragile X syndrome
b fetal alcohol syndrome
c diabetes mellitus
d congenital toxoplasmosis
e uncontrolled maternal phenylketonuria

6.36 *Congenital dislocation of the hips occurs more frequently in*

a children with a positive family history
b in boys than in girls
c in babies born by breech delivery
d the right hip than the left hip
e Chinese people than white people

6.37 *Which of the following laboratory findings in the cerebrospinal fluid support the diagnosis of bacterial meningitis?*

a turbid appearance
b 100/mm^3 of lymphocytes
c CSF glucose of 4.5 and a blood glucose of 6
d protein level of more than 20 g/litre
e gram negative diplococci seen on gram stain

6.38 *Organisms which characteristically cause meningitis in the neonatal period include*

a streptococcus pneumoniae
b meningococci
c Group B haemolytic streptococci
d Listeria monocytogenes
e Escherichia coli

6.39 *Which of the following statements about febrile convulsions is/are true?*

a they often occur below 6 months of age
b they affect about 0.5% of all children
c children with one febrile convulsion have an increased risk of another
d they may occur after measles, mumps, rubella (MMR) vaccination
e children with 1 episode of a typical febrile convulsion lasting 2 min have a 20% risk of developing epilepsy subsequently

6.40 *Which of the following statements about breath-holding attacks is/are true?*

a they usually occur in infancy
b the child may be cyanosed during the attacks
c the child should be admitted to hospital for investigations
d the risk of developing epilepsy subsequently is about 10%
e sodium valproate is useful in preventing further episodes

6.41 *Precocious puberty*

a has an equal sex incidence
b has an underlying organic cause in the majority of the cases in boys
c has an underlying organic cause in the majority of the cases in girls
d may be caused by a craniopharyngioma
e may be caused by granulosa cell of the ovary in girls

6.42 *Which of the following statements about atopic eczema in children is/are true?*

a it affects about 0.5% of all children
b the onset of symptoms is usually after 3 years old
c affected children often have a positive family history
d more than 50% of the cases persist in adulthood
e infection with herpes simplex virus may give rise to Kaposi varicelliform eruption

6.43 *Infantile spasms*

a usually occur above the age of 2 years
b are a form of tonic-clonic epilepsy
c characteristically occur in clusters
d are associated with mental retardation
e are associated with characteristic EEG appearances

6.44 *Which of the following neonatal skin lesions usually disappear spontaneously within 1 month?*

a milia
b peeling skin in postmature babies
c erythema toxicum
d strawberry naevi
e harlequin colour change

6.45 *Which of the following statements about intussusception is/are true?*

a it usually occurs between 1 and 2 years of age
b the associated pain is characteristically continuous
c 'redcurrant jelly' is a characteristic late sign

d a sausage shaped mass may be palpable in the left lower quadrant
e a laparotomy is required to treat the condition in over 95% of cases

6.46 *Oesophageal atresia*

a is characteristically associated with oligohydramnios
b is often associated with a tracheoesophageal fistula
c may be diagnosed by a plain radiograph after passing a firm radio-opaque tube into the upper pouch
d may be associated with congenital heart disease
e is excluded by the presence of air in the stomach on an abdominal radiograph

6.47 *Which of the following are appropriate management for status epilepticus in a 2 year old child?*

a ensure airway is patent
b administer intramuscular diazepam
c administer rectal diazepam
d administer intravenous paraldehyde
e measure blood glucose and administer intravenous dextrose if hypoglycaemic

6.48 *Which of the following statements about short stature in a 13 year old girl is/are true?*

a the previous weights and heights are important in the assessment
b the height of the parents are important in the assessment
c an organic cause can be found in over 90% of the children
d turner's syndrome may be a cause
e pubertal development is important in the assessment

6.49 *Which of the following statements about Duchenne muscular dystrophy is/are true?*

a it is autosomal recessive in inheritance
b there is excessive dystrophin in the muscle cells of affected individuals
c onset of symptoms usually occurs after 7 years old
d prominence of the calf muscles is a characteristic early feature
e affected subjects characteristically have low level of creatinine kinase

6.50 *Causes for cerebral palsy include*

a neonatal meningitis
b antenatal anoxia
c Wilson's disease
d congenital malformation of the brain
e subacute sclerosing panencephalitis

6.51 *Which of the following are appropriate management within the first few hours of a 4 year old child presenting with diabetic ketoacidosis?*

a encourage oral fluid intake
b administer intravenous dextrose saline
c measure urea, electrolyte, and glucose levels
d administer a bolus of Monotard insulin
e ECG monitoring

6.52 *Which of the following findings in a 3 day old infant are abnormal and should be further investigated?*

a blood pressure of 75/45
b pulse rate of 120/min
c respiratory rate of 35 breaths/min
d haemoglobin 18.0 g/dl
e failure to pass meconium since birth

6.53 *Which of the following statements about sudden infant death syndrome is/are true?*

a postmortem studies show that respiratory infection is the commonest cause
b it is the commonest cause of death of infants between 1 month and 1 year old
c it occurs more frequently in infants sleeping in supine than prone position
d it occurs more frequently in male than females
e it occurs more frequently during summer than winter

6.54 *Which of the following statements about chickenpox is/are true?*

a the skin lesions characteristically appear in crops
b it is caused by the same virus which causes herpes zoster
c cerebellar ataxia is a recognized complication
d the skin lesions characteristically first appear as vesicles
e subacute sclerosing panencephalitis is a recognized complication

6.55 *Which of the following statements about hypospadias is/are true?*

a the urethra opens into the dorsal aspect of the penis
b it may be associated with ventral curvature of the penis
c circumcision may be indicated in the first week of life
d socially unacceptable urinary stream is an indication for surgical treatment
e potential sexual difficulties in future years is an indication for surgical repair

6.56 *With respect to consent to treatment, which of the following situations would justify proceeding with the proposed treatment to a child in United Kingdom?*

a consent is obtained from the mother to perform appendectomy on her 15 year old son
b consent is obtained from a 7 year child to perform a laparotomy for intestinal obstruction
c consent is obtained from the mother to perform a laparoscopy on her 19 year old daughter
d no consent can be obtained to explore a suspected subdural haematoma in an unconscious 10 year old boy, if the parents are unavailable
e consent is obtained from both parents of a 18 year old mentally handicapped girl (with a mental age of 4) for sterilization

6.57 *Which of the following statements about bronchiolitis is/are true?*

a influenza virus is the commonest causative organism
b the peak incidence is between the ages of 12 and 18 months
c feeding difficulty is a common presenting symptom
d more than 90% of those affected require hospital admission
e more than 90% of those affected respond to nebulised salbutamol

6.58 *Contraindications to pertussis immunization include*

a cerebral palsy
b Down's syndrome
c a family history of convulsions
d prematurity
e a family history of adverse reactions following pertussis immunization

6.59 *Which of the following statements about childhood asthma is/are true?*

a it affects about 0.5% of all children
b nocturnal cough is often the only symptom
c an inhaler with spacer cannot be used for a 5 year old child
d a 3 year old child can use a peak flow meter
e it occurs more commonly in those whose parents smoke in the house

6.60 *Which of the following statements about neural tube defects is/are true?*

a they include anencephaly
b folic acid supplements before conception and during the early part of pregnancy reduce the risk in the fetus
c the risk is higher in a subsequent pregnancy if a previous pregnancy is affected

d the diagnosis is excluded by a normal antenatal maternal alpha-fetoprotein
e the diagnosis is excluded by a normal antenatal ultrasound

6.61 *Conduct disorders include*

a persistent school refusal
b persistent truancy
c autism
d fire setting
e separation anxiety

6.62 *Which of the following statements about childhood accidents is/are true?*

a the commonest childhood accidents are road traffic accidents
b the commonest fatal accidents are accidental poisoning
c it is impossible to prevent accidents in children below the age of 3 years
d they constitute the commonest cause of death between the ages of 1 month and 1 year
e legislation has a role to play in their prevention

6.63 *Which of the following features suggest a diagnosis of truancy rather than school refusal?*

a onset at 11 years of age
b association with abdominal pain
c association with headache
d parents' lack of knowledge of their child's non-attendance at school
e previous history of good behaviour at school

6.64 *Pertussis vaccines should be avoided for children with*

a a family history of febrile convulsions
b a personal history of febrile convulsions
c spina bifida
d asthma
e diabetes mellitus

Answers

6.1 a **False** b **True** c **False** d **True** e **False**
A 9 month old child can sit unsupported, but is unable to walk with a hand held until the age of a year. He or she can pass an object from one hand to another from the age of 6 months, and most develop a thumb-finger grasp from 9 months. Most 9 month olds would be able to say 'mum' or 'dad', but would not be able to say other words with meaning or put two words together.

6.2 a **True** b **True** c **True** d **False** e **False**

An average 18 month old can walk alone steadily, but is not able to walk upstairs, two feet per step, until about 2 years of age. He or she is able to scribble with a pencil, but is unable to copy a circle until 3 years of age. He or she can say up to 10 recognizable words.

6.3 a **True** b **False** c **True** d **True** e **True**

The average 3 year old child can walk upstairs one foot per step, but is unable to walk downstairs one foot per step until 4 years of age. He or she is able to build a tower of 6 cubes from 2 years of age and copy a circle from 3 years of age, but is unable to copy a square until 4 years of age, and a triangle until 5 years of age. A child can give his or her own name at the age of 3.

6.4 a **False** b **True** c **True** d **False** e **False**

Most diseases involving enzyme deficiencies are recessive in inheritance. Galactosaemia and phenyketonuria are autosomal recessive, whilst Hunters' syndrome is sex-linked recessive in inheritance. Both tuberose sclerosis and neurofibromatosis are autosomal dominant in inheritance.

6.5 a **False** b **True** c **True** d **True** e **False**

Down's syndrome occurs in 1 every 600 live births. It occurs more frequently with increasing maternal age, but paternal age has little effect on the risk of Down's syndrome. As the basic defect is trisomy 21, it occurs with equal frequency in males and females. Triple test screening may be carried out in mothers over the age of 35, and amniocentesis may be carried out for antenatal diagnosis. Adults with Down's syndrome have an increased risk of developing Alzheimer's dementia.

6.6 a **True** b **True** c **False** d **True** e **True**

Characteristic features of Down's syndrome include general features such as short stature and mental retardation; facial features such as epicanthic folds, upward sloping palpebral fissures, squints, low set ears; limb features such as incurving of the fifth fingers, single palmar crease, wide gap between the first and second toe; and associated systemic features such as congenital heart disease, anal atresia, duodenal atresia, increased incidence of leukaemia, and increased incidence of Alzheimer's disease.

6.7 a **False** b **True** c **False** d **True** e **True**

Clinical features of Turner's syndrome include short stature, oedema of the feet in the newborn, low hairline, increased carrying angles at the elbows, widely spaced nipples, primary amenorrhoea, and infertility in early adult life. Coarctation of the aorta occurs in about a fifth of all cases. Renal abnormalities may also occur. Rocker-bottom feet is a feature of Edward's syndrome (trisomy 18).

6.8 a **True** b **True** c **False** d **True** e **True**

Organisms which may cross the placenta to infect the fetus include the TORCHS infection (*Toxoplasmosis*, rubella, cytomegalovirus, hepatitis, syphilis). Other organisms which may also cross the placenta include parvovirus (which causes 'slapped cheek' disease in children, but which may also cause increased risk of abortion in fetuses), chickenpox, and HIV. Neonates may be infected with group B streptococcus as they pass through the birth canal.

6.9 a **True** b **True** c **True** d **False** e **False**
Pre-term infants are more likely than term infants to have idiopathic respiratory distress syndrome (due to lack of surfactant), apnoeic attacks (due to variation of respiratory drive), hypoglycaemia (due to lack of glycogen storage), jaundice (due to liver immaturity and deficiency of gluconryl transferase), infections (due to immature immunological development), intraventricular haemorrhage, necrotising enterocolitis, and retinopathy of prematurity.

6.10 a **False** b **False** c **False** d **True** e **True**
The commonest cause of jaundice within the first 24 h is excess haemolysis. This include rhesus incompatibility or ABO incompatibility, red cell enzyme deficiencies such as glucose-6-phosphate dehydrogenase deficiency, or congenital spherocytosis. Congenital infection (e.g. rubella, cytomegalovirus) may also cause jaundice in the first 24 h of life. Physiological jaundice usually occurs at 3–5 days, and breast milk jaundice usually presents with prolonged jaundice beyond 10 days.

6.11 a **False** b **True** c **True** d **False** e **True**
Breast-feeding is especially advantageous in developing countries, and may result in reduced risk of malnutrition, gastrointestinal infection, and infant mortality. Breast milk is less likely than cow's milk to cause hypernatraemia and hypocalcaemia, and has less curd protein. Other advantages of breast-feeding include reduced risk of atopic diseases, gastrointestinal infections, necrotizing enterocolitis, and sudden infant death syndrome.

6.12 a **False** b **False** c **True** d **True** e **True**
Gastro-oesophageal reflux in the first year of life is common, and is due to immaturity of the lower oesophageal sphincter. Infants present with regurgitation of feeds or vomiting. In most cases, the infants gain weight satisfactorily, and the condition resolves spontaneously as they become older. However, oesophagitis may occur in more severe cases, leading to iron deficiency anaemia. Aspiration pneumonia may also occur in severe cases. Conservative treatments such as sitting the infants upright and thickening feeds with Carobel may relieve the symptoms. Surgical intervention is rarely required.

6.13 a **False** b **False** c **False** d **False** e **True**
Congenital hypertrophic pyloric stenosis is due to hyperplasia and hypertrophy of the circular fibres of the pyloric muscle. It occurs most frequently in firstborn male infants. It characteristically presents in the first 4–6 weeks with projectile vomiting. The infants are characteristically hungry. Examination may reveal peristalsis and a pyloric tumour in the right upper quadrant. Ultrasound has replaced barium study in confirming the diagnosis.

6.14 a **True** b **True** c **True** d **False** e **True**
Rickets is due to vitamin D deficiency. The sources of vitamin D are from the diet and

from the action of ultraviolet light on the ergosterols in the skin. Hence lack of sunshine, dietary deficiency, and malnutrition may contribute to the development of rickets. Vitamin D is converted to 25-hydroxycholecalciferol in the liver, and then to 1,25-hydroxycholecalciferol in the kidneys. Hence, both chronic liver disease and chronic renal failure may cause rickets. Another cause of ricket is vitamin D resistant rickets, which is due to a defect in the renal tubular reabsorption of phosphate.

6.15 a **True** b **True** c **False** d **False** e **False**
The vaccines which are usually given below 6 months of age include toxoids (i.e. diphtheria and tetanus vaccines) and killed vaccines (i.e. pertussis and haemophilus type B vaccine). BCG may be given at birth to newborns of high-risk families. Live vaccines which result in the production of antibodies are generally ineffective before 9 months of age, as the maternal antibodies interfere with the development of immunity. Hence, MMR is not given until 1 year of age at the earliest. Meningococcus Type B vaccine is currently not yet available.

6.16 a **True** b **True** c **False** d **True** e **True**
Infection with mumps may be asymptomatic. Clinical features of mumps include general features such as fever and malaise; enlargement of parotid glands (which may cause difficulty in swallowing) and aseptic meningitis. Other rarer features include sensorineural deafness, epididymo-orchitis, and pancreatitis.

6.17 a **False** b **False** c **True** d **True** e **False**
Acute laryngotracheobronchitis (croup) is caused by viruses such as para-influenza virus, influenza virus, or respiratory syncytial virus. It occurs most frequently in winter. The characteristic symptoms are tachypnoea and inspiratory stridor after a cold. Hoarseness is frequent in older children. Very sudden onset, high pyrexia, drooling saliva, and difficulty in swallowing are more characteristic of acute epiglottitis, which is caused by *Haemophilus influenzae* type B. The throat must not be examined if acute epiglottitis is suspected, but a 'cherry red' epiglottis may be seen during intubation.

6.18 a **True** b **True** c **True** d **True** e **True**
In late childhood, general clinical features of cystic fibrosis include short stature, respiratory symptoms such as bronchiectasis, pneumothorax, bronchospasm, lobar collapse leading to cor pulmonale, and pancreatic insufficiency causing malabsorption. Other complications which may occur from late childhood include destruction of islet cells causing diabetes mellitus; biliary cirrhosis, portal hypertension, gallstones, delayed puberty, and infertility in the male.

6.19 a **True** b **True** c **False** d **False** e **True**
Common symptoms of heart failure in infancy include tachypnoea and feeding difficulties. Common signs include tachycardia, intercostal and subcostal recession, tachypnoea, gallop rhythm (due to the presence of a third heart sound), and an enlarged liver. Oedema of the ankles, which occurs in adults, is very rarely seen in infancy. Raised jugular venous pressure is almost impossible to detect in infancy.

6.20 a **True** b **False** c **True** d **False** e **True**

Congenital heart diseases may be divided into cyanotic and acyanotic types. Common cyanotic heart diseases include transposition of the great arteries and Fallot's tetralogy. Common acyanotic heart diseases include left to right shunts such as atrial septal defect, ventricular septal defect, and patent ductus arteriosus and obstructive lesions such as coarctation of the aorta, aortic stenosis, and pulmonary stenosis.

6.21 a **True** b **False** c **True** d **True** e **False**

Ventricular septal defects are the commonest congenital heart lesions. Small defects are usually asymptomatic, and a pansystolic murmur at the left lower sternal edge may be found on routine examination. Large lesions usually present early in infancy with symptoms and signs of heart failure (i.e. feeding difficulties, tachycardia, tachypnoea, recession, hepatomegaly). The risk of bacterial endocarditis is proportional to the blood flow across the defect, and hence is higher in ventricular septal defects than in atrial septal defects.

6.22 a **False** b **True** c **False** d **True** e **True**

Coarctation of the aorta is a localized narrowing in the descending aorta. Blood may bypass the narrowing by collateral vessels. If the lesion is severe, it may present in infancy with symptoms and signs of heart failure. If the lesion is mild, it may be asymptomatic, or present later with increased blood pressure in the upper limbs. The femoral pulses may be absent or weak, and there may be radio-femoral delay. Chest radiograph may show notching of the ribs by collateral vessels.

6.23 a **False** b **True** c **True** d **True** e **True**

Clinical signs of dehydration may be deceptive, as they may be absent in hypertonic dehydration. However, characteristic signs of dehydration include dry mucous membranes, loss of skin turgor, poor capillary return, depressed fontanelles, sunken eye, tachycardia, and coma in the late stages.

6.24 a **False** b **False** c **True** d **False** e **True**

Hirschprung's disease is a condition of failure of migration of ganglion cells to the nerve plexuses of the large bowel. The aganglionic segment becomes tonically contracted. About four-fifths of all cases present in the first month of life with failure to pass meconium in the first 24 h, abdominal distension, and vomiting in the late stages. They are of the 'long segment' type. However, a significant minority presents after the neonatal period with failure to thrive and intermittent abdominal distension. The rectum is characteristically empty on rectal examination. The diagnosis may be confirmed by rectal biopsy (which may show aganglionic segments), barium enema, or anorectal manometric studies.

6.25 a **False** b **True** c **False** d **False** e **False**

Rotavirus is responsible for most gastroenteritis in infancy, and occurs most frequently in winter. Common clinical features include vomiting, diarrhoea, abdominal tenderness, and dehydration. Management depends on the severity of the clinical features and especially on the degree of dehydration. However, most infants can be managed at home with medical supervision. Treatment consists mainly of oral rehydration therapy with fluids containing glucose and electrolytes. It has been found that glucose in the rehydration therapy enhances the effectiveness of rehydration. Antidiarrhoeal agents should not be given, as they reduce the transit time. Antibiotics should not be given for viral gastroenteritis, as they may cause diarrhoea and vomiting.

6.26 a **True** b **False** c **True** d **True** e **True**
In Potter's syndrome, there is complete renal agenesis. Hence, the fetus fails to produce urine, and there is oligohydramnios. As a result, the fetus is compressed, and leg deformities, especially talipes, may be present. Other features include characteristic facial features such as low set ears and receding chin, and pulmonary hypoplasia.

6.27 a **False** b **True** c **True** d **True** e **False**
Posterior urethral valves occur in the male, and are the commonest causes for obstruction in the lower urinary tract. They may be diagnosed antenatally by the appearance of bladder distension on ultrasound examination, or may present in the neonatal period with bladder distension. Milder cases may present later with urinary infection or with overflow incontinence of urine. The definitive diagnosis may be made on micturating cystourethrogram. Most cases can be treated by ablation of the valves on endoscopy.

6.28 a **False** b **False** c **True** d **False** e **True**
The commonest cause for more than 10^5 organisms/ml of bag urine to be cultured in infancy is skin contamination. Hence, the test should be repeated with either a clean catch specimen of urine or from suprapubic aspiration. Urinary tract infection usually presents in infancy with non-specific symptoms, such as poor feeding, pyrexia, vomiting, diarrhoea, or prolonged jaundice in the neonatal period. In any infants suspected of urinary tract infection, urine samples must be sent for culture. All infants with a confirmed urinary tract infection should be investigated with ultrasound, plain abdominal radiograph to exclude urinary calculi, and either micturating cystourethrogram or an radioisotope scan to exclude vesicoureteric reflux and renal scarring. Infants with vesicoureteric reflux should be given prophylactic antibiotics.

6.29 a **False** b **True** c **True** d **False** e **True**
Nephrotic syndrome occurs more frequently in Asian than in white children. This is partly because nephrotic syndrome secondary to other diseases (e.g. hepatitis B) occurs more frequently. The syndrome occurs more frequently in males than females. It is due to minimal change glomerulonephritis in about four-fifths of cases. These cases respond to corticosteroid treatment, and renal biopsy is only indicated if the child fails to respond to corticosteroid treatment. Children with nephrotic syndrome are susceptible to both pneumoccoccal and meningococcal infection in the active phase of the disease, and prophylactic penicillin should be given.

6.30 a **True** b **True** c **True** d **False** e **False**
Clinical features of Henoch-Schönlein purpura include skin symptoms (e.g. urticaria,

vasculitic lesions especially on the buttocks), joint symptoms (e.g. arthralgia and arthritis in the large joints), gastrointestinal symptoms (e.g. malaena, abdominal pain, and occasionally intussusception), and renal symptoms (e.g. haematuria, proteinuria, hypertension). Henoch-Schönlein purpura is associated with a normal platelet count. If the platelet count is low, the purpuric rash may be due to idiopathic thrombocytopenia purpura or acute leukaemia.

6.31 a **False** b **False** c **False** d **False** e **True**
Thalassaemia occurs in Mediterranean and Asian countries, and is associated with failure to produce either α or β haemoglobin chains. In β thalassaemia there is failure of β chain production. Hence, HbA ($\alpha_2\beta_2$)is reduced, but HbA_2 ($\alpha_2\delta_2$) is slightly increased. The characteristic haematological features are severe haemolytic anaemia with hypochromic microcytic picture. Children require repeat blood transfusions, and this may lead to iron overload. Desferrioxamine subcutaneous infusion may reduce the degree of iron overload, and children must not be given iron supplements. Antenatal diagnosis is possible by analysis of the fetal DNA on chorionic villous biopsy.

6.32 a **False** b **True** c **True** d **False** e **False**
Vitamin K is required in the extrinsic coagulation pathway, and vitamin K deficiency results in prolonged prothrombin time (or increased INR). Factors VIII and IX are required for the intrinsic pathway, and deficiency results in prolonged partial thromboplastin time (PTT; kaolin cephalin clotting time). Prolonged bleeding time is either due to a reduction in the number of platelets (e.g. due to idiopathic thrombocytopenic purpura), platelet function disorders, or Von Willebrand disease (due to reduced platelet adhesiveness).

6.33 a **False** b **False** c **False** d **False** e **True**
Idiopathic thrombocytopenic purpura is the commonest cause for thrombocytopenia in children. It often follows a viral infection, and is thought to be autoimmune. Most cases present with generalized petechiae and bruises. The condition often resolves spontaneously in less than 6 months. However, bleeding into the viscera or the brain occurs rarely. Hence, the child must be carefully observed and the platelet level monitored. Full blood count characteristically shows a normal haemoglobin and white cell count, but the platelet number is severely reduced. The diagnosis is confirmed by finding a normal or increased number of megakaryocytes in the bone marrow. If the symptoms or platelet level suggest a significant risk of bleeding into a solid organ or into the brain, corticosteroids or intravenous human normal immunoglobulins may be given to produce a temporary elevation of the platelet level. Splenectomy is very rarely required.

6.34 a **True** b **True** c **False** d **False** e **True**
Child physical abuse may present in many different ways. Localized bruising, especially fingertip bruises or slap marks, are common in child physical abuse, but generalized petechiae suggest platelet or clotting abnormalities. Multiple fractures of different ages, spiral fractures (suggesting rotating injury), epiphyseal separation,

and periosteal bleed are all characteristic of child physical abuse. Torn frenulum may be caused by a milk bottle forced into the child's mouth. Mongolian blue spots are congenital and are especially common in infants of dark-skinned ethnic origin. They usually disappear after the first year of life.

6.35 a **False** b **True** c **False** d **True** e **True**
Fragile X syndrome is associated with mental retardation, large ears, long face, and large testes. However, microcephaly is not a characteristic feature. Causes of microcephaly include fetal alcohol syndrome, congenital infections (by the TORCHS organisms), maternal uncontrolled phenylketonuria, perinatal asphyxia, and congenital microcephaly.

6.36 a **True** b **False** c **True** d **False** e **False**
Congenital dislocation of the hips occur less frequently in Africans and Chinese infants who are carried with their legs astride on the mother's back. Firstborn girls, those with a positive family history, and infants born by breech delivery are at increased risk. Congenital dislocation of the hips occurs more often in the left than in the right hip, a fact which is still unexplained.

6.37 a **True** b **False** c **False** d **True** e **True**
The typical findings in the cerebrospinal fluid in bacterial meningitis are turbid appearance, polymorphs, CSF glucose less than two-thirds of the blood glucose level, a high protein level (of more than 1.5 g/litre, say), organisms seen on gram stain, and a positive culture. Gram negative diplococci seen on microscopy suggests meningococcal meningitis. Lymphocytes in the CSF suggests either viral or tuberculous meningitis.

6.38 a **False** b **False** c **True** d **True** e **True**
Organisms which characteristically cause meningitis in the neonatal period include group B haemolytic streptococci, *Escherichia coli* and other gram negative bacilli, and *Listeria monocytogenes*. *Streptococcus pneumoniae* meningitis usually occurs in the older child. Although meningococcal meningitis occurs more frequently in those below 5 years of age than in other age groups, it does not characteristically occur in the neonatal period.

6.39 a **False** b **False** c **True** d **True** e **False**
Febrile convulsions occur between the age of 6 months and 5 years, and the peak incidence is in the second year of life. Children with febrile convulsions often have a positive family history. Febrile convulsions are characteristically symmetrical tonic/clonic generalized seizures lasting less than 10 min with no focal features, and usually occur when the temperature rises rapidly in febrile illness. They may occur after pertussis or MMR vaccination. Parents should be encouraged to cool the child and to administer paracetamol during a febrile illness. About a third of children with one febrile convulsion have a recurrence, and parents may be taught to use give rectal diazepam either during a febrile illness or during a seizure. The risk of epilepsy after an episode of uncomplicated febrile convulsion is about 1–2%.

6.40 a **False** b **True** c **False** d **False** e **False**
Breath-holding attacks occur in toddlers, usually after a temper tantrum. The child cries, and then holds his breath and becomes cyanosed. Very occasionally, there may be a few jerks in the limbs or the child may go unconsciously for a very short time. The child then rapidly recovers. The parents should be reassured that this is totally benign and does not require any drug treatment or investigations.

6.41 a **False** b **True** c **False** d **True** e **True**
Puberty before the age of 9 in boys and 8 in girls may be defined as precocious. It occurs about 4 times more frequently in girls than in boys. No organic causes are found in most cases in girls, but they are usually present in boys. Organic causes for precocious puberty include CNS causes (e.g. hypothalamic tumours, craniopharyngioma, post meningitis, hydrocephalus, tuberous sclerosis), ovarian causes for girls (e.g. granulosa cell tumour), testicular tumours in boys, and other endocrine causes (e.g. virilising congenital adrenal hyperplasia, hypothyroidism).

6.42 a **False** b **False** c **True** d **False** e **True**
Atopic eczema occurs in about 3% of all children, and symptoms often start in infancy. Affected children often have a positive family history of atopic eczema, asthma, or hayfever. Breast-feeding may reduce the risk of developing atopic eczema. About 90% of atopic eczema in childhood resolves at puberty. Atopic eczema is usually symmetrical and affects the face and the flexor surfaces of the limbs. Herpes simplex infection in the presence of atopic eczema may give rise to a life-threatening condition, Kaposi varicelliform eruption. Hence, herpes infection should be treated with acyclovir.

6.43 a **False** b **False** c **True** d **True** e **True**
Infantile spasms are a form of myoclonic epilepsy. The symptoms usually start between the ages of 3 months and 9 months, with typical flexion of the trunk and limbs, each spasm lasting between 2–3 s. They characteristically appear in clusters, and may occur more than 100 times a day. Causes include tuberous sclerosis, untreated metabolic disorders (e.g. phenylketonuria) or intracranial malformations, although no causes may be detected in a significant proportion of the cases. The EEG characteristically shows hypsarrythmia. Most infants with infantile spasms, especially those caused by underlying neurological causes, will develop mental retardation.

6.44 a **True** b **True** c **True** d **False** e **True**
Milia are tiny sebaceous cysts on the nose which usually disappear. Peeling skin in postmature babies is common, which usually disappear. However, olive oil may be used to prevent skin cracking. Erythema toxicum are red blotches in the neonate which usually disappear within 24 h. Harlequin colour changes are said to occur when one side of the body suddenly becomes redder than the other. These are vasomotor phenomena, and are usually short-lived. Strawberry naevi may enlarge after birth, although they usually resolve at the age of 5 years.

6.45 a **False** b **False** c **True** d **False** e **False**
Intussusception occurs when a segment of bowel invaginates into another below it. The usual site is the terminal ileum or the ileocaecal valve, resulting in a ileocolic intussusception. It characteristically occurs between 6 and 12 months of age. The characteristic symptoms are paroxysmal colicky pain and vomiting. In the late stages, there may be abdominal distension and rectal bleeding, 'redcurrant jelly'. A sausage shaped mass may be palpable in the right upper quadrant. If the infant presents within the first 24 h, a barium enema may confirm the diagnosis, and hydrostatic reduction may be successful in reducing the intussusception without laparotomy in the majority of the cases.

6.46 a **False** b **True** c **True** d **True** e **False**
In oesophageal atresia, the fetus cannot swallow and is therefore associated with polyhydramnios. It is often associated with a tracheoesophageal fistula, and therefore air may be present in the stomach. It is also associated with other congenital abnormalities such as anorectal abnormalities and congenital heart disease. The diagnosis should be suspected if there is a history of polyhydramnios, or if the baby froths at the mouth and appears unable to swallow saliva. The diagnosis can be excluded if a wide-bored tube can be passed through the oropharynx to the stomach. The diagnosis can be made by the appearance of a coiled tube on a plain radiograph after a firm radio-opaque tube is passed through the oropharynx.

6.47 a **True** b **False** c **True** d **False** e **True**
The first priority in the treatment of status epilepticus is to ensure a patent airway, good respiratory effort, and good circulation. Pulse and blood pressure should be monitored if possible. Oxygen may be given via a face mask. Blood glucose should always be measured and intravenous dextrose given if hypoglycaemia is present. If facilities are available, blood calcium and magnesium should also be measured. The first drug of choice is either intravenous or rectal diazepam. Rectal diazepam is particular suitable if the child is at home, or if venous access is difficult. Diazepam may be repeated once if there is no response after 5 min. Intramuscular (or rectal) paraldehyde may be used if there is no response after another 5 min. Thereafter, intravenous phenytoin, phenobarbitone, chlormethiazole, or clonazepam may be tried. In the last resort, paralysis and artificial ventilation will be needed. Intramuscular diazepam is poorly absorbed, and should not be used in status epilepticus.

6.48 a **True** b **True** c **False** d **True** e **True**
The commonest causes for short stature in a 13 year old girl are constitutional short stature or delayed puberty. In constitutional short stature, the parents also tend to be short. Organic causes are seldom found. The mid-parental height is a good indicator for the child's potential height. Previous heights and weights of the child is important in assessing whether the child has always been short for her age, or whether there has been a recent fall in height centiles. Pubertal assessment, together with bone age if indicated, is important in assessing whether short stature is due to delayed puberty. Other causes for short stature include any chronic illnesses, malabsorption, or

endocrine causes such as hypothyroidism or growth hormone deficiency, Turner's syndrome, and psychological deprivation.

6.49 **False** b **False** c **False** d **True** e **False**
Duchenne muscular dystrophy is the commonest type of muscular dystrophy, and is sex-linked recessive in inheritance. In about three quarters of the cases, there is a gene deletion in the X chromosome, resulting in deficiency in the production of dystrophin in muscle cells. The onset of symptoms usually occurs before 5 years of age with delayed walking, frequent falls, and difficulty in climbing stairs. Characteristic signs include prominence of calf muscles (termed 'pseudohypertrophy', as the muscles are actually weak), and positive Gower's sign (the child climbs up his legs as he gets up from a lying position). The creatinine kinase level is characteristically greatly elevated, and there are characteristic EMG and muscle biopsy appearances.

6.50 a **True** b **True** c **False** d **True** e **False**
Cerebral palsy is a permanent non-progressive neurological disorder which may be caused by congenital malformation of the brain, antenatal causes (e.g. anoxia), perinatal causes (e.g. birth-related cerebral trauma), and postnatal causes (e.g. meningitis, non-accidental injury, and accidental head injury). Wilson's disease and subacute sclerosing panencephalitis are both progressive neurological disorders.

6.51 a **False** b **False** c **True** d **False** e **True**
The appropriate initial assessment and management of a 4 year old child presenting with diabetic ketoacidosis include taking relevant history, assessing the circulatory status and degree of dehydration, excluding signs of infection, and obtaining a baseline weight of the child. The child should be kept nil by mouth and a nasogastric tube should be inserted, to prevent risk of vomiting followed by aspiration. ECG monitoring should be performed to detect signs of hypo- or hyperkalaemia, and signs of cardiovascular collapse. Urea, electrolytes, blood glucose, and blood gases should be measured. The child should be resuscitated with either intravenous plasma or normal saline to replace fluid losses. Short-acting insulin (e.g. actrapid) should be given both as a bolus and as an infusion, and the rate of infusion should be adjusted according to blood glucose levels. Potassium supplements may be needed if the serum potassium level is low or normal, and there is adequate urine output.

6.52 a **False** b **False** c **False** d **False** e **True**
The newborn infant has a higher pulse rate and respiratory rate, and a lower blood pressure than the older child. The haemoglobin level is also higher, sometimes as high as 20.0 g/dl. However, this usually decreases within the next few weeks. Failure to pass meconium within 24 h should raise the suspicion of large-bowel obstruction such as anorectal agenesis, Hirschprung's disease, or meconium ileus due to cystic fibrosis.

6.53 a **False** b **True** c **False** d **True** e **False**
Sudden infant death syndrome is defined as unexpected death of an infant in whom postmortem examination fails to reveal an adequate cause of death. It is the

commonest cause of death between the ages of 1 month and 1 year. It occurs more frequently in males, in premature babies, in winter, in low social class, in those whose parents smoke, and in babies who sleep prone.

6.54 a **True** b **True** c **True** d **False** e **False**
Chickenpox is caused by the same virus which causes herpes zoster, and shingles is a reactivation of the dormant virus in the posterior root ganglion. The condition may be asymptomatic apart from low-grade fever. The characteristic rash appears in crops, progressing from macule to papule to vesicles, which then dry and crust. Complications include cerebellar ataxia and pneumonia. Subacute sclerosing panencephalitis is a complication of measles.

6.55 a **False** b **True** c **False** d **True** e **True**
In hypospadias, the urethra opens into the ventral aspect of the penis. If the urethra opens into the dorsal aspect of the penis, it is known as epispadias. Hypospadias may be associated with ventral curvature of the penis. Circumcision must not be performed in the presence of hypospadias, as the foreskin may be required for future surgical repair. Socially unacceptable urinary stream and potential future sexual difficulties are well-established indications for surgical intervention. Nowadays, even cosmetic appearance may sometimes be regarded as valid indication for surgery.

6.56 a **True** b **False** c **False** d **True** e **False**
As a general rule, in the United Kingdom, treatment of children aged under 16 requires the consent from a parent with parental responsibility, but children aged above 16 can give valid consent themselves. For young people aged between 17 and 18, either consent from the young person or his or her parents would be valid. However, if a proposed emergency treatment is required to save live, the doctors may proceed to treatment under common law if none of those parental responsibility are available to give consent. Unfortunately, for a mentally handicapped person above the age of 18 who cannot give valid informed consent, neither the person nor the parents can give consent. For routine elective treatments in such cases, application should be made to the High Court to declare that such treatments are not illegal. In the Gillick case, the prescription of oral contraceptives to girls under the age of 15, who either are sexually active or are shortly becoming sexually active, but who refuse to inform their parents or allow the doctor to inform the parents, was debated. The case established that children who are under the age of 16 but are judged sufficiently mature by the doctor to understand the proposed treatment may be able to give valid consent.

6.57 a **False** b **False** c **True** d **False** e **False**
Bronchiolitis is most often caused by respiratory syncytial virus, and usually affects infants under 1 year of age, and especially those under the age of 6 months. Characteristic symptoms include fever, coryza, feeding difficulties, and respiratory difficulties. Characteristic signs include tachypnoea, intercostal and subcostal recession, and rhonchi. Cyanosis may occur in severe cases. Most cases can be managed at home under medical supervision. However, if there are significant feeding difficulties or

significant tachypnoea, the infant should be admitted for observation. Oxygen may be given via a headbox. In moderate or severe cases, blood gases should be monitored. Feeding may be given via a nasogastric tube, or intravenous dextrose may be given. Rarely, the infant may need artificially ventilation. Unlike asthma in the older child, bronchiolitis does not usually respond to β-agonist such as salbutamol. Nebulized ribavirin (an antiviral agent) may be used in those with greatest risk of mortality from bronchiolitis, such as those with congenital heart disease or cystic fibrosis.

6.58 a **False** b **False** c **False** d **False** e **False**
Pertussis immunization should not be given to those with a history of severe local or general reaction to a preceding dose. If the child is suffering from an acute illness, immunization should be postponed until the child has recovered. Stable neurological conditions (e.g. cerebral palsy, Down's syndrome), a family history of convulsions or adverse reactions following immunization and prematurity are not contraindications to immunization.

6.59 a **False** b **True** c **False** d **False** e **True**
Childhood asthma affects at least 5% of all children, and a fifth of all children wheeze at some time. Children with a family history of atopy, those whose mothers smoke during pregnancy, those exposed to passive smoking, and those with a history of bronchopulmonary dysplasia are at particular risk. Cough may be the only symptom, and nocturnal cough is particularly common. Other symptoms include dypsnoea and wheeze. Peak flow meters can only be used by children of 5 years or older. An inhaler with spacer can be used from about 3 years of age.

6.60 a **True** b **True** c **True** d **False** e **False**
Neural tube defects include anencephaly, spina bifida, and encephalocele (part of the brain protruding through the skull). Spina bifida is an incomplete vertebral arch, and include a spectrum of conditions ranging from spina bifida occulta to myelomeningocele, where the spinal cord's central canal is exposed. Mothers who have a previous pregnancy affected by neural tube defects have a 10-fold increased risk of recurrence over the general population. It has been shown by a Medical Research Council study that folic acid supplements before conception and in the early part of pregnancy reduces the risk of recurrence of neural tube defects in subsequent pregnancies. This is the only known method for primary prevention. Secondary prevention methods include screening by antenatal ultrasound and maternal alphafetoprotein measurements. However, none of these methods is 100% sensitive and specific. Closed neural tube defects are not associated with an elevated maternal alfafetoprotein level. Similarly, some mild neural tube defects may not be detected on antenatal ultrasound.

6.61 a **False** b **True** c **False** d **True** e **False**
Conduct disorders and emotional disorders are the two major categories of childhood psychological disorders. Conduct disorders are commoner, and occur more frequently in boys than in girls. They are characterized by persistent inappropriate antisocial and

aggressive behaviour for their age. Examples are persistent truancy, fire setting, stealing, etc. Separation anxiety is an example of emotional disorder.

6.62 a **False** b **False** c **False** d **False** e **True**
Childhood accidents only constitute about 2% of all childhood accidents, but over a half of all fatal accidents. Accident is the commonest cause of deaths in children over the age of 1 year. However, sudden infant death syndrome is the commonest cause of death below the age of 1 year. Childhood accidents may be prevented by education of children and their parents, and appropriate legislation (e.g. seat belts for children).

6.63 a **False** b **False** c **False** d **True** e **False**
Truancy usually occurs in older children at the end of their secondary education, whilst school refusal usually occurs either in the primary school or during the transition between primary and secondary education. Children with school refusal are usually conscientious and have a good behavioural and academic record, whereas children with truancy often have antisocial and aggressive behaviour. School refusal is an emotional disorder, and may be associated with somatic symptoms such as headaches and abdominal pain. School refusers usually refuse to leave home, whereas truants leave home but do not attend school.

6.64 a **False** b **False** c **False** d **False** e **False**
The only valid contraindications for pertussis vaccines are evolving neurological disorders, generalized or local adverse reactions to a previous dose, and a current acute systemic illnesses (when immunization should be postponed). Children with either a family or personal history of febrile convulsions have a slightly increased risk of febrile convulsion following pertussis vaccine, but this may be minimized by advice to parents on preventing fever. Spina bifida and cerebral palsy are stable neurological disorders, and are not contraindications to pertussis immunization.

7 *Psychiatry*

Questions

7.1 *Which of the following statements about delusions is/are true?*

a they are always false
b they may be caused by a lack of education
c they may disappear if evidence to the contrary is explained to the person
d they may be caused by unusual cultural upbringing
e they cannot be shared by others who live with the person

7.2 *Symptoms of generalized anxiety disorder often include*

a tension headaches
b hallucinations
c palpitation
d breathlessness
e excessive inappropriate worries about possible future accidents

7.3 *Examples of primary delusions include the belief*

a by a depressed man that he is dead
b by a woman suffering from mania that she is the Queen
c by a man that he will be killed as a result of auditory hallucinations telling him so
d by a woman on hearing the sound of rain that her son has been abducted
e by a man on remembering a game of football played 10 years ago that he is being followed

7.4 *Predictors of good outcome for schizophrenia include*

a insidious onset
b older age of onset
c married
d the predominance of negative symptoms
e good social relationships

7.5 *Which of the following thought abnormalities are characteristic of schizophrenia?*

a primary delusion
b thought insertion

c thoughts of self-harm
d grandiose delusion
e delusion of passivity

7.6 *Which of the following are catatonic symptoms?*

a stupor
b waxy flexibility
c chorea
d social isolation
e bizarre rigid posture

7.7 *Negative symptoms of schizophrenia include*

a loss of drive
b auditory hallucinations in the third person
c social isolation
d paranoid delusions
e blunted affect

7.8 *Recognized treatments for acute paranoid schizophrenia include*

a psychodynamic psychotherapy
b group therapy
c oral neuroleptic drug (e.g. chlorpromazine)
d intramuscular antipsychotic depot injection
e electroconvulsive therapy (ECT)

7.9 *Causes for delirium include*

a withdrawal from alcohol
b withdrawal from drugs
c encephalitis
d liver failure
e hypoglycaemia

7.10 *Characteristic features of delirium include*

a impairment of consciousness
b inability to concentrate (e.g. in counting from 20 backwards)
c symptoms being worse at night
d disorientation of time
e impairment of recall (e.g. inability to recall a four-digit number immediately after presentation)

7.11 *Which of the following are more likely to occur in Alzheimer's dementia than in vascular dementia (multiple-infarct dementia)?*

a previous history of transient ischaemic attacks
b hypertension

c abrupt onset
d stepwise progression
e abnormal neurological signs

7.12 *Recognized causes of dementia include*

a Huntington's chorea
b human immunodeficiency virus disease
c vitamin B_{12} deficiency
d excess alcohol intake
e hyperthyroidism

7.13 *Which of the following psychiatric features may be caused by alcohol misuse?*

a psychosis predominated by paranoid symptoms
b psychosis predominated by hallucinations
c delirium on withdrawal
d amnesic state
e anorexia nervosa

7.14 *Characteristic symptoms of hypomania include*

a irritability
b inability to concentrate on one's work
c exaggerated feelings of well-being
d increased sleepiness
e tiredness

7.15 *Characteristic signs of mania on mental state examination include*

a grandiose delusions
b nihilistic delusions
c clang associations
d loosening of associations
e flights of ideas

7.16 *Which of the following statements about schizophrenia is/are true?*

a it is more common in those with one parent suffering from the disease
b patients with schizophrenia often have non-progressive structural brain lesions
c it is more common in those born in summer than in winter
d the age of onset is earlier in men than women
e patients with schizophrenia have a deficiency of dopaminergic neurones

7.17 *Clozapine*

a is used in the treatment of schizophrenia resistant to other antipsychotic drugs
b frequently causes extra-pyramidal side-effects
c may cause neutropenia
d is not effective in relieving negative symptoms of schizophrenia
e is a phenothiazine

7.18 *Completed suicide is commoner in*

a winter than summer months
b men than women
c the medical professional than the general population
d the divorced than the married
e people belonging to social class II than social class I

7.19 *Factors indicating a higher risk of suicide include*

a a statement by the patient of suicidal intent
b a past history of alcohol abuse
c a diagnosis of a personality disorder
d a diagnosis of schizophrenia
e a past history of drug dependence

7.20 *Clinical features of delirium tremens include*

a electrolyte disturbances
b disorientation in time
c severe agitation
d visual hallucinations
e impairment of recent memory

7.21 *Signs and symptoms of withdrawal from opiates include*

a excessive sleep
b intense craving
c constipation
d abdominal cramps
e constricted pupils

7.22 *Recognized treatments for anorexia nervosa include*

a supportive counselling
b cognitive psychotherapy
c family therapy
d behavioural programme
e carbimazole

7.23 *Clinical features of anorexia nervosa include*

a self-induced vomiting
b self-induced purging
c reduced exercise
d amenorrhoea
e underestimate by the subject of his/her own weight

7.24 *ECT is effective in the treatment of*

a depressive psychosis
b mania following childbirth
c obsessive compulsive behaviour
d acute catatonia
e severe generalized anxiety state

7.25 *Obsessive compulsive disorder may take the form of*

a recurrent thoughts of the same theme
b recurrent impulses
c repeated handwashing
d repeated hallucinations commanding the subject to repeat certain actions
e recurrent delusions

7.26 *Specific treatments for obsessive compulsive disorder include*

a imipramine
b clomipramine
c fluoxetine (Prozac)
d lithium
e phenelzine (a monoamine oxidase inhibitor)

7.27 *Dissociative disorders may take the form of*

a fugue
b amnesia
c multiple personality disorder
d post-traumatic stress disorder
e trance

7.28 *Which of the following statements about dissociative disorder is/are true?*

a the subject is often greatly distressed by the symptoms
b the subject may deliberately fake the symptoms for personal gains
c it may be caused by physical pathology
d the disorder often confers benefits on the subject
e it occurs more frequently in men than in women

7.29 *Mood-congruent delusions of depression include*

a delusion that one is suffering from cancer
b nihilistic delusion
c grandiose delusion
d primary delusion
e delusion of guilt

7.30 *Causes of delusion of persecution include*

a obsessive compulsive disorder
b generalized anxiety disorder
c schizophrenia
d severe depression
e mania

7.31 *Which of the following statements about Huntington's chorea is/are true?*

a the pathological changes occur mainly in the occipital lobe
b it occurs much more commoner in men than in women
c it is associated with involuntary movements of the arms and shoulders
d it is autosomal recessive in inheritance
e it is commonly associated with depression

7.32 *Which of the following statements about simple phobias is/are true?*

a they usually start after the age of 30
b the prognosis is better the earlier the age of onset
c the subject often deliberately expose himself/herself to the feared objects
d the subject often experiences anxiety symptoms at the prospect of encountering the feared objects
e the subject is never totally free from anxiety

7.33 *Which of the following statements about agoraphobia is/are true?*

a it is more likely than simple phobia to be associated with depression
b it is more likely than simple phobia to be associated with panic attacks
c it commonly starts in childhood
d the subject is more likely to experience anxiety symptoms in a park than in a cinema
e it occurs more commonly in men than women

7.34 *Symptoms of panic attacks include*

a shortness of breath
b palpitations
c tingling sensations

d fear of dying
e fear of going mad

7.35 *Which of the following statements about behaviour therapy for phobias is/are true?*

a relaxation must be taught before the exposure treatment
b social phobia responds to simple behaviour therapy better than simple phobia
c in exposure techniques, the subject must be actually placed in the feared situation
d flooding treatment is significantly more effective than hierarchical exposure
e the fundamental underlying principle of the therapy is conditioning

7.36 *Depersonalization*

a is an alteration of self-awareness so that the subject feels unreal
b may occur in normal subjects
c is associated with generalised anxiety disorders
d is associated with temporal lobe epilepsy
e may occur with sleep deprivation

7.37 *Which of the following statements about personality disorder is/are true?*

a all of those who have committed murder suffer from a personality disorder
b the diagnosis is usually made by interviewing the patient alone
c the diagnosis of mental illness excludes the diagnosis of a personality disorder
d the diagnosis can be made from standardized psychological tests alone
e it may be caused by head injury

7.38 *Features of antisocial (dissocial) personality disorder include*

a pronesness to blame oneself
b excessive sensitivity to punishment
c irresponsible behaviour
d impulsive actions
e inability to maintain loving relationships

7.39 *Features of borderline personality disorder include*

a emotional instability
b excessive doubt and caution
c perfectionism
d chronic feelings of emptiness
e recurrent suicidal threats

7.40 *Which of the following statements about post-traumatic stress disorder is/are true?*

a it may occur without a particularly threatening event
b previous neurotic disorder predisposes to the development of post-traumatic disorder
c the subject often deliberately seeks reminder of the stressful event
d subjects should be encouraged to express associated emotions immediately after the stressful event
e the disorder often occurs more than a year after the original stressful event

7.41 *Features of post-traumatic stress disorder include*

a irritability
b insomnia
c intrusive memories ('flashbacks')
d numbness of feelings
e persistent anxiety

7.42 *Which of the following statements about Munchausen's syndrome (factitious disorder) is/are true?*

a it is a dissociative disorder
b the subject often has numerous admissions to hospitals
c the motive for the complaints is nearly always for financial gain
d it occurs more frequently in women than men
e the subject often gives a false name and address to health professionals

7.43 *Symptoms given by subjects with Munchausen's syndrome may include*

a abdominal pain
b auditory hallucinations
c fits
d severe headache
e rectal bleeding

7.44 *Which of the following are at an increased risk of alcohol misuse compared with the general population?*

a women
b age over 45
c Orientals
d barmen
e doctors

7.45 *Clinical features indicating alcohol dependence include*

a physical withdrawal symptoms when alcohol intake is reduced
b evidence of a increasing effect with the same intake of alcohol

c progressive neglect of alternative interests
d persistent drinking in spite of liver disease
e difficulties in controlling the level of alcohol consumption

7.46 *Compared to tricyclic antidepressants, selective serotonin reuptake inhibitors (SSRI) are*

a more cardiotoxic
b more dangerous in overdose
c more likely to cause nausea and vomiting
d more likely to cause weight gain
e more likely to cause insomnia

7.47 *Foods which must be avoided when a non-selective monoamine oxidase inhibitors (MAOI) is taken include*

a most cheese
b fresh chicken
c beer
d apples
e Marmite

7.48 *For which of the following disorders is the incidence higher in elderly people than in younger adults?*

a depressive disorder
b mania
c personality disorder
d dementia
e delirium

7.49 *Which of the following statements about paraphrenia (paranoid states in elderly people) is/are true?*

a admission to a psychiatric ward due to paraphrenia is rare
b it has an equal sex distribution
c affected subjects often have auditory hallucinations
d affected subjects are more likely to have a poorly adjusted personality
e affected subjects should be treated with antipsychotic drugs

7.50 *Deliberate self-harm occurs more frequently among*

a females than males
b those aged over 30 than those aged between 16 and 30
c the divorced than the married
d those suffering from personality disorders
e social class II than social class V

7.51 *Which of the following statements about psychodynamic psychotherapy is/are true?*

a it is a form of insight-oriented psychotherapy
b the main aim is to convey non-possessive warmth and empathy to the client
c the therapist explains the psychodynamic theory to the client from the outset
d the therapist may interpret the client's feeling towards him/her
e the therapist needs to understand the client's psychological defence mechanisms

7.52 *Which of the following statements about consent to psychiatric treatment is/are true?*

a emergency treatment cannot be given before the relevant mental health legislation procedures have been completed, even if the patient's life is at immediate risk
b patients with mental illness cannot validly consent to any psychiatric treatment
c patients with mental illness cannot validly consent to any physical treatment
d the degree of risk to self and others should be taken into account in the application for a treatment order
e attempts should be made to contact the nearest relatives before compulsory order for admission for treatment

7.53 *Compared with truants, school-refusers are more likely to*

a be younger
b have poor academic records
c display antisocial behaviour
d have overprotective parents
e have separation anxiety

7.54 *Recognized management measures for functional nocturnal enuresis (enuresis not due to a physical cause) include*

a restriction of fluids before bedtime
b use of star charts
c use of an enuresis alarm
d oral chlorpromazine
e oral desmopressin

7.55 *Which of the following statements about nocturnal enuresis is/are true?*

a it occurs in less than 5% of 5 year old children

b it occurs more frequently in girls
c a significant proportion of the children has a positive family history amongst first degree relatives
d urinary tract infection should be excluded
e it may be precipitated by stress

7.56 *Which of the following statements about narcolepsy is/are true?*

a it usually starts after the age of 40
b it occurs more frequently in females than males
c affected subjects often have a positive family history
d affected subjects may have sudden episodes of paralysis (cataplexy)
e amphetamine is a recognized treatment

7.57 *Insight is characteristically absent in*

a obsessive compulsive disorder
b simple phobias
c mania
d advanced Alzheimer's dementia
e an acute episode of schizophrenia

Answers

7.1 a **False** b **False** c **False** d **False** e **False**
A delusion is an irrational unshakeable belief, which is not explained by educational, cultural, or religious upbringing. The characteristic feature is the irrational mental process for the belief. A delusion may occasionally be shared by others who have a close relationship with the person (*folie à deux*, or induced psychosis). Separation of the persons involved often results in disappearance of the delusion in the non-dominant partner.

7.2 a **True** b **False** c **True** d **True** e **True**
Unlike phobic anxiety disorders, generalized anxiety disorders are persistent and not restricted to any particular environment. The symptoms comprise three main groups. The first group is inappropriate apprehension such as worries and foreboding about possible future accidents and generally feeling 'on edge'. The second group is due to autonomic overactivity such as tachycardia, palpitations, sweating, or dry mouth. Patients may hyperventilate and complain of dizziness. The third group is due to motor tension such as tremor, restlessness, and tension headaches. Hallucinations are not a feature of generalized anxiety disorders.

7.3 a **False** b **False** c **False** d **True** e **True**
Secondary delusions arise as a result of preceding abnormal experience, such as

hallucinations, abnormal mood (e.g. depression or mania), or other pre-existing delusions, and secondary delusions can be understood from the previous abnormal mental experience. Primary delusions appear suddenly without any preceding mental events. This may be a result of attributing false meaning to a normal perception (delusional perception), such as the belief of a woman on hearing the sound of rain that her son has been abducted. This may also be a result of attributing false meaning to a normal memory (delusional memory), such as the belief by a man on remembering a game of football played 10 years ago that he is being followed. Primary delusion may also be preceded by a change in mood (delusional mood), a feeling that some sinister event is about to happen.

7.4 a **False** b **True** c **True** d **False** e **True**
Prediction of the outcome of schizophrenia in individual patients is often difficult, and the known factors are only of moderate predictive value. Known predictors of good outcome for schizophrenia include older age at onset, married, good social relationships and work record, no previous psychiatric history, sudden onset, predominant affective (mood) symptoms, good previous personality, and good compliance with treatment.

7.5 a **True** b **True** c **False** d **False** e **True**
Thought abnormalities which are included in Schneider's first rank symptoms include thought withdrawal, thought insertion, thought broadcasting, delusional perception (a type of primary delusion), and delusions of control, influence, or passivity. Other first rank symptoms include hearing one's own thoughts spoken aloud, auditory hallucinations in the third person, hallucinations in the form of a commentary, and somatic hallucinations. Grandiose delusions are more common in the manic phase of manic-depressive psychosis, and thoughts of self-harm are probably more characteristic of severe depression.

7.6 a **True** b **True** c **False** d **False** e **True**
Catatonic symptoms are psychomotor disturbances. They vary from extremes such as stupor (marked decrease in reactivity to the environment) or mutism to episodes of violent excitement. Responses to commands may vary from negativism (resistance to all instructions) to command automatism (automatic compliance to all commands). The posture may be rigid and resist all attempts to move, or waxy flexibility. Inappropriate bizarre postures are also catatonic symptoms.

7.7 a **True** b **False** c **True** d **False** e **True**
Schizophrenic symptoms are often divided into positive and negative symptoms. Positive symptoms are the prominent symptoms usually seen in the acute phase such as hallucinations, delusions, thought insertion, withdrawal, and broadcasting. They respond to typical neuroleptics such as phenothiazines (e.g. chlorpromazine) and butyrophenones (e.g. haloperidol). Negative symptoms are the residual symptoms seen in the chronic form of the disease, such as blunting of affect, loss of drive, social withdrawal, and decline in social functioning and daily living skills. They

do not respond to typical neuroleptics. Atypical neuroleptics (e.g. sulpride, clozaril) are thought to improve negative symptoms, but this is still not firmly established.

7.8 a **False** b **False** c **True** d **True** e **False**
Treatment for acute paranoid psychosis is mainly by treatment with and antipsychotic drug, either orally or intramuscularly. Psychodynamic psychotherapy or group therapy are not suitable as these patients often misinterpret what is said. ECT is generally unsuitable for schizophrenia except the catatonic type. There is now some evidence that cognitive therapy may be effective if used in conjunction with drug therapy.

7.9 a **True** b **True** c **True** d **True** e **True**
Delirium is characterized by impairment of consciousness, attention, thinking, and cognition. It is distinguished from dementia in that there is no impairment of consciousness in dementia. It is important to diagnose this condition early, as urgent physical treatments may be indicated. The causes include drug intoxication (e.g. digoxin, anticholinergic drugs), withdrawal from alcohol or drugs, metabolic disease (e.g. liver or renal diseases), CNS infection (e.g. meningitis or encephalitis), intracranial lesions, and vitamin deficiencies (e.g. thiamine deficiency).

7.10 a **True** b **True** c **True** d **True** e **True**
Delirium is characterized by impairment of consciousness, attention, thinking, and cognition. The impairment of consciousness may vary from slight clouding of consciousness to coma. Attention is impaired, and patients often cannot focus on one task. Thinking is often muddled. There may be perceptual distortions (e.g. mistaking a clock for a human face), or even visual hallucinations. Cognition is affected, and recall and recent memory are often affected. Disorientation in time is common, and disorientation in place and person may occur in severe cases. The sleep-wake cycle is often disturbed, and insomnia, reversal of the sleep-wake cycle, nocturnal worsening of symptoms are common. It is distinguished from dementia in that there is no impairment of consciousness in dementia.

7.11 a **False** b **False** c **False** d **False** e **False**
Vascular dementia occurs more frequently in men than Alzheimer's disease. Vascular (multi-infarct) dementia is more likely than Alzheimer's dementia to be associated with previous history of strokes or transient ischaemic attacks, presence of hypertension, and carotid bruits. Definite neurological signs are more frequent in multi-infarct dementia. Vascular dementia usually has an abrupt onset and stepwise progression, probably separate small cerebrovascular accidents. On the other hand, the onset and progression of Alzheimer's dementia is usually gradual and insidious. Personality and insight are more likely to be preserved in vascular dementia. However, the distinction between Alzheimer's dementia and vascular dementia is often clinically difficult to make.

7.12 a **True** b **True** c **True** d **True** e **False**
Alzheimer's disease and vascular dementia are the commonest causes of dementia, but

it may also be caused by a number of other causes. Other degenerative causes include Huntington's chorea, Pick's disease, and Lewy body disease. Metabolic causes include alcoholic dementia, liver failure, uraemia, hypercalcaemia, and vitamin B_{12} deficiency. Endocrine causes include acquired hypothyroidism. Infective causes include encephalitis, neurosyphilis, and HIV disease. Intracranial causes include intracranial tumours and subdural haematoma.

7.13 a **True** b **True** c **True** d **True** e **False**
Chronic alcohol misuse causes serious social, physical, and psychiatric disorders. It may cause a wide range of psychiatric disorders such as depression, psychosis (predominated by hallucinations, delusions, jealousy, or paranoid symptoms), suicide, dementia, delirium on withdrawal, and suicide. Korsakov's psychosis is an amnesic state (chronic impairment of recent memory) usually caused by alcohol misuse.

7.14 a **True** b **True** c **True** d **False** e **False**
Hypomania is a lesser degree of mania, and is usually not accompanied by delusions or hallucinations. The characteristic symptoms are persistent elevation of mood or irritability, increased energy and activity with inability to concentrate on work or leisure activities, and increased feelings of wellbeing. The subject may overspend or consume more cigarettes or alcohol than usual. There is a decreased need for sleep.

7.15 a **True** b **False** c **True** d **False** e **True**
Subjects with mania are overactive, with decreased need for sleep, and overfamiliar. They are easily distracted and cannot concentrate on any one activity. Their mood may range from elation to irritability. They have pressure of speech. There may be also flights of idea. Although the thoughts and speech move quickly from one topic to another, the links between the topics are understandable. Sometimes, the link may be two words of similar sound (clang association), e.g. 'train' and 'pain'; or they may be the same word with different meanings (punning). This is different from derailment or loosening of associations, when there are no understandable links between different topics.

7.16 a **True** b **True** c **False** d **True** e **False**
The aetiology of schizophrenia is still unclear. It is more common in those with a family history in their first degree relatives. Also, both twin and adoption studies showed that genetic factors play a significant role. On the other hand, there has recently been evidence that patients with schizophrenia have abnormalities in brain structure and psychological performance deficits associated with abnormal patterns of cerebral blood flow. Moreover, schizophrenia is commoner in those born in winter months than summer months. Men have an earlier age of onset of schizophrenia than women, with more severe relapses. This gives rise to the neurodevelopmental hypothesis of schizophrenia, in which pathological changes occur early in life. It is generally thought that there is an overactive dopamine activity in schizophrenia.

7.17 a **True** b **False** c **True** d **False** e **False**
Clozapine is a dibenzodiazepine and not a phenothiazine. It is an atypical neuroleptic,

and has been shown to be effective in treating positive and negative symptoms of schizophrenia. It rarely causes extrapyramidal side-effects. Unfortunately, it may occasionally cause neutropenia or fatal agranulocytosis. Hence, the blood count must be frequently monitored. This is usually performed by the manufacturer of the drug.

7.18 a **False** b **True** c **True** d **True** e **False**
Completed suicide is commoner in men than women; in the married than the never-married, widowed, and divorced; in certain professions such as veterinary and medical professionals and farmers; in social classes I and V than other social classes, and in cities than in rural areas.

7.19 a **True** b **True** c **True** d **True** e **True**
In suicidal risk assessment, the past medical and psychiatric history, social situation, and current mental state should all be taken into account. A history of chronic illness, a past history of depression, personality disorder, schizophrenia, drug or alcohol misuse, and deliberate self-harm are all high risk indicators. A open statement of suicidal intent and feelings of hopelessness are important risk indicators on mental state examination.

7.20 a **True** b **True** c **True** d **True** e **True**
Delirium tremens is a serious condition resulting from withdrawal after prolonged excessive drinking. The patient is characteristically severely agitated, disorientated in time, place, and person, and there is impairment of recent memory. Misinterpretations and visual hallucinations are often present. The hands are often tremulous, and there may be sweating, tachycardia, and dilated pupils. The patient is often dehydrated with electrolyte disturbances. Urgent admission under joint medical and psychiatric care is required.

7.21 a **False** b **True** c **False** d **True** e **False**
The withdrawal symptoms from opiates are opposite to the effect of opiates. Characteristic symptoms include intense craving, runny eyes and nose, vomiting, diarrhoea, abdominal cramps, and muscle pain. Characteristic signs include tachycardia, pyrexia, and dilated pupils.

7.22 a **True** b **True** c **True** d **True** e **False**
The treatments for anorexia nervosa remains controversial. Regular monitoring of weight and diet intake, nursing supervision with eating, and behavioural programme are frequently used. Supportive counselling, cognitive psychotherapy, and family therapy have all been used. It is generally thought that intensive psychoanalytic psychotherapy is not helpful. Tricyclic antidepressants is also sometimes used, especially if there are symptoms of depression. Serotonin reuptake inhibitors such as fluoxetine are sometimes used for bulimia nervosa.

7.23 a **True** b **True** c **False** d **True** e **False**
In anorexia nervosa, the body-mass index is 17.5 or less. The weight loss is self-induced (by self-induced vomiting, self-induced diarrhoea, use of appetite-suppressants, or excessive exercise). There is a distortion of body-image, and the

patient frequently overestimates his or her weight. There is an unreasonable fear of fatness. There is widespread disturbance of the hypothalamic-pituitary-gonadal system, and women frequently have amenorrhoea.

7.24 a **True** b **True** c **False** d **True** e **False**
Conditions which electroconvulsive therapy has been shown to be effective include severe depression (especially depressive psychosis), severe mania, and acute catatonic states. The effectiveness of treating acute schizophrenia with positive symptoms is debatable. It is not effective in treating obsessive compulsive disorder and generalized anxiety state.

7.25 a **True** b **True** c **True** d **False** e **False**
Obsessive compulsive disorders may take the form of obsessional thoughts, ruminations, impulses (urges to perform certain acts), and rituals (e.g. handwashing) unlike psychosis. The patient regards these thoughts as his or her own, and often actively resists them.

7.26 a **False** b **True** c **True** d **False** e **False**
It has been found that drugs with serotonin uptake blocking effects are effective treatments for obsessive compulsive disorder. This include clomipramine and specific serotonin uptake inhibitors such as fluvoxamine and fluoxetine. Imipramine has little serotonin uptake blocking effect.

7.27 a **True** b **True** c **True** d **False** e **True**
In dissociative disorders, the mental or physical symptoms are caused by unconscious psychological mechanisms, and are unaccompanied by any physical pathology. This may take the form of fugue, amnesia, multiple personality disorder, or trance. The patient may also have physical symptoms such as paralysis, convulsion, or sensory loss, and are often known as conversion disorders.

7.28 a **False** b **False** c **False** d **True** e **False**
Dissociative disorders are caused by unconscious psychological mechanisms and not by physical pathology. They occur more frequently in women than in men. Although the symptoms often confer advantages for the patient (secondary gains), this is not a conscious attempt to deceive. Deliberate attempts to fake the symptoms would be termed malingering. The subject with dissociative disorder often shows less concern than expected from the apparent severity of the symptoms (*la belle indifference*).

7.29 a **True** b **True** c **False** d **False** e **True**
Mood-congruent delusions of depression are delusions related to ideas which commonly occurs in depression of lesser severity. These ideas include worthlessness, guilt, ill-health, death, and poverty. Grandiose delusions are mood-congruent delusions of mania, and primary delusions characteristically occur in schizophrenia.

7.30 a **False** b **False** c **True** d **True** e **True**
Delusion of persecution may be caused by organic illness, severe depression, mania, and schizophrenia. It may also occur in isolation (persistent paranoid psychosis). In

severe depression, the subject may believe that he or she is persecuted due to misdeeds on his or her own part. In mania, the subject may believe that he or she is persecuted due to jealousy on the part of others. In schizophrenia, the subject may have bizarre explanations of why he or she is persecuted. Delusion is not a feature in obsessive compulsive disorder or in generalized anxiety disorder.

7.31 a **False** b **False** c **True** d **False** e **True**
Huntington's chorea is an autosomal dominant disorder, and occurs men and women equally. The pathological changes are mainly in the frontal lobe and the basal ganglia. The gamma-aminobutyric acid (GABA) concentration is reduced, and the dopamine concentration is increased in the basal ganglia. The clinical symptoms start with choreiform movements of face and the upper limbs, and these gradually progress to other parts with the body with rigidity and ataxia. Dementia occurs later. All types of psychiatric symptoms may occur, especially depression and paranoid symptoms.

7.32 a **False** b **False** c **False** d **True** e **False**
In phobias, the subject has anxiety symptoms only when provoked by particular situations or with objects. The subject is totally free of anxiety in the absence of these situations or objects. This contrasts with generalized anxiety disorders. The subject often avoids the feared situations or objects, and may become anxious at the prospect of encountering these objects or situations. Simple phobias (e.g. spider phobia, phobia of heights) are usually continuation of childhood phobias. The prognosis is better in those with onset in adult life precipitated by stress.

7.33 a **True** b **True** c **False** d **False** e **False**
Agoraphobic patients are anxious when they are in crowded places where they cannot leave easily. It commonly starts in adult life, and is more commonly than other types of phobia to be associated with depression and depersonalization experiences. Panic attacks are common. It occurs more frequently in women than men.

7.34 a **True** b **True** c **True** d **True** e **True**
Panic attacks are episodes of severe anxiety symptoms unrelated to any particular set of situations. Subjects often have autonomic symptoms (e.g. palpitations, sweating), and fear (especially of dying, going mad, or loss of control). Hyperventilation is common, and the subject complains of shortness of breath, dizziness and numbness, or tingling sensation.

7.35 a **True** b **False** c **False** d **False** e **True**
The fundamental underlying principle of behaviour therapy is a combination of classical and operant conditioning. The subject learns to associate relaxation with the feared situations. Hence, relaxation techniques must be successfully taught before exposure treatment. Exposure treatment may be performed either in imagination or in practice. In flooding treatment, the patient experiences the situation which will produce the most anxiety. There is no evidence that this is any more effective than gradual exposure treatment, and is definitely more unpleasant. Simple phobia is most

effectively treated by simple behaviour therapy. Social phobia is best treated by a combination of behaviour and cognitive therapy.

7.36 a **True** b **True** c **True** d **True** e **True**
Depersonalization is an alteration of self-awareness so that the subject feels unreal. Derealization is said to occur if the environment feels unreal. It may occur transiently in normal people, especially when they are tired. It may also occur in generalized anxiety disorder, panic attacks, depression, temporal lobe epilepsy, and schizophrenia.

7.37 a **False** b **False** c **False** e **False** e **True**
Personality disorder refers to persistent patterns in a person's behaviour which are abnormal and are nearly always associated with considerable personal and social disruption. It can be either constitutional or acquired as a result of brain injury or disease. The diagnosis should be made only after obtaining information from as many sources as possible. The diagnosis cannot be made from standardized psychological testing, as psychological tests measure traits which are different from those important in clinical practice. Personality disorder can coexist with mental illness, and often makes treatment of the mental illness more difficult.

7.38 a **False** b **False** c **True** d **True** e **True**
Those with antisocial (dissocial) personality disorder persistently disregard of the feeling of others and display persistent irresponsible attitudes. Although they have little difficulty in establishing relationships, they cannot maintain enduring relationships. They are often impulsive with low threshold to discharge aggression or violence. They often blame others, have little sense of guilt, and fail to learn from experience and punishments.

7.39 a **True** b **False** c **False** d **True** e **True**
Those with borderline personality disorder act impulsively without consideration of the consequences of their actions, and they have mood instability. They often have difficulties in controlling their anger, and are unable to form stable relationships. They have a chronic feelings of emptiness with unclear self-identity and aims. They try hard to avoid abandonment, and often threaten or commit episodes of self-harm.

7.40 a **False** b **True** c **False** d **True** e **False**
Post-traumatic stress disorder is a intense and prolonged reaction to an extremely stressful event (e.g. natural disasters, serious accidents, victims of violence) which nearly anyone would find stressful. There may be a delay between the stressful event and the onset of the disorder, but it seldom exceeds 6 months. Subjects with previous neurotic disorders or certain personality traits may be more likely to develop the disorder. The subject often complains of intrusive memories ('flashbacks'), and deliberately avoids reminders.

7.41 a **True** b **True** c **True** d **True** e **True**
Features of post-traumatic stress syndrome include autonomic hyperarousal (e.g. irritability, insomnia, poor concentration, anxiety), intrusive memories, and recurring

unpleasant dreams, and avoidance behaviours (e.g. avoidance of reminders of the stressful events, emotional detachment, numbness of feelings).

7.42 a **False** b **True** c **False** d **False** e **True**
Münchausen's syndrome is a factitious disorder in which the subject feigns symptoms repeatedly. The motivation for this behaviour is almost always unclear, and secondary gain is not obvious. It differs from dissociated disorder in that the behaviour appears to be conscious, and it also differs from malingering in that the motive is unclear. It occurs more frequently in men than women. The subject often has numerous episodes of admissions to hospitals, and numerous unnecessary investigations and treatments are often performed. The subject often gives a false name and address to avoid detection, and discharges himself prematurely before the doctors and nurses can obtain further information about him.

7.43 a **True** b **True** c **True** d **True** e **True**
A wide variety of physical and psychiatric symptoms can be shown by subjects of Münchausen's syndrome. Severe abdominal pain, fits, bleeding are common physical symptoms. All kinds of psychiatric symptoms may occur.

7.44 a **False** b **False** c **False** d **True** e **True**
Men below the age of 30 have a higher risk of alcohol misuse. People of certain occupation such as barmen, chefs, executives, salesmen, and doctors are also at an increased risk of alcohol misuse. People of certain religions such as Hinduism and Islam are at a lower risk. Asians and Orientals also have a lower risk. Some of them have a variant of the isoenzyme aldehyde dehydrogenase, which will render them susceptible to unpleasant side-effects when exposed to alcohol.

7.45 a **True** b **False** c **True** d **True** e **True**
Clinical features indicating alcohol dependence include a strong desire or sense of compulsion to take alcohol, difficulties in controlling the level of consumption of alcohol, a physical withdrawal state when the level of alcohol consumption is reduced, evidence of tolerance (i.e. a higher level of alcohol intake is required to give the same effect), progressive neglect of alternative pleasures and interests, persistence in drinking despite clear harmful effects, and narrowing of the personal repertoire of patterns of alcohol intake (e.g. need to drink irrespective of the day of the week or time of the day).

7.46 a **False** b **False** c **True** d **False** e **True**
The main side-effects of tricyclic antidepressants are anticholinergic side-effects (e.g. dry mouth, tachycardia, blurred vision), α-adrenergic and histamine antagonism (e.g. drowsiness, postural hypotension), cardiac arrhythmias, and seizures. Cardiotoxicity is the most dangerous side-effect in an overdose. On the other hand, the side-effects of selective serotonin reuptake inhibitors (e.g. fluoxetine, paroxetine) are gastrointestinal (e.g. nausea and vomiting, diarrhoea or constipation, weight loss), and central nervous system (e.g. headache, dizziness, insomnia), and rarely extrapyramidal reaction.

7.47 a **True** b **False** c **True** d **False** e **True**
Subjects taking a MAOI should avoid foodstuffs containing tyramine and certain drugs. Otherwise, the free tyramine which is not broken down by MAOI may act as an indirect sympathomimetic and release noradrenaline, causing a dangerous increase in blood pressure. Foods which should be avoided include all cheese (except cream and cottage cheese), most alcohol, yeast products (e.g. Marmite), sausages, and aged food.

7.48 a **True** b **False** c **False** d **True** e **True**
The incidence of the major types of dementia (Alzheimer's, vascular, and Lewy body types) is higher in the elderly than younger adults. Delirium is also commoner in the elderly. They are more likely to have pre-existing dementia and visual and hearing deficit which predispose to delirium, and serious physical illnesses which may precipitate delirium. Depression is commoner in the elderly, but there is no increase in the incidence of mania. New presentation of personality disorder in the elderly is rare.

7.49 a **False** b **False** c **True** d **True** e **True**
Paraphrenia describes elderly patients' chronic delusions and hallucinations, but without the typical decline due to negative symptoms. Affected subjects are more likely than the general population to have a family history of schizophrenia, to have a previous poorly adjusted personality, and to be socially isolated. Females are much more likely to be affected than males. Characteristic symptoms are delusions of persecution (e.g. that neighbours are plotting to harm the subject) and hallucinations, usually auditory. Treatment with antipsychotic drugs is usually effective, although delusions may not entirely disappear.

7.50 a **True** b **False** c **True** d **True** e **False**
Deliberate self-harm is commoner in women than men, among those aged between 16 and 30 than older patients, among the divorced than single people or the married, and among the lower social classes. It also occurs more frequently in those with personality disorders.

7.51 a **True** b **False** c **False** d **True** e **True**
Psychodynamic psychotherapy is a form of insight-oriented psychotherapy. The main aims are to help the patient to understand how the past experience influences his or her present behaviour, the psychological defence mechanisms used; and to change these pattern of behaviour where appropriate. There are different schools of psychodynamic theories, but most originate initially from the theories put forward by Freud. The client is often encouraged to free associate (talk freely about anything that comes to mind), or to bring dreams and fantasies into the session, which may help to unravel the unconscious mental processes. The therapist may form hypothesis about the connection between the client's past experience and present behaviour, or between past experience and the present relationship between the therapist and the client. The therapist may convey this hypothesis to the client in the form of interpretations.

7.52 a **False** b **False** c **False** d **True** e **True**
The mental health legislation varies widely in different countries, although there are

certain common principles. Patients with mental disorders are in generally able to consent to both psychiatric and physical treatments, as long as they are able to understand the general nature and purpose of the proposed treatments, and their side-effects. Exceptions are specialized or potentially irreversible treatments such as psychosurgical treatments, hormone treatment to reduce sex drive, or ECT. In appropriate circumstances, patients should be encouraged to receive the treatment voluntarily without the use of mental health legislation. When the patient's life is at risk and emergency treatment is needed, this should be given before completing the necessary mental health legislation. In the U.K., this is covered by the common law. In deciding whether to apply for a compulsory order for admission or treatment, it is necessary to balance depriving the patient of his or her autonomy (self-determination) against the potential benefits of the proposed treatment. The degree of risk to self and others must be taken into account. In general, it is good practice to contact the patient's nearest relatives before deciding on the application for compulsory order for assessment or treatment. In England and Wales, this is enshrined in the Mental Health Act 1983.

7.53 a **True** b **False** c **False** d **True** e **True**
School refusers may miss school because they have separation anxiety, they have specific fears about the school, or they may be kept at home by their parents. Truants often miss school as a form of rebellion, and stay away from home at school time. School refusal often occurs when the child moves from primary to secondary school, but may also occur during primary school or in adolescents. Truancy usually occurs during secondary school. School refusers are more likely to have separation anxiety, have better academic records and behaviour, and have overprotective parents. They are also more likely to have physical symptoms such as abdominal pain or headache.

7.54 a **True** b **True** c **True** d **False** e **True**
In the management of functional enuresis, general advice about lifting the child during the night, and fluid restriction before bedtime should be given. Star charts may also be used as a form of behavioural therapy to reward success. If these measures are ineffective, enuresis alarm may be used. This can either be the traditional pad and bell method or the more modern enuresis sensors. Tricyclic antidepressants such as imipramine have been used as a short term measure. Desmopressin (synthetic antidiuretic hormone) at bedtime can also be used, although some children relapse when this is stopped.

7.55 a **False** b **False** c **True** d **True** e **True**
About 10% of 5 year old children have nocturnal enuresis, but this decreases to about 5% at 7 years and 1% at 15 years of age. It occurs more frequently in boys than girls. There is a genetic component, and more than half of all children have a positive family history in a first degree relative. Psychological stress may also precipitate enuresis in a child who was previously dry. Physical causes such as urinary tract infection and diabetes mellitus should be excluded.

7.56 a **False** b **False** c **True** d **True** e **True**
Narcolepsy is a condition in which the subject have sudden uncontrolled episodes of falling asleep. The condition usually starts between the age of 10 and 25. It occurs more frequently in males than females, and affected subjects often have a positive family history. The subject may also have cataplexy (sudden transient episodes of flaccid paralysis) or hypnagogic hallucinations (hallucinations on falling to sleep). Recognized treatments include amphetamine (which may reduce the frequency of narcoleptic episodes) and tricyclic antidepressants (which may reduce the frequency of attacks of cataplexy).

7.57 a **False** b **False** c **True** d **True** e **True**
Insight is generally absent in major psychosis such as schizophrenia, mania, and severe depression. Insight is generally present in neurosis such as phobias, anxiety states, and obsessive compulsory disorders. Insight may be present in early dementia, especially in vascular dementia, but it is lost in advanced dementia.

8 *Postgraduate specialties*

Questions

Ear, nose and throat

8.1 *Which of the following statements regarding the Rinne test is/are true?*

a the base of a tuning fork is held on the vertex of the head
b a positive result occurs if the air conduction is better than bone conduction
c a positive result implies that the outer and middle ear is functioning properly
d a positive result implies that the cochlear is functioning properly
e It may give a positive result in one ear and a negative result in the other

8.2 *Examples of sensorineural deafness include*

a Menière's disease
b injury to the tympanic membrane
c chronic otitis media
d noise-induced deafness
e presbycusis (deafness of old age)

8.3 *Wax in the ear*

a only occurs in the elderly
b usually results from abnormalities of the hair follicles
c often causes severe ear pain
d may be softened by the use of olive oil
e should be removed by syringing with water at room temperature

8.4 *Signs of acute otitis media in a child may include*

a pyrexia
b tenderness of the pinna
c increased shiny appearance of the tympanic membrane
d redness of the tympanic membrane
e perforation of the tympanic membrane

8.5 *Which of the following statements about otitis media with effusion (glue ear) is/are true?*

a it affects less than 10% of all children in some time of their lives

b it occurs most frequently in children aged 12 or above
c parental smoking is a predisposing factor
d all cases require medical or surgical intervention
e the impedance curve (of middle ear pressure) is characteristically flat

8.6 *Recognized causes of earache include*

a acute otitis externa
b impacted molar tooth
c tonsillitis
d carcinoma of the larynx
e post-tonsillectomy

8.7 *Which of the following statements about Menière's disease is/are true?*

a there is distension of the membranous labyrinth
b it commonly starts before the age of 30
c it almost always affects both ears
d it is associated with fluctuating level of deafness
e tinnitus may be the only symptom in the early stages

8.8 *Which of the following statements about epistaxis is/are true?*

a the source of bleeding is usually from high up the nose in children
b the source of bleeding is often from the Little's area in the elderly
c bleeding from the Little's area is the most difficult to control
d epistaxis in the elderly is sometimes associated with hypertension
e electric cautery may be performed if the source of bleeding is the Little's area

8.9 *Characteristic symptoms and signs of acute sinusitis include*

a tenderness over the maxillary antrum
b pyrexia
c swelling of the cheek
d tenderness on percussion of the lower teeth
e maxillary pain aggravated by bending

8.10 *Which of the following statements about nasopharyngeal carcinoma is/are true?*

a it is commoner in South East Asia than in the United Kingdom
b adenocarcinoma is the commonest type
c it may be caused by Herpes simplex virus
d unilateral serous otitis media may be a feature
e it may present with cranial nerve palsy or enlarged cervical lymph nodes

8.11 *Characteristic symptoms of allergic rhinitis include*

a nasal obstruction
b prolonged sneezing attacks
c rhinorrhoea with mucopus
d conjunctival lacrimation
e shortness of breath

8.12 *Recognized adverse effects of enlarged adenoids include*

a mouth breathing
b sinusitis
c recurrent acute otitis media
d chronic suppurative otitis media
e snoring

8.13 *Which of the following statements about acute tonsillitis is/are true?*

a staphylococcus is the cause in more than 30% of the cases
b it occurs most frequently in summer
c it may be complicated by acute otitis media
d dysphagia may be a symptom
e there are often tender enlarged cervical lymph nodes

8.14 *Which of the following statements about peritonsillar abscess (quinsy) is/are true?*

a it is a collection of pus within the capsule of the tonsil
b it occurs more frequently in children than adults
c the uvula is often very oedematous
d trismus is a characteristic symptom
e drainage can be performed under local anaesthetic in adults

8.15 *Valid indications for tonsillectomy include*

a a recent history of quinsy
b sleep apnoea
c a recent episode of glandular fever
d suspected tonsillar malignancy
e hyperactivity in a child

Orthopaedics

8.16 *Causes for restriction of the active movements of the knee joint include*

a torn meniscus
b knee effusion
c paralysis of the muscles

d knee pain
e Marfan's syndrome

8.17 ***Which of the following statements about different types of fractures is/are true?***

a a spiral fracture is caused by direct force to the bone
b a greenstick fracture frequently occurs in children
c a comminuted fracture results in more than two bone fragments
d an impacted fracture is unstable
e a transverse fracture is often caused by traction

8.18 ***Compared to applying traction, internal fixation after reduction of a fracture***

a allows more accurate maintenance of position
b is associated with a longer hospital stay
c is more likely to delay rehabilitation
d is less likely to require further surgery
e is more likely to be complicated by infection

8.19 ***Which of the following statements about whiplash injuries is/are true?***

a cervical radiograph usually shows fracture of one of the cervical vertebrae
b they characteristically occur when the subject is in a stationary car struck by another car from behind
c they are caused by the sudden flexion of the neck after the neck is extended
d the patient should be operated on immediately
e nearly all patients recover completely after a month

8.20 ***Which of the following statements about fracture of the clavicle is/are true?***

a it seldom occurs in young adults
b it often occurs following a fall on the outstretched hand
c the commonest site of fracture is in the medial third of the clavicle
d it almost always requires internal fixation
e non-union of the fracture is common

8.21 ***Which of the following statements about anterior dislocation of the shoulder is/are true?***

a it is the commonest type of dislocation of the shoulder
b there is usually obvious abnormal contour of the shoulder
c it may be associated with sensory loss over the insertion of the deltoid
d reduction is always carried out under general anaesthesia
e the arm should be immobilised for a period of time after reduction of the dislocation

8.22 *A Colles' fracture*

a is almost always produced by a fall on the outstretched hand
b is a fracture of the lower end of the radius
c commonly occurs in children
d characteristically causes the 'dinner-fork deformity'
e may be associated with median nerve symptoms

8.23 *Which of the following statements about fractures of the femur is/are true?*

a they occur most frequently in the young adults
b inter-trochanteric fractures have a better prognosis than intracapsular fractures
c the affected leg is characteristically internally rotated
d the affected leg is characteristically adducted
e intracapsular fracture may be complicated by ischaemic necrosis of the femoral head

8.24 *Bony metastatic tumours*

a are commoner than primary bone tumours
b may cause pathological fractures
c may be associated with a raised alkaline phosphatase level
d are always associated with radiolucency on radiographs
e in the thoracic vertebrae commonly originate from the thoracic vertebrae

8.25 *Paget's disease of bone*

a occurs most frequently in African countries
b may be associated with thickening of the skull bones
c may be associated with bowing of the femur
d is nearly always associated with pain
e has an increased risk of primary bone tumour

8.26 *Which of the following statements about lumbar disc prolapse is/are true?*

a It occurs most frequently in the elderly
b Insidious onset is characteristic
c The commonest level is L2–L3
d The 'straight leg raising' test is characteristically positive
e A prolapse at L5–S1 level may be associated with a loss of ankle jerk

8.27 *Which of the following statements about tennis elbow is/are true?*

a it is synonymous with golfer's elbow
b it occurs more frequently in car mechanics than the general population
c it is associated with pain on the medial side of the elbow

d radiography of the elbow is diagnostic
e surgery is indicated in more than 50% of cases

8.28 *Meniscus tears of the knee*

a occur most frequently in the elderly
b are frequently asymptomatic
c are sometimes associated with haemarthrosis
d can be diagnosed on a plain radiograph
e almost always require open surgical intervention

8.29 *Acute septic (suppurative) arthritis*

a is most commonly caused by streptococcus
b is often asymptomatic
c is excluded by a normal plain radiograph
d may be diagnosed by microscopic examination of joint aspirate
e occurs more frequently in rheumatoid patients receiving steroid intra-articular injection

8.30 *Which of the following statements about total replacement of the hips is/are true?*

a it is indicated for patients with severe hip pain due to osteoarthritis
b sepsis is extremely rare after the operation
c it should not be used in patients below the age of 65
d prosthesis complicated by sepsis should be removed
e the operation seldom results in complete relief of symptoms

Accident and emergency

8.31 *Which of the following are appropriate treatments for acute stable ankle sprains*

a non-steroidal anti-inflammatory drugs
b ice
c elevation of leg
d non-weight bearing exercises
e compression by strapping

8.32 *Which of the following statements about acute carbon monoxide poisoning is/are true?*

a the incidence has been increasing
b inadequately ventilated heating appliances are a source of carbon monoxide
c headache and confusion are characteristic signs
d almost all patients present with cherry red appearance
e hyperbaric oxygen is the treatment of choice for clinically severe poisoning

8.33 *Which of the following are appropriate management for thyroid crises?*

a fluid restriction
b ECG monitoring
c administration of intravenous β-antagonists
d administration of propylthiouracil
e administration of antipyretics

8.34 *Which of the following statements about whiplash injuries is/are true?*

a the incidence has decreased since seat belts have become compulsory
b it occurs more commonly in front impact collision than rear impact collision in a road traffic accident
c cervical pain and stiffness are characteristic symptoms
d application of a soft collar is a recognized treatment
e over 98% of patients are symptom-free a year after injury

8.35 *Which of the following are appropriate management for a 25 year old man with 20% full thickness burns, including the arms and the face?*

a intravenous fluid replacement
b preparation for blood transfusion
c transfer to a burns unit
d humidified high flow oxygen
e analgesia

8.36 *Characteristic clinical features of severe hypothermia (with core temperature of 29°C) include*

a shivering
b hypertension
c tachycardia
d hyperventilation
e arrhythmias

8.37 *Which of the following statements about paracetamol poisoning is/are true?*

a clinical features may include progressive jaundice
b clinical features may include encephalopathy
c those with chronic alcohol problems are at less risk of its toxic effects
d a serum level of 100 mg/litre is more serious 4 h after ingestion than it is 12 h after ingestion
e N-acetylcysteine should be not be given if the patient presents 8 h after ingestion

Ophthalmology

8.38 *Differential diagnoses of a 45 year old man presenting with an acute painful red eye include*

a viral conjunctivitis
b angle closure glaucoma
c open angle glaucoma
d iritis
e a foreign body under the upper lid

8.39 *A 25 year old woman presents with an unilateral acute painful red eye and photophobia. Examination with slit-lamp reveals a small irregular pupil. Flare and inflammatory cells were seen in the anterior chamber*

a the most likely diagnosis is acute angle closure glaucoma
b intensive gentamicin eye drops should be given
c intensive steroid eye drops should be given
d posterior synechiae (iris adhesion to lens) may be present
e cyclopentolate or atropine eye drops should be given to the affected eye

8.40 *A 7 month old boy has had a history of bilateral watery eyes for quite some time. On examination, the conjunctiva was not inflamed*

a it is due to congenital excessive secretion of tears
b a likely diagnosis is foreign bodies under the upper lids
c the infant should be admitted immediately for examination under general anaesthetic
d the condition may resolve spontaneously
e a simple surgical procedure may be required in future

8.41 *Symptoms of a dry eye often include*

a itchiness
b loss of vision
c burning sensation in the eyes
d flashing lights in front of the eyes
e red eyes

8.42 *Causes of conjunctivitis include*

a viral infection
b bacterial infection
c allergy
d contact lens
e chlamydia infection

8.43 *A superficial dendritic ulcer*

a is a disease of the cornea
b is caused by mechanical trauma
c is easier visualized after staining with fluorescein
d may be treated by steroid eye drops
e usually heals spontaneously with no ill effects with appropriate treatment

8.44 *Recognized treatments for chronic open angle glaucoma include*

a topical β-blocker (e.g. timolol)
b topical cyclopentolate
c topical adrenaline
d argon laser trabeculoplasty
e trabeculectomy

8.45 *A 35 year old woman presents with a month history of seeing coloured haloes in the evening, and 3 h history of severe pain in the right eye. On examination, the distant vision was reduced to less than 6/60, the cornea was cloudy, and the pupil was non-reactive in mid-dilated position*

a the most likely diagnosis is episcleritis
b intensive cyclopentolate eye drops should be given immediately
c intravenous or oral acetazolamide should be given immediately
d a peripheral iridectomy will be required in the right eye
e a peripheral iridectomy will be required in the left eye

8.46 *Symptoms of cataracts include*

a gradual reduction in visual acuity
b recent increase in myopia
c ocular pain
d glare
e watery eyes

8.47 *Which of the following statements about measurement of visual acuity is/are true?*

a a visual acuity of 6/12 is better than 6/9
b the visual acuity of an eye cannot be better than 6/6
c it is not possible for person with a visual acuity of less than 6/60 to count the number of fingers of a hand placed 60 cm (2 feet) in front of him
d it is not possible for a person who cannot count the number of fingers of a hand placed 2 feet in front of him to detect hand movement

e it is not possible for a person who cannot detect the presence of light to detect hand movement

8.48 *Signs of background diabetic retinopathy include*

a cottonwool spots (soft exudate)
b new vessels at the optic disc
c dot and blot haemorrhages
d microaneurysms
e vitreous haemorrhages

8.49 *A 4 year old child suffers from amblyopia in the right eye*

a the visual acuity of the right eye is reduced
b it may be treated by occluding the right eye
c structural abnormalities can be found in the right eye in almost all cases
d the visual acuity in the right eye is normal with the appropriate glasses
e amblyopia is usually also present in the fellow eye

8.50 *Causes of amblyopia include*

a large differences of refractive errors between the two eyes
b a unilateral cataract
c unilateral ptosis
d a convergent squint
e a unilateral retinoblastoma

8.51 *Causes of a 65 year old man presenting with sudden onset of complete blindness in the right eye include*

a central retinal artery occlusion
b chronic open angle glaucoma
c age-related macular degeneration
d branch retinal vein occlusion
e temporal arteritis

8.52 *Which of the following statements about reading spectacles/lenses is/are true?*

a the lenses are more concave than in spectacles for distance
b the strength of the lenses required increases with age
c myopic subjects are more likely to require reading spectacles at an earlier age than normal-sighted subjects
d hypermetropic (long-sighted) subjects are more likely to require reading spectacles at a later age than normal-sighted subjects
e they are often incorporated into the lower segments of bifocal lenses

Answers

Ear, nose, and throat

8.1 a **False** b **True** c **True** d **False** e **True**

In the Rinne test, a vibrating tuning fork is held close to the subject's ear (i.e. air conduction), and the subject compares the intensity of the sound when placed with the base of the tuning fork on the mastoid process (i.e. bone conduction). The test is then repeated in the other ear. If air conduction is better than bone conduction, the subject is Rinne positive. This implies that the conduction function (outer and middle ear) is functioning properly. However, it is not a test of cochlear function.

8.2 a **True** b **False** c **False** d **True** e **True**

Causes of conductive deafness include disease of the outer and middle ear, injury to the tympanic membrane, and disease of the ossicles. Presbyacusis, noise-induced deafness, and Menière's disease are common causes of sensori-neural deafness.

8.3 a **False** b **False** c **False** d **True** e **False**

Wax is a normal body secretion by ceruminous glands in the outer meatus. It usually migrates laterally and needs to be removed only if it causes hearing loss or irritation of the ear. Impacted wax is usually removed by softening with olive or almond oil for a few days, and then syringing the ear with water at 38°C. Syringing the ear with water at other temperatures results in severe vertigo.

8.4 a **True** b **False** c **False** d **True** e **True**

The main symptoms of acute otitis media are earache, deafness, and general systemic effects associated with the infection. The child is usually pyrexic, and there may be tenderness of the mastoid. Signs on otoscopy may include loss of lustre of the tympanic membrane, blood vessels in the periphery and redness at the centre of the tympanic membrane, bulging tympanic membrane, or perforated tympanic membrane with bloodstained discharge.

8.5 a **False** b **False** c **True** d **False** e **True**

Otitis media with effusion (glue ear) is due to accumulation of fluid within the middle ear, resulting in conductive deafness. About a third of all children will have the condition some time in their lives. Predisposing conditions include nasopharyngeal obstruction (e.g. large adenoid), recurrent acute otitis media, inadequately treated acute otitis media, allergic rhinitis, and parental smoking. Otoscopic examination may reveal fluid in the middle ear and retraction of the tympanic membrane. The impedance curve of middle ear pressure is characteristically flat. The condition frequently resolves spontaneously, although some may require surgical intervention of myringotomy and grommet insertion with or without adenoidectomy.

8.6 a **True** b **True** c **True** d **True** e **True**

Earache may be caused by diseases of the ear (e.g. otitis media, otitis externa), but it may also be referred pain via auricular branches of other cranial nerves. It may be referred from diseases of teeth (e.g. dental caries, impacted molar tooth), from diseases of the tonsils (e.g. tonsillitis, post-tonsillectomy), from diseases of the larynx (e.g. laryngeal carcinoma) or piriform fossa, and from the temporomandibular joint.

8.7 a **True** b **False** c **False** d **True** e **True**
In Menière's disease, the membranous labyrinth is distended by endolymph. It frequently starts after the age of 40. The disease usually starts in one ear, and may become bilateral in a quarter of all cases. The symptoms include vertigo, deafness, and tinnitus. Vertigo occurs intermittently, usually lasting for a few hours each time. There are often fluctuations in the level of deafness, but it often deteriorates progressively with time. Tinnitus may be the only symptom in the early stages of the disease.

8.8 a **False** b **False** c **False** d **True** e **True**
The commonest causes are spontaneous bleeding in children and young adults are spontaneous bleeding from the Little's area in children and young adults, and bleeding from high up the nose associated with hypertension. Bleeding from the Little's area may be precipitated by minor trauma, and is usually easy to control. The bleeding point can usually be visualized and cauterized by silver nitrate stick or by electric cautery. Bleeding from far back or higher up the nose often requires admission to the hospital for nasal packing and sedation.

8.9 a **True** b **True** c **False** d **False** e **True**
Characteristic symptoms of acute sinusitis include a recent history of upper respiratory infection or dental infection, and throbbing maxillary pain aggravated by bending or coughing. Characteristic signs include pyrexia, tenderness on percussion of the maxillary antrum or upper teeth, and mucopus in the nose or nasopharynx.

8.10 a **True** b **False** c **False** d **True** e **True**
Nasopharyngeal carcinoma is commoner in south-east Asia than other parts of the world. It is almost always squamous cell carcinoma. It may be caused by the Epstein-Barr virus. Local symptoms (e.g. nasal obstruction, blood-stained discharge) often occur late. The disease may present with unilateral serous otitis media (due to eustachian tube obstruction), cranial nerve palsies, and cervical lymph node enlargement.

8.11 a **True** b **True** c **False** d **True** e **False**
The characteristic symptoms of allergic rhinitis are nasal obstruction, clear watery rhinorrhea, prolonged sneezing, and conjuctival lacrimation. Shortness of breath is not a symptom unless there is associated asthma. Signs may include oedematous nasal mucosa and clear discharge from the nose, but often signs may be minimal.

8.12 a **True** b **True** c **True** d **True** e **True**
The adenoids are lymphatic tissue in the posterior wall of the nasopharynx. Atrophy starts to occur from about 7 years of age, and ill-effects from adenoid enlargement usually occur at 1–4 years of age. Ill-effects may result from nasal obstruction

(e.g. mouth breathing, sinusitis, snoring, or even sleep apnoea) or from eustachian tube obstruction (e.g. recurrent otitis media, chronic suppurative otitis media).

8.13 a **False** b **False** c **True** d **True** e **True**
Tonsillitis is often caused by streptococcal infection or viral infection. It occurs most frequently in winter and spring. Symptoms of acute tonsillitis include sore throat, dysphagia, referred ear pain, and systemic effects such as fever, headache, malaise, and anorexia. There are often enlarged tender cervical lymph nodes. Complications include acute otitis media and quinsy.

8.14 a **False** b **False** c **True** d **True** e **True**
A peritonsillar abscess is a collection of pus outside the capsule of the tonsil, usually in above the tonsil. It occurs more frequently in adults than children. The characteristic symptoms are pyrexia, severe sore throat and dysphagia, and trismus. The tonsil is often displaced medially downwards, and the uvula is often grossly oedematous. Drainage can be performed under local anaesthesia (lignocaine spray) in adults, or under general anaesthesia for children.

8.15 a **True** b **True** c **False** d **True** e **False**
There are considerable debate about the indications for tonsillectomy. Strong indications include suspected malignancy, sleep apnoea, and a recent history of quinsy. Other valid indications include recurrent tonsillitis causing acute or chronic otitis media and recurrent tosillitis. However, the threshold for tonsillectomy in recurrent tonsillitis is debatable.

Orthopaedics

8.16 a **True** b **True** c **True** d **True** e **False**
Restriction of the active movements of any joints may include mechanical block (e.g. torn meniscus), effusion, paralysis of the muscle, pain, or contracture of the soft tissues. In Marfan's syndrome, the soft tissue is lax and the range of active movements is increased.

8.17 a **False** b **True** c **True** d **False** e **False**
A fracture is comminuted if there are more than two bone fragments. A transverse fracture usually results from direct force to the bone, whilst a spiral fracture usually results from an indirect force. In greenstick fracture, the bone bends but the break is incomplete. This usually occurs in children when the bones are soft and compliant. An impacted fracture occurs when the bone fragments are driven into one another. They are unlikely to displace, and the fracture is said to be stable.

8.18 a **True** b **False** c **False** d **False** e **True**
Internal fixation allows better maintenance of position than traction, allows more mobility and promotes early rehabilitation. It also results in shorter hospital stay. However, it requires a more complicated operative procedure, and may be complicated by infection or delayed union. Further surgery is required to remove the internal fixation device.

8.19 a **False** b **True** c **True** d **False** e **False**
Whiplash injuries usually occur when the subject is sitting in a stationary car which is struck from the back by another car. This causes extension of the neck followed by sudden flexion. The injuries are to the ligaments and soft tissues of the cervical spine. The characteristic symptoms are painful stiff neck, but radiation of pain down the arm and numbness of the arms and hands may occur. Cervical radiograph is usually normal. The treatment is conservatively with a cervical collar, followed by gradual mobilization with physiotherapy. Some patients recover completely; in others the symptoms may persist for a long time.

8.20 a **False** b **True** c **False** d **False** e **False**
Fracture of the clavicle is common in children and in young adults. It typically occurs following a fall on the outstretched hand. The commonest site of fracture is in the junction between the middle and the lateral third of the clavicle. Supporting the weight of the arm with a sling is the usually treatment, and internal fixation is seldom required. The fracture usually heals wells with little loss of function.

8.21 a **True** b **True** c **True** d **False** e **True**
Dislocation of the shoulder is usually in the anterior direction, although it can also be in the posterior or inferior direction. In the anterior dislocation, there is usually an abnormal contour of the shoulder with flattening of the deltoid. The axillary nerve may be damaged causing paralysis of the deltoid and sensory loss over the insertion of the deltoid. Reduction may be carried out either under an analgesic injection or under general anaesthesia. The arm should be immobilized for 3–4 weeks after reduction to allow capsular healing to occur. This will minimize the risk of recurrent dislocation in future.

8.22 a **True** b **True** c **False** d **True** e **True**
A Colle's fracture is a fracture at the distal radial head. It is commonest in the elderly with osteoporosis, and almost always occurs after a fall on the outstretched hand. A 'dinner-fork' deformity is characteristic. Median nerve compression is a recognized complication after reduction of the fracture.

8.23 a **False** b **True** c **False** d **True** e **True**
Fractures of the femur characteristically occur in the elderly whose bones are frequently osteoporotic. As the blood supply reaches the femoral head via the femoral neck, intracapsular fracture may be associated with ischaemic necrosis of the femoral head. The affected leg in fracture of the femur is characteristically externally rotated and adducted.

8.24 a **True** b **True** c **True** d **False** e **True**
Bony metastatic tumours are much commoner than primary tumours of the bone. The commonest primary sites are breast, bronchus, kidneys, prostate, and thyroid. Carcinoma of the breast often spreads to the clavicles, ribs, and thoracic vertebrae. Carcinoma of the prostate often spreads to the pelvis and lumbo-sacral spine. While most secondary bone tumours are associated with radiolucency, metastasis from

carcinoma of the prostate are often bone-forming and cause increased radiodensity on a radiograph. Symptoms may include pain and pathological fractures.

8.25 a **False** b **True** c **True** d **False** e **True**
Paget's disease of the bone occurs most frequently in the United Kingdom and other European countries, and is extremely rare in African countries. The aetiology is unknown. The characteristic features are kyphosis, enlarged skull, and bowing of the long bones of the legs. Stress fractures or pathological fractures may occur. It may also be associated with blindness due to compression of the optic nerve, or deafness due to compression of the auditory nerve. There is an increased risk of developing primary bony tumour.

8.26 a **False** b **False** c **False** d **True** e **True**
Intervertebral disc prolapse frequently occur between the ages of 30 and 50. The onset is characteristically sudden after lifting a heavy weight. The commonest levels are L4–L5 and L5–S1. The characteristic signs are spine tenderness, restriction of movements of the spine, and pain down the leg on lifting the leg with the knee straight (the straight leg raising test). Neurological signs depend on the level of the prolapse. A prolapse at L5–S1 level causes compression of the S1 root resulting in loss of ankle jerk.

8.27 a **False** b **True** c **False** d **False** e **False**
Tennis elbow affects the origin of the extensor muscles of the wrist. It typically gives rise to pain on the lateral side of the elbow and the forearm, especially when gripping. It occurs more frequently in those whose work involves gripping, such as tennis players and car mechanics. It is not associated with radiological changes. The condition often recovers spontaneously, but local hydrocortisone injection may provide symptomatic relief. Surgery is very seldom indicated. Golfer's elbow is a similar condition, but affects the medial side of the elbow.

8.28 a **False** b **False** c **True** d **False** e **False**
Meniscus tears of the knee occur most frequently in the young male. They usually occur after a twisting injury, and the symptoms are usually severe. Locking of the knee may occur, and haemarthroses are common. A plain radiograph does not directly confirm or exclude meniscus tears. MRI scans or arthroscopy are needed. Most meniscus surgery is carried out through the arthroscope.

8.29 a **False** b **False** c **False** d **True** e **True**
Acute septic arthritis is a serious acute condition. It is most commonly caused by staphylococcus. It may arise from osteomyelitis or blood spread. Rheumatoid patients receiving steroid injection are particular liable. The characteristic clinical features are high fever, and acutely painful and swollen joints with severe limitation of movements of the joints. There may be no radiograph changes in the early stages, but microscopic examination of joint aspirate may be diagnostic.

8.30 a **True** b **False** c **False** d **True** e **False**
Severe symptoms due to osteoarthritis are the commonest indications for total hip replacement. Late sepsis occasionally occurs, and is difficult to manage. Removal of the prosthesis is often necessary. However, as complete relief of symptoms can be achieved in many patients, the operation is often carried out in younger patients.

Accident and emergency

8.31 a **True** b **True** c **True** d **True** e **True**
An ankle sprain is an acute rupture of ankle ligaments. The lateral ligament is most commonly affected. Appropriate treatments include rest, ice, and non-steroidal inflammatory drugs to reduce inflammation. Elevation of the leg and compression are useful in reducing swelling. Weight bearing is usually associated with pain, but non-weightbearing exercises may be given. Surgical treatment is seldom needed unless there is complete rupture of a ligament, or for top athletes.

8.32 a **False** b **True** c **True** d **False** e **True**
Carbon monoxide is produced by incomplete combustion of carbon-containing compounds. The incidence of carbon monoxide poisoning has been declining since the introduction of natural gas as a domestic fuel. Important sources include car exhaust fumes and inadequately ventilated heating appliances. Clinical features of acute carbon monoxide poisoning include headaches, confusion, and coma. Cherry-red appearance is an unreliable sign. Treatment involves delivery of a very high level of oxygen, either by delivering 100% oxygen by face mask or endotracheal tube, or by administering hyperbaric oxygen.

8.33 a **False** b **True** c **True** d **True** e **True**
Thyroid crisis occurs in a patient poorly controlled thyrotoxicosis, may be precipitated by infection, trauma, or other factors and is potentially life-threatening. The characteristic clinical features are those of severe hyperthyroidism. Appropriate management include general measures such as adequate fluid replacement, antipyretics, treatment of arrhythmia and congestive heart failure, and treatment of the underlying precipitating factors. Specific treatment include β-antagonists to protect the cardiotoxic and neurological effects of excessive thyroid hormones, carbimazole, or propylthiouracil to block thyroid hormone synthesis, oral iodine solution to block hormone release, and intravenous hydrocortisone to treat relative adrenal insufficiency.

8.34 a **False** b **False** c **True** d **True** e **False**
Whiplash injury describes the mechanism of injury of hyperextension of the neck followed by forward flexion. The incidence has increased since the introduction of seat belts, as they protect the head but not the neck from injury. It occurs more commonly in rear impact collision. Characteristic symptoms include cervical pain and stiffness, headache, and parasthesia of the arms. Treatment may include non-steroidal anti-inflammatory drugs and application of a soft collar for a short time, but early passive

mobilization of the neck is encouraged. About a quarter of the patients still have symptoms a year after the injury.

8.35 a **True** b **True** c **True** d **True** e **True**
Facial burns should raise the suspicion of smoke inhalation, and patients should be given humidified high flow oxygen. For full-thickness burns exceeding 10%, intravenous fluid replacement is immediately required, and blood transfusion is likely to be needed in the near future. Opioid analgesia may be given. As a general rule, burns exceeding 15% or facial burns require transfer to the burns unit.

8.36 a **False** b **False** c **False** d **False** e **True**
Characteristic clinical features of severe hypothermia include bradycardia, other arrhythmias, hypotension, hypoventilation, and loss of consciousness. Shivering usually occurs in mild hypothermia with a core temperature above 32°C. Arrhythmias include bradycardia, prolongation of the PR and QT intervals, characteristic J waves, atrial fibrillation, and ventricular fibrillation.

8.37 a **True** b **True** c **False** d **False** e **False**
Clinical features of paracetamol poisoning include nausea and vomiting, right upper quadrant abdominal pain, progressive jaundice, prolongation of prothrombin time, and features of encephalopathy. Hyperglycaemia or hypoglycaemia may also occur. The patient should be considered for stomach emptying if the presentation is within 4 h of ingestion. Intravenous *N*-acetylcysteine should be given if the concentration of paracetamol is above a line joining 200 mg/litre at 4 h and 50 mg/litre at 12 h in a log concentration vs time plot. If the patient has a chronic alcohol problem, this threshold should be lowered, as they are more at risk of the toxic effects of paracetamol. A serum level of 100 mg/litre is more serious if it is taken 12 h than if it is taken 4 h after ingestion. *N*-acetylcysteine should be given if the patient presents within 15 h of ingestion. If the presentation if after 15 h of ingestion, treatment may still be useful, and specialist advice should be sought.

Ophthalmology

8.38 a **False** b **True** c **False** d **True** e **True**
Differential diagnoses of an acute painful red eye include a foreign body under the upper lid, a corneal abrasion, iritis, and acute angle closure glaucoma. Acute angle closure glaucoma occurs in eyes with shallow anterior chamber, and closure of the angle by peripheral iris causes obstruction to the aqueous outflow and an acute increase in intraocular pressure. By contrast, in primary chronic open angle glaucoma, the increased intraocular pressure is caused by increased resistance of the aqueous drainage channels in the trabecular meshwork. It does not usually cause pain. Viral conjunctivitis is also usually painless.

8.39 a **False** b **False** c **True** d **True** e **True**
The presence of flare and inflammatory cells in the anterior chamber is diagnostic of acute iritis. The small irregular pupil suggests that posterior synechiae (iris adhesion

to the lens) have developed. The immediate treatment should be pupil dilating agents (e.g. cyclopentolate or atropine eye drops) which would reduce the ciliary spasm and minimize the development of posterior synechiae. Intensive steroid eye drops would reduce the inflammation and the severity of the symptoms. Antibiotic drops are not indicated unless there are signs of infection.

8.40 a **False** b **False** c **False** d **True** e **True**
An infant presenting with a long history bilateral watery eyes is likely to have congenital obstruction of the nasolacrimal duct due to non-canalization. This may be confirmed by detecting reflux of secretions from the lacrimal sac on gently pressing over the lacrimal sac. With conservative treatment, canalization will occur in the vast majority of the infants before 12 months of age. Hence, the usual treatment may consist of educating the parents to massage the nasolacrimal duct. If canalization does not occur by 12 months of age, probing may be carried out under general anaesthetic.

8.41 a **True** b **False** c **True** d **False** e **True**
Symptoms of a dry eye include a uncomfortable, red, itchy eye with a burning sensation. Loss of vision, and flashing lights in front of the eye do not occur.

8.42 a **True** b **True** c **True** d **True** e **True**
Conjunctivitis is simply inflammation of the conjunctiva. Although the commonest causes is viral infection, other causes include bacterial, fungal, and parasite infections, allergy, chemicals, and mechanical trauma. *Chlamydiae* are intracellular parasites. They may cause trachoma (the world's second major blinding condition), and neonatal conjunctivitis. This infection must be treated urgently with topical tetracycline and systemic erythromycin.

8.43 a **True** b **False** c **True** d **False** e **True**
A superficial dendritic ulcer is caused by herpes simplex infection. It has a characteristic branching pattern appearance, and is much easier visualized after staining with either fluorescein or rose bengal. This condition must be treated seriously, as the ulcer may heal with scarring which may impair vision. Steroids must not be given alone, as they may aggravate the condition. The appropriate treatment is topical antiviral agent (e.g. acyclovir). The majority of dendritic ulcers heal with no adverse effects with this treatment.

8.44 a **True** b **False** c **True** d **True** e **True**
Chronic open angle glaucoma is caused by changes in the trabecular meshwork which may impede aqueous outflow. Hence, the intraocular pressure is increased. Topical β-blockers (e.g. timolol) are usually the initial treatment. If this is insufficient, topical pilocarpine or adrenaline may be added. Acetazolamide (carbonic anhydrase inhibitor) may be taken orally. In cases where drug treatment is ineffective or if there are problems with compliance, argon laser trabeculoplasty or trabeculectomy may be performed to improve aqueous outflow.

8.45 a **False** b **False** c **True** d **True** e **True**
The history of recently seeing coloured haloes in the evenings, sudden onset of severe pain in the eye with reduced visual acuity, cloudy cornea, and a non-reactive mid-dilated pupil is characteristic of acute angle closure glaucoma. The intraocular pressure is almost certainly raised, and the anterior chamber shallow. Immediate treatment includes intravenous acetazolamide and/or osmotic agents (e.g. mannitol), intensive pilocarpine drops, and topical steroids. Once the acute episode is resolved, peripheral iridectomy may be performed on that eye either by laser or by surgery. As it is likely that the other eye also has a narrow angle and is predisposed to angle closure, a laser peripheral iridectomy should also be performed on the other eye at a later date.

8.46 a **True** b **True** c **False** d **True** e **False**
The commonest symptom of cataracts is gradual progressive reduction in visual acuity. Nuclear sclerosis is often associated with increasing myopia. Other types (e.g. posterior subcapsular type) may give rise to glare. Ocular pain and watery eyes are not symptoms of cataracts.

8.47 a **False** b **False** c **False** d **False** e **True**
A Snellen chart placed 6 m away is usually used to measure visual acuity. The numerator denotes the distance between the examinee and the chart, and the denominator denotes the maximum distance which a standard 'normal' subject would be able to just read the last line achieved by the examinee. Hence, a visual acuity of 6/12 is worse than 6/9. Many people are able to achieve a visual acuity of 6/4. If the visual acuity is less than 6/60, the ability to count the number of fingers of a hand placed 60–90 cm (2–3) feet in front of the subject should be tested. If this cannot be achieved, the ability to detect hand movement should be tested. If the subject cannot detect hand movement, the ability to detect the presence of light and its direction should be tested.

8.48 a **False** b **False** c **True** d **True** e **False**
Diabetic retinopathy is often classified into background retinopathy, maculopathy, preproliferative retinopathy, proliferative retinopathy, and advanced diabetic eye disease. Signs of background retinopathy include microaneurysms, dot and blot haemorrhages, flame-shaped haemorrhages, and hard exudates. Signs of diabetic maculopathy include exudates and oedema at the macula. Signs of preproliferative diabetic retinopathy include cottonwool spots, venous dilatation, and arteriolar narrowing. Signs of proliferative diabetic retinopathy include neovascularization and vitreous traction with retinal detachment.

8.49 a **True** b **False** c **False** d **False** e **False**
Amblyopia ('lazy eye') is defective vision in the non-dominant eye which occurs after a period of disuse, and which persists even after correction of any refractive errors and any structural abnormalities in the eye. Squint is a common cause, and there are no structural abnormalities in the eye. It may be treated by partially or totally occluding the other eye, or by dilating the pupil of the dominant eye.

8.50 a **True** b **True** c **True** d **True** e **True**
Amblyopia may be caused by stimulus deprivation (e.g. ptosis, retinoblastoma, cataract), squints, large differences in refractive errors between the two eyes, or high refractive errors in both eyes.

8.51 a **True** b **False** c **False** d **False** e **True**
Causes for sudden onset of complete blindness include central retinal artery occlusion and temporal arteritis. Chronic open angle glaucoma usually has an insidious onset over many years. Age-related macular degeneration has an insidious onset, and the blindness is never complete. Branch retinal vein occlusion usually causes loss of part of the field of vision.

8.52 a **False** b **True** c **False** d **False** e **True**
Reading spectacles are often required from middle age due to presbyopia (age-related loss of ability to accommodate due to hardening of the crystalline lens in the eye). Convex lenses are required, and the strength of the lenses required increases with age. Myopic subjects are less likely to require reading spectacles at an early age, as they have an excess of convex power in the refractive system in their eyes. Conversely, hypermetropic subjects are more likely to require reading spectacles at an early age, as there is a deficit of convex power in the refractive system in their eyes. Reading lenses are often incorporated into the lower segment of bifocal lenses. In a varilux lens the strength of the lenses increase progressively from the upper to the lower segment.

9 *Public health and health services*

Questions

9.1 *Which of the following is/are examples of primary prevention?*

a use of condoms to prevent pregnancy
b immunization against measles, mumps and rubella
c amniocentesis to detect Down's syndrome
d adding fluoride to drinking water to prevent dental caries
e improved diabetic control

9.2 *Which of the following is/are examples of positive health promotion?*

a a club encouraging local people to increase physical exercise
b a health education programme highlighting the importance of cervical screening
c regular meetings to teach relaxation methods such as yoga and self-hypnosis
d setting up a national trust to disseminate good clinical practice in the management of cystic fibrosis
e a scheme which provides healthy food at a low price

9.3 *Which of the following statements about screening is/are correct?*

a they are mostly examples of primary prevention
b all screening tests with both sensitivity and specificity above 99% should be implemented
c no harm is done to those who receive a false positive result
d all screening tests currently performed have been proven to be cost-effective
e if a screening test for a disease is not cost-effective in one country, it is not suitable in other countries

9.4 *Which of the following parameters of a specified screening test remain constant when the prevalence of a disease increases?*

a sensitivity
b specificity

c positive predictive value
d negative predictive value
e reliability (how repeatable the screening test is)

9.5 *A screening test performed on 100 subjects yielded 15 true positives, 70 true negatives, and 5 false negatives*

a the prevalence of the disease is 20%
b the sensitivity of the test is 60%
c the specificity of the test is 87.5%
d the positive predictive value of the test is 75%
e the negative predictive value of the test is 93% (to the nearest%)

9.6 *Whibc of the following statements about a screening test is/are true?*

a a reduction in the sensitivity of the test will result in an increase in the number of false positives
b a reduction in the specificity of the test will result in an increase in the number of false negatives
c a reduction in the sensitivity of the test will result in an increase in the cost per case detected, if all costs are taken into account
d a reduction in the specificity of the test will result in an increase in the cost per case detected, if all costs are taken into account
e a test with a high sensitivity nearly always has a high specificity

9.7 *Compared to the population screening strategy, the strategy of screening high risk groups is more likely to*

a have a higher benefit to cost ratio
b attract higher motivation from those screened
c attract higher motivation from the staff
d benefit a higher proportion of the individuals screened
e result in larger benefits to the community overall

9.8 *Which of the following statements about health protection is/are true?*

a a change in the attitude of the people targeted are necessary for health protection to be effective
b it always involves prohibition of certain actions by certain groups of people
c the health protection plan must be communicated to those which the plan is intended to benefit
d all health protection schemes should be implemented if it can be demonstrated that some people can benefit from them
e they may involve legislation, economic policies, and use of new technologies

9.9 *The degree of herd immunity required to inhibit spread increases if*

a the frequency of new introduction of the infection to the population increases
b the degree of mixing of individuals within the population increases
c the infective period of the disease increases
d the infectivity of the disease increases
e the severity of the symptoms of the disease increases

9.10 *Which of the following is/are recognized appropriate management for three cases of meningococcal disease caused by group B meningococcus in the same school over a period of 3 days?*

a a letter is sent to the parents of all children in the school, advising them to be vigilant of the symptoms of the disease
b all children in the school are offered vaccination
c rifampicin or ciprofloxacin is offered to household contacts of the three affected children
d rifampicin is offered to all children in the school
e all teachers found to be nasal carriers of meningococcus should be excluded from work

9.11 *Which of the following is/are very significant factors for the decline of tuberculosis in the last century in developed countries (e.g. the UK)?*

a improvements in nutrition and housing conditions
b pre-employment chest radiograph for all teachers
c introduction of BCG
d use of surgically-induced pneumothorax
e introduction of suitable antituberculous chemotherapy

9.12 *Which of the following is/are significant reasons for the emergence of drug-resistant tuberculosis in the developing countries?*

a genetic differences amongst different ethnic groups
b use of single rather than combination chemotherapy
c the prevalence of bovine infection in developing countries
d failure of the patients to complete the whole course of treatment
e excessive doses of antituberculosis drugs prescribed

9.13 *The human immune deficiency virus may be transmitted*

a via blood transfusion
b during male homosexual intercourse

c during heterosexual intercourse
d from mother to fetus via the placenta
e via breast milk

9.14 *For the which of the following infections are vaccines currently available?*

a cholera
b hepatitis c
c typhoid
d malaria
e HIV

9.15 *If a member of the family is diagnosed to have the following infections, the whole family should be treated*

a scabies
b herpes simplex
c head lice
d enterobiasis (threadworms)
e giardiasis

9.16 *Five people out of 80 who attended a buffet developed diarrhoea and vomiting within 48 h. Which of the following is/are recognized immediately appropriate responses?*

a the kitchen where the buffet was prepared should be closed down
b any remaining food samples should be sent for microbiological investigations
c the Environmental Health Officer should interview those who prepared the food and inspect the kitchen
d questionnaires should be administered to symptomatic individuals about the food they ate on the menu
e questionnaires should be administered to asymptomatic individuals about the food they ate on the menu

9.17 *Which of the following statements about causes of death throughout the world are true?*

a over 80% of all deaths in children younger than 15 years of age are in the developing world
b the proportion of deaths due to communicable (infectious) diseases is higher in developing countries than in developed countries
c the probability of a person dying from a non-communicable disease is lower in developing countries than in developed countries
d HIV infection is amongst the top 5 leading causes of death worldwide
e carcinoma of the breast causes more death than diarrhoeal diseases of childhood worldwide

9.18 *Which of the following is/are appropriate public health messages on diet?*

a use butter rather than sunflower margarine
b eat fried food rather than baked food
c eat white rather than wholemeal bread
d use skimmed or semi-skimmed milk rather than whole milk
e eat pork rather than chicken

9.19 *Health for All by the Year 2000*

a emphasizes on providing access to health care for treatment of diseases
b is promoted by the World Health Organization
c aims for more equitable health status amongst different countries
d makes national health targets unnecessary
e consists of outcome, but not process, targets

9.20 *Population health needs*

a can be measured precisely by the existing workload of hospitals
b can be measured precisely by the existing workload of GPs
c are always in excess of demands
d are always known to the health professionals working in the area
e are a better guide to the planning of future health services than demands

9.21 *Which of the following criteria are essential in assessing the health needs of a population?*

a the prevalence of chronic conditions
b the incidence of acute conditions
c the existence of an effective intervention
d the research interests of the health professionals in the area
e the cost-effectiveness of the available interventions

9.22 *In a certain district health authority, CABG operations were found to be cheaper and associated with a better clinical outcome compared to other alternative treatments (e.g. drugs). However, the criteria for offering patients these operations were inconsistent, and patients of lower social classes were more likely to be refused the operation compared with those of higher social classes with the same clinical parameters*

a the operations were effective
b the operations were cost-effective
c the operations had a high efficacy
d the allocation of the services were equitable
e the accessibility was high for those in the lower social class

9.23 *QALY gained by a certain new treatment*

a is a measure of the cost
b is a measure of the health gain
c may be negative
d is increased if the length of life gained is increased and the quality of life is unchanged by the new treatment
e is decreased if the quality of life gained is increased, and the length of life is unchanged by the new treatment

9.24 *Using the World Health Organization's definition of impairment, disability and handicap, which the following statements is/are true?*

a all patients with diabetes mellitus are handicapped
b red-green colour blindness constitutes handicap for the shopkeeper
c red-green colour blindness constitutes disability for the aspiring pilot
d all impairment causes disability
e the given impairment may cause handicap to a person in one society, but not to another in a different society

9.25 *Rationing of health care does not take place in health care systems financed predominantly by*

a central government directly through tax revenue
b fees paid by individuals seeking health care
c compulsory employer insurance schemes
d central government indirectly through the internal market (purchaser-provider) system
e individuals health insurance schemes

9.26 *Which of the following statements about the use of QALY in rationing health care is/are true?*

a it does not involve any value judgement
b it generally discriminates against older people
c it gives priority to equity as an objective over and above efficient allocation of resources
d the quality of the evidence on which estimates of benefits are based is taken into account
e the objective is to maximize the cost per QALY gained

9.27 *The incidence of cot deaths (number of cot deaths per 1000 live births in a given period of time) is higher in country A than in country B. Which of the following is/are possible reasons?*

a the general fertility rate of country A is lower than in country B
b country B has better expertise in diagnosing rare causes of infant deaths

c the definition of cot deaths is different between the two countries
d the stillbirth rate is higher in country A than in country B
e the usual sleeping positions of infants in the two countries are different

9.28 Compared with the use of measures of clinical outcome as indicators of the quality of health care, measures of clinical process

a are less reliable
b are more difficult to interpret
c almost always provide less information on how improvements may be made
d require more support by research evidence that the relevant indicator is important
e are relatively more useful for general practice

9.29 A certain cohort study showed that patients with acute myocardial infarct who received immediate administration of low dose aspirin had a lower mortality rate over the next 6 months than those who did not, with a p value of 0.05

a it is important to ensure that the characteristics of the patients in the study and control groups are similar
b the 6 month survival probability of a patient who received aspirin immediately after an acute myocardial infarct is 95%
c the 6 month survival probability of a patient who did not receive aspirin immediately after an acute myocardial infarct is 5%
d the probability of the result arising by chance when there is no actual difference in outcome between the two groups of patients is 95%
e the result of the study is more conclusive than if the p value were 0.01

9.30 Which of the following statements is/are associated with the 'iceberg principle' of health care?

a people may demand treatment which is not regarded as necessary by the health professionals
b ill people may not have any desire to seek help from health professionals
c health professionals may provide treatments which are harmful
d people who seek help from health professionals may have to wait a considerable length of time before their first consultation
e ill people who wish to seek help from health professionals may be prevented from doing so by geographical distance

9.31 According to the 'triangle of causation' for diseases, examples of host factors in the causation of chest infection include

a age

b housing conditions
c nutritional status
d winter seasons
e emergence of new types of bacteria

9.32 ***In a primary school with 1200 children, 6 children had meningitis caused by a specific bacterium from 1 April 1994 to 31 September 1994. All children are susceptible and no vaccines are available for this type of bacterium. None of these cases occurred within the same calendar month. Out of these 6 children, 3 died within 24 h of the disease, and the other 3 cases recovered within 5 days.***

a the risk for the disease within the six months was 0.5%
b the incidence for the disease was 0.5% per children-year
c the crude mortality rate was 30%
d the case fatality rate for the disease was 50%
e the prevalence of the disease was more than 0.5% on 1 August 1995

9.33 ***Which of the following factors will increase the prevalence of a disease?***

a increase in the incidence of the disease
b increase in the mortality rate of the disease
c increase in the recovery rate of the disease
d immigration of healthy individuals to the population
e emigration of diseased individuals from the population

9.34 ***Which of the following statements about different types of studies is/are true?***

a the prevalence of a disease can be deduced from studying a case series
b the incidence of a disease can be deduced from a cohort study
c the causation of a disease can be deduced from a cross-sectional study
d the prevalence of a disease can be calculated from a case-control study
e the effectiveness of a treatment may be evaluated in an intervention study (clinical trial)

9.35 ***50 consecutive patients with lung cancers were identified from the Cancer Registry. Data were obtained from their relatives about their age, sex, address, smoking and alcohol habits, occupation, and other details. These were compared to the data obtained from 200 other people who died of other conditions***

a this was a cohort study

b the incidence of lung cancers can be calculated from this study
c the prevalence of lung cancers can be calculated from this study
d this study may demonstrate whether certain occupations are associated with lung cancers
e this study may show conclusively whether smoking causes lung cancers

9.36 *Types of studies which may confirm whether an association between a risk factor and a disease exist include*

a a repeat cross-sectional study
b a case series
c a cross-sectional study
d a cohort study
e an intervention study

9.37 *Out of a total of 1000 patients with a mental illness in an intervention study, 600 patients were treated with the conventional treatment, and the rest were given both a new drug. In the group receiving conventional treatment, 18 patients developed a neurological side-effect within 6 months, whereas in the group receiving the new drug 24 patients developed the neurological side-effect within 6 months*

a the risk of developing the side-effect within 6 months amongst those receiving conventional treatment is 3%
b the incidence of developing the side-effect amongst those receiving conventional treatment is 3 per 100 patient-years
c comparing those who received the new drug and those who do not, the relative risk of developing the side-effect is 2
d the attributable risk of the new drug for acquiring the side-effect within 6 months comparing the groups is 1%
e the prevalence of the side-effect amongst the 1000 patients can be calculated from the above data

9.38 *It is claimed that a case-control study shows that excess alcohol intake is associated with liver cancer. Possible confounding variables which might be taken into account include*

a age
b the level of alcohol intake
c diet
d sex
e the diagnosis of liver cancer

9.39 A case-control study appears to show that patients with schizophrenia (a mental illness) are more likely to be from a lower social class than the general population. Which of the following is/are possible explanations for this finding?

a the cases and the controls were drawn from population in different geographical situations
b this is a chance finding, as the number of cases and controls was small
c schizophrenia causes unemployment which causes the patient to drift into a lower social class
d a lower social class is a risk factor for precipitating schizophrenia
e doctors are more likely to diagnose schizophrenia in a person from a lower social class

9.40 A new drug is suspected to be associated with anaemia if used over a period of months. Which of the following observations would support that the anaemia is caused by the new drug?

a the risk of anaemia is the same irrespective of the dose of the drug given
b the risk of anaemia increases if the drug is given over a longer period of time
c the risk of anaemia remains the same when the drug is stopped
d laboratory experiments show that the drug inhibits the synthesis of haemoglobin
e experiments on guinea pigs show that the new drug is associated with anaemia

Answers

9.1 a **True** b **True** c **False** d **True** e **False**

Primary prevention refers to measures designed to prevent diseases before they develop. Amniocentesis to detect Down's syndrome is an example of secondary prevention, as a fetus with Down's syndrome has already been conceived when amniocentesis is carried out. Good control of blood glucose to prevent complications is an example of tertiary prevention, as both disease and symptoms have already developed.

9.2 a **True** b **False** c **True** d **False** e **True**

Positive health promotion seeks to improve the physical, social, and psychological wellbeing of the population. Negative health promotion mainly seeks to prevent or treat diseases.

9.3 a **False** b **False** c **False** d **False** e **False**
Screening tests seek to detect diseases before symptoms develop, and are examples of secondary prevention. Screening tests should only be implemented if most of the Wilson criteria are fulfilled.* High sensitivity and specificity are only two of the many criteria. Those who receive a false positive result may suffer both from psychological harm and from possibly unnecessary investigations and treatment. Many of the screening tests currently performed, such as school medical examinations and antenatal urine testing, have not been proven to be cost-effective. Whether a test is cost-effective or not depends partly on the prevalence of the disease in the population screened. Hence, a test may not be cost-effective in a country with a low prevalence of the disease, and yet may be cost-effective in another country where the prevalence is high.

9.4 a **True** b **True** c **False** d **False** e **True**
The sensitivity, specificity, and reliability are characteristics of the test, and remain constant irrespective of the prevalence of the disease. Positive predictive value increases, and the negative predictive value decreases when the prevalence of the disease increases.

9.5 a **True** b **False** c **True** d **False** e **True**
The number of false positives is 100 – 15 – 5 – 70 = 10.
Hence:

prevalence of the disease
= number of people in the population with disease/total population
= (15 + 5)/100 = *20%*.

sensitivity of the test
= proportion of those with the disease who correctly receive a positive test
= 15/(15 + 5) = *75%*

specificity of the test
= proportion of those without the disease who correctly receive a negative test
= 70/(70 + 10) = *87.5%*

positive predictive value
= proportion of those with a positive test who have the disease
= 15/(15+10) = *60%*

negative predictive value
= proportion of those with a negative test who do not have the disease
= 70/(70 + 5) = *93%*

9.6 a **False** b **False** c **True** d **True** e **False**
A reduction in the sensitivity of the result will result in an increase in the number of false negatives, while a reduction in the specificity of the test will result in an increase in the number of false positives. A reduction in the sensitivity of the test will result in less cases being detected, and hence an increase in the cost per case detected. A

* Wilson criteria include: the disease must be an important health problem; there is an early symptomatic stage; the disease is treatable; the test is acceptable to patients, reliable, and cost-effective.

reduction in the specificity of the test will result in an increase in the number of false positives, which will require diagnostic tests. Hence, the total cost per case detected is also increased if the cost in further diagnostic tests is included. A test may have a very high sensitivity but a very low specificity, if a low threshold of the screening test is lowered.

9.7 a **True** b **True** c **True** d **False** e **False**
The population screening strategy usually results in larger benefits to the community. However, the benefit to cost ratio is lower, as a lower proportion of the individuals from the lower risk group would benefit from a true positive screening test. The motivation of the staff would be lower with the population screening strategy, as the disease screened may not be a major health problem in the general population. The motivation of those screened would also be lower with the population screening strategy, as those not at a high risk may not perceive the screening to be relevant to them.

9.8 a **False** b **False** c **False** d **False** e **True**
Health protection measures may result in change in people's behaviour of without a change of attitude. An example is seatbelt legislation. It may involve either prohibition (e.g. smoking in public places) or encouragement/enforcement of certain activities (e.g. food labelling to encourage healthy eating). The health protection plan may or may not be communicated those intended to benefit. For example, adding fluoride to drinking water prevents dental caries in children. Health protection schemes should be evaluated taking into account both the benefits to certain groups of people and the possible harm or restriction of freedom for other groups of people. Health protection may involve legislation (e.g. speed limits), economic measures (e.g. taxation on alcohol or cigarettes) or use of new technologies (e.g. new vaccines).

9.9 a **True** b **True** c **True** d **True** e **False**
Herd immunity is the resistance of a population to the spread of infection due to a high proportion of the population being immune to the disease. An infection cannot spread in a population if each existing case spreads to less than one other individuals in the population. Hence, the degree of herd immunity required to inhibit spread is often less than 100%, and depends on many factors. The degree of herd immunity required to inhibit spread increases if the frequency of new introduction of the infection to the population increases; the degree of mixing of individuals within the population increases, the infective period of the disease increases, and the infectivity of the disease increases. The severity of the symptoms does not affect the spread of the disease.

9.10 a **True** b **False** c **True** d **True** e **False**
Three cases of meningococcal disease caused by the same group of organisms in the same school over a period of 3 days definitely constitute an outbreak. A letter should be sent to all parents, advising them to be vigilant of the symptoms of meningococcal diseases, and to seek medical advice if appropriate. As with all cases of meningococcal disease, all household and kissing contacts should be offered antibiotic prophylaxis (i.e. either rifampicin or ciprofloxacin for adults, and rifampicin for children). Most but not all public health doctors would agree that the whole school should receive

chemoprophylaxis. Vaccines are not available for meningococcal group B, they are only available for groups A and C. Nasal carriers are common, in up to about a fifth of the population. Hence, exclusion of teachers who are nasal carriers is unjustified.

9.11 a **True** b **False** c **True** d **False** e **True**
There has been a dramatic decline in the incidence of tuberculosis in developed countries in the last hundred years. The frequency was already declining before the introduction of chemotherapy, owing to improved nutrition and housing condition. The introduction of chemotherapy in late 1940s and the introduction of BCG vaccination in the 1950s led to further decline. Although pre-employment screening for teachers was important in the past, it was not a significant reason for the decline. Surgically-induced pneumothorax was used in the past, before the introduction of chemotherapy, although it was not a significant reason for the decline in the incidence of tuberculosis. There has been a slight increase in the incidence of tuberculosis and drug-resistant tuberculosis recently, due to AIDS infection.

9.12 a **False** b **True** c **False** d **True** e **False**
Significant reasons for the emergence of drug-resistant tuberculosis in the developing countries include failure to use appropriate combination therapies, inadequate dosage prescribed, and failure of the patients to complete the whole course prescribed. Some patients misinterpret the alleviation of symptoms after a short time as the cure of the disease, and stop the treatments inappropriately. The problem is tackled by ensuring the patients complete their courses of treatment by direct supervision.

9.13 a **True** b **True** c **True** d **True** e **True**
The human immune deficiency virus (HIV) is transmitted via the blood stream. Important routes of transmission include male homosexual intercourse, heterosexual intercourse, sharing of needles amongst drug misusers, and blood transfusion. Vertical transmission from mother to baby occurs. Transmission via breast milk is rare, but has been documented. In developed countries, mothers with HIV infection should be advised against breast feeding. However, in developing countries, the risk of malnutrition and gastroenteritis far outweighs the risk of HIV infection, and the mother should be encouraged to breast-feed her baby.

9.14 a **True** b **False** c **True** d **False** e **False**
Cholera and typhoid vaccines are killed vaccines. Cholera vaccine is given as a single dose, whilst typhoid vaccine is given in two separate doses. Unfortunately, they are not 100% effective. Hepatitis B vaccine is currently available, and is given in three separate doses. However, there are currently no vaccines available for hepatitis C or HIV. Chemoprophylaxis but not vaccines are available for malaria.

9.15 a **True** b **False** c **True** d **True** e **False**
Scabies is caused by a small mite, *Sarcoptes sabiei*. It causes a very itchy rash, especially on the wrist and between the fingers. Transmission is by close personal contact. It is advisable to treat all family contacts simultaneously to minimize the risk of reinfection. Head lice are found only on the scalp of human beings. They cause

itchiness and excoriation, and the eggs (nits) can usually be seen firmly attached to the hair. The reservoir is usually in the family, and treatment of the whole family is again desirable. Enterobiasis (threadworms) live in the bowel, and usually affect the children. Infection may be symptomless, but it may also cause itchiness around the anus. Eggs may be laid around the peri-anal skin, and carried to another individuals via fingers. Again, simultaneous treatment of the whole family is important. Treatment of other asymptomatic members of the family is unnecessary for both herpes simplex and giardiasis.

9.16 a **False** b **True** c **True** d **True** e **True**
The fact that five people developed gastrointestinal symptoms within a short time after the buffet suggests strongly, though not conclusively, that an infective agent was responsible. Identification of the food source, the process responsible for unkilled microorganisms to be present in the cooked food, and the microorganisms responsible, are essential to control the infection. To identify the food source, the food items on the menu should be listed. Questionnaires on the food items consumed must be administered to *both* symptomatic *and* asymptomatic individuals, and a chi-squared statistical test may be carried out. To identify the process responsible for the infection, the environmental health officer should inspect the kitchen and interview those who prepared the food regarding the cooking procedures. If necessary, the relevant food retailers (e.g. supermarkets, butchers) could also be inspected. To identify the relevant microorganisms, any remaining food specimen and stool and vomitus specimen from symptomatic individuals should be sent for microbiological examination.

9.17 a **True** b **True** c **False** d **False** e **False**
The Global Burden of Disease Study has provided valuable data on the global causes of mortality and morbidity. The developing countries have a much younger age distribution in the population, and a higher mortality rates for children. As a result, about 98% of all deaths in children younger than 15 years are in the developing world. The proportion of communicable diseases (such as lower respiratory diseases, diarrhoeal diseases, tuberculosis, and measles) is much higher in developing than in developed countries. However, the probability of a person dying from non-communicable diseases is still higher in developing than in developed countries. Hence, they cannot be regarded as diseases of the affluent. The 10 leading causes of death are ischaemic heart disease, cerebrovascular accidents, lower respiratory infections, diarrhoeal disease, perinatal disorders, chronic obstructive pulmonary disease, tuberculosis, measles, road-traffic accidents, and lung cancer. Deaths resulting from HIV infection are small compared with these causes.

9.18 a **False** b **False** c **False** d **True** e **False**
Increased consumption of saturated fats and cholesterol increase the risk of cardiovascular diseases. Hence, the public should be advised to use polyunsaturated margarines and oils instead out saturated fats (e.g. butter, lard). Fried food tends to contain more saturated fats than grilled or baked food. Red meat (e.g. pork) contains more cholesterol and saturated fats than white meat (e.g. chicken, turkey, fish). Skimmed

or semi-skimmed milk contains less saturated fats than whole milk. A high fibre diet is also beneficial. The public should be encouraged to consume more fruits, and wholemeal bread rather than white bread. Salt intake should be minimized.

9.19 a **False** b **True** c **True** d **False** e **False**
The 'Health for All by the Year 2000' is a form of health targets adopted by the World Health Organization in 1981. The aims were to emphasize the promotion of health through prevention and promotion of healthy lifestyles rather than the cure of diseases, and to achieve more equitable health outcomes for people within and between countries. The 38 targets consist of structural targets (e.g. the organization of health services), process targets (e.g. introduction of screening, improvement of the quality of drinking water, etc.), and outcome targets (e.g. eradication of infectious diseases such as measles). These targets may then be monitored. Many countries have in addition, implemented national targets to improve the health of the population. For example, targets contained in the 'Health of the Nation' document were introduced in the United Kingdom, with the chosen key target areas in ischaemic heart disease and strokes, cancers, mental illness, HIV and sexual health, and accidents.

9.20 a **False** b **False** c **False** d **False** e **True**
People who believe that they would benefit from medical intervention seek advice and treatment from health professionals. This creates health demand, which may be measured by the existing workload of the health services. However, this demand may not be the same as health needs for three reasons. Firstly, there are some health needs (e.g. screening services which patients are unaware of; treatment for mental illness which the patient has no insight into) which are perceived to be necessary by health professionals, but not by the patients themselves. Secondly, patients who are unaware of their health needs will not consult health professionals. Hence, health professionals do not always know about the health needs of the population. Thirdly, patients may demand treatments which are unnecessary (e.g. antibiotic treatment for a common cold). Hence, epidemiological data are needed to measure health needs. Health needs may be in excess, or may be less than health demands. Health needs are a better guide to the planning of health services than demands.

9.21 a **True** b **True** c **True** d **False** e **True**
The evaluation of how common diseases are in the population, the existence and cost-effectiveness of effective interventions, and the current health service provision are central to health needs assessment. How common diseases are may be measured by prevalence for chronic diseases, and incidence for acute diseases. The commoner certain conditions are in the population, the higher the level of health needs. Health needs occur only if there are effective interventions. For example, the health needs for total knee replacement only existed after it was proved to be an effective treatment. The relative cost-effectiveness compared to other treatments is also important. The evaluation of the current health service provision is essential to assess how the identified needs may be provided. The perspectives of the health professionals and the public are also important.

9.22 a **True** b **True** c **True** d **False** e **False**
In evaluating the quality of provision of health care, a number of different criteria are used. *Efficacy* is the capability of the treatment to produce the desired effect (e.g. the alleviation of angina symptoms for a CABGoperation). *Effectiveness* is the measurement of the clinical outcome (e.g. reduction of mortality and increase in the quality of life after a CABG operation). *Cost-effectiveness* is the measure of the amount of benefits produced per unit of money invested, relative to other available interventions (e.g. drug treatment). *Equity* is the concept of fairness. However, the precise definition is highly controversial. For example, definitions such as equal treatment for equal clinical condition, equal clinical outcomes for all, equal accessibility of health services etc. are all problematic. *Accessibility* is the measure of the barriers to obtaining the treatment.

9.23 a **False** b **True** c **True** d **True** e **False**
In cost-utility analysis, the total costs required to yield a common unit of health gain are compared for different alternative treatments. QALY is often used as the common unit of health gain. It takes into account the length of life gained, adjusted for the quality of life gained. If the quality of life is plotted against time, the area under the graph would be a measure of QALY. QALY gained is negative if the new treatment yields less benefit than the current conventional treatment. If the length of life is increased but the quality of life is unchanged, the QALY gained is increased. Similarly, if the quality of life is increased but the length of life is unchanged by the new treatment, the QALY is also increased.

9.24 a **False** b **False** c **True** d **False** e **True**
According to the World Health Organization, an *impairment* is a disturbance of the normal structure or functioning of the body. *Disability* is loss or restriction in functional ability as a result of impairment. However, not all impairment causes *disability*. For example, red-green colour blindness is an impairment. It causes disability only to those whose intended occupation require precise colour discrimination (e.g. pilots, train drivers). Shopkeepers with red-green colour blindness are not impaired. *Handicap* is a disadvantage for a given individual, resulting from an impairment or a disability that limits or prevents his or her fulfilment of a role that would be expected for a group of which that individual is a member. Not all patients with diabetes mellitus are handicapped. Many patients are able to fulfil their full role in society. A given impairment may cause handicap to one person in one society, but not to another in a different society. For example, a person who fully recovers from an episode of psychotic illness may function normally in one society, but may be handicapped by stigma and stereotypic assumptions in another.

9.25 a **False** b **False** c **False** d **False** e **False**
Rationing of health care occurs in all health care systems. It may take different forms in different systems, and rationing may be either explicit or implicit. In a predominantly private health care system financed by fee-paying individuals, rationing is on the basis of the ability to pay. In health care systems financed by compulsory employer insurance schemes, rationing is based on employment status. In health care systems

financed by individual insurance schemes, rationing is on the basis of the ability and willingness to pay the insurance premium. In tax-funded health care systems, rationing may be either explicit (e.g. based on cost-effectiveness) or implicit (e.g. through waiting lists and health professionals' decision-making process).

9.26 a **False** b **True** c **False** d **False** e **False**
QALY takes into account the length of life gained, adjusted for the quality of life gained. Estimating the improved quality of life due to a certain treatment involves value judgement. As the length of life gained from a given treatment is shorter for older than younger people, use of QALY in rationing health care generally discriminates against older people. The objective of using QALY in rationing is to minimize the cost the cost per QALY gained, and to provide greatest total health gain to the population. However, it does not take equity into account. Another criticism of QALY is that it does not weigh the quality of the evidence on which estimates of benefits are based.

9.27 a **False** b **True** c **True** d **False** e **True**
Cot deaths are sudden deaths of infants for which no apparent causes are found at postmortem examination. The difference in the incidence of cot deaths between the two countries may be real or apparent. Apparent causes include different definitions of cot death and different postmortem detection rates of the rarer causes of infant deaths. As the denominator is the number of live births, differences in stillbirth rates and general fertility rates between the countries have no effect on the incidence of cot deaths. Real causes include different infant sleeping positions (e.g. infants who sleep in supine position are less at risk than those in prone position), different prevalence of parental smoking, and difference in room temperature.

9.28 a **False** b **False** c **False** d **True** e **False**
Quality of health care may be measured by structure, process, or outcome. Clinical process measures are about what has been done to patients, and when and how it was done. Outcome measures are about the extent to which the desired outcome has been achieved (e.g. reduction in mortality rate, improvement in quality of life, patient satisfaction). Apart from unambiguous outcomes such as death, process can be more rapidly and reliably measured and interpreted more easily than outcome. Process measure requires more support from research evidence that the relevant indicator is important. However, once this is established, measures of clinical process may provide more information on what actions should be taken to improve the quality of health care delivered. In general, outcome measures are more useful in specialties where death rates are important (e.g. neurosurgery, cadiothoracic surgery), but process measures are more useful in specialties where death is a relatively rare event (e.g. psychiatry, general practice).

9.29 a **True** b **False** c **False** d **False** e **False**
In a cohort study, one must ensure that the characteristics (e.g. age and sex distribution) of the patients in the study and control group are similar. Otherwise, the difference detected may simply be due to differences in these confounding variables rather than the variable under study (i.e. aspirin). A p value of 0.05 means that the

probability of the result arising purely by chance when there is no actual difference in outcome between the two groups of patients is 5% (1 in 20). The result of this study is less conclusive than if the *p* value had been 0.01 (i.e. a 1 in 100 chance of arising by chance).

9.30 a **False** b **True** c **False** d **True** e **True**
The iceberg principle of health care is that only a small proportion of people who need health care are known to the health professionals, and an even smaller proportion actually receive such care. There are many reasons for this. Ill people may not have any desire to seek health care, because of their perception of their ill health, culture, or ignorance. Even if they wish to seek help, they may be prevented from doing so by geographical distance or financial consideration. Even if they make appropriate demand for health care, they may have to wait a considerable length of time.

9.31 a **True** b **False** c **True** d **False** e **False**
The three elements in the 'triangle of causation' are host, environmental, and agent factors. In chest infection, for example, host factors include factors in the individual subjects such as age, immune system, nutritional status, etc. Environmental factors include housing conditions, seasonality, etc. Agent factors are microorganisms such as bacteria, viruses, etc.

9.32 a **True** b **False** c **False** d **True** e **False**
The *risk* for the disease developing within the six months is 6/1200 × 100% = *0.5%*
Total person-time at risk in the 6 months is (1200 × 0.5) = 600 children-year.

Incidence
= number of new cases/total person-time at risk for disease
= 6/600
= *1% per children-year.*

Crude mortality rate
= number of deaths/size of population in the middle of the period
= 3/1200 (approximately)
= *0.25%*

Case fatality rate for the disease
= number of deaths in a period/number of diagnosed cases in the same period
= 3/6
= *50%*

The number of children with the disease at any time was at most 1. Hence, the *prevalence* was less than 1/1200 < 0.1%

9.33 a **True** b **False** b **False** d **False** e **False**
Factors which will increase the prevalence of a disease include increase in the incidence of the disease, decrease in mortality rate or recovery rate of the disease, immigration of diseased individuals to the population, and emigration of healthy individuals from the population.

9.34 a **False** b **True** c **False** d **False** e **True**
The prevalence of a disease can be calculated from a cross-sectional study. The incidence of a disease can be deduced both from cohort and intervention studies. The effectiveness of a treatment may also be evaluated from an intervention study. The causation of a disease cannot be deduced from a cross-sectional study.

9.35 a **False** b **False** c **False** d **True** e **False**
This was a case-control study, comparing various risk factors between those with lung cancers and those without. Neither the incidence nor the prevalence can be directly deduced from the study. This may show possible association between certain risk factors and the development of lung cancer. However, evidence of consistency, specificity, dose-response, etc. are needed before causation can be demonstrated.

9.36 a **False** b **False** c **False** d **True** e **True**
Studies which may show whether an association between a risk factor and a disease exist include cohort studies, case-control studies, and intervention studies.

9.37 a **True** b **False** c **True** d **False** e **False**
The risk of developing the side-effect within 6 months amongst those receiving conventional treatment is $18/600 \times 100\% = 3\%$. The risk of developing the side-effect within 6 months amongst those receiving the new drug is $24/400 \times 100\% = 6\%$. Hence, the relative risk is $6/3 = 2$. The attributable risk of the new drug is $6\% - 3\% = 3\%$. The prevalence of the side-effect depends on how long the side-effect lasts, which is not indicated in the question.

9.38 a **True** b **False** c **True** d **True** e **False**
Confounding variables are possible factors which are associated with both the risk factor (alcohol intake in this case) and the outcome (liver cancer in this case). Age, sex, and diet are all possible confounding variables. However, alcohol intake is the risk factor under consideration, and the diagnosis of liver cancer is the outcome.

9.39 a **True** b **True** c **True** d **True** e **True**
An apparent association between a risk factor and a disease in a case-control study may have several possible explanations. The cases and controls may be drawn from different populations. The numbers of cases and controls may be small, and it may be a chance finding. Doctors may be more likely to diagnose a mental illness in a subject from a lower social class. Finally, schizophrenia may cause the patient to drift into a lower social class, or a lower social class may precipitate schizophrenia.

9.40 a **False** b **True** c **False** d **True** e **True**
Once an association has been demonstrated, criteria which support causality include a strong association; consistency (e.g. animal experiments also show the same effects); a dose-response relationship between exposure and severity of the outcome (e.g. the risk of anaemia increases with either the dose of the drug or the length of time it is given); plausibility (e.g. the discovery of a biochemical explanation); reversibility (e.g. stopping the drug would reduce the risk of anaemia); and specificity.

10 General practice

Questions

10.1 ***Which of the following statements regarding treatment of asymptomatic adult patients with an abnormal blood pressure reading found on opportunistic screening is/are true?***

a patients with a single diastolic blood pressure reading of 110 mm Hg should be treated with an antihypertensive agent immediately

b patients with three consecutive systolic blood pressure readings of 150 mm Hg should be treated with an antihypertensive agent

c asymptomatic elderly patients above the age of 80 should never be treated irrespective of their blood pressure readings

d patients with a single diastolic blood pressure of 135 mm Hg should have their blood pressure rechecked two more times within the next 2 weeks before commencing therapy

e patients with three consecutive diastolic blood pressure readings of 115 mm Hg should be treated with an antihypertensive agent

10.2 ***Which of the following statements is/are true regarding hypertension in general practice?***

a about 5% of all patients above 40 years of age are hypertensive

b 20% of all cases are secondary to other known diseases

c all hypertensive patients should have chest radiography

d all hypertensive patients should have their weights and smoking habits recorded

e it is particularly important to treat those with a strong family history of ischaemic heart disease

10.3 ***Which of the following should be performed at least annually on all diabetic patients?***

a blood pressure

b check sensory function in the feet

c fundoscopy

d liver function tests

e glycosylated haemoglobin

10.4 ***Common presentations of depression in general practice include***

a chronic tiredness
b multiple physical symptoms with no organic causes found
c hoarse voice for over three months
d morning headaches exacerbated by cough
e insomnia

10.5 ***Which of the following are recognized appropriate management for mild to moderate depression presented to a GP for the first time?***

a prescription of amitriptyline (a tricyclic antidepressant)
b referral to a psychological counsellor
c referral for cognitive therapy
d prescription of paroxetine (a 5-hydroxytryptamine reuptake inhibitor)
e prescription of phenelzine (a MOAI)

10.6 ***Recognized appropriate management for a 60 year old patient with insomnia include***

a reassurance that this is common
b advice for learning self-hypnosis
c advice to alter activities just before bedtime
d prescription of barbiturates
e prescription of carbamazepine

10.7 ***Patients with alcohol problems***

a are almost always known to the practice
b may present with recurrent epigastric pain
c have a higher incidence of marital problems
d often deny their problems
e may be helped by self-referral to Alcoholics Anonymous

10.8 ***Which of the following statements about ear syringing for wax in the general practice is/are true?***

a it can only be carried out by a qualified medical practitioner
b asymptomatic wax seen with the auroscope should be removed by syringing
c the wax should be softened by ear drops instilled an hour before the procedure
d the water used for syringing should be at the room temperature
e the water jet should be directed horizontally

10.9 ***Which of the following groups of patients should routinely receive influenza vaccination annually?***

a patients with chronic renal failure

b patients resident at nursing homes
c patients with a history of epilepsy
d patients with diabetes mellitus
e health care workers in hospitals

10.10 *Which of the following diseases are notifiable in the UK?*

a meningococcal septicaemia
b tuberculosis
c measles
d Haemophilus influenzae pneumonia
e malaria

10.11 *Which of the following statements about cervical screening is/are true?*

a the proportion of 'inadequate' smears can be reduced by improved smear-taking techniques
b the smear must be taken by a qualified medical practitioner
c all women should commence having smear tests from 16 years of age
d women with normal smears should be recalled every 2 years
e a women with an abnormal smear should be informed that she has cervical cancer

10.12 *Which of the following may be attributable to combined oral contraceptives?*

a severe migraine
b hypertension
c mid-cycle bleeding
d hypoglycaemia
e deep vein thrombosis

10.13 *A 10 weeks old pregnant mother brought in her previously healthy 7 year old daughter with 1 day history of a rash, which is diagnosed as chickenpox. The mother did not have a past history of chickenpox*

a advise her mother that the rash will evolve in crops, before drying to form scabs
b the child should be isolated from her healthy twin sister
c an urgent blood test should be performed on the mother
d administering varicella zoster immunoglobulin (VZIG) to the mother will prevent the fetus from being infected
e the child should be given a dose of VZIG

10.14 *Recognized appropriate management of patients with moderately severe ocular and nasal symptoms from hayfever include*

a sodium cromoglycate eye drops
b steroid eye drops
c sodium cromoglycate nasal drops
d steroid nasal drops
e oral antihistamine

10.15 *Which of the following procedures may be performed by most GPs in well-equipped premises*

a steroid injection for tennis elbow
b colonoscopy
b cryocautery of verrucae
c excision of a lipoma
d renal biopsy

10.16 *Compared to the non-fundholders, the fundholders in a general practice*

a have the role as purchaser as health care in additional to their providing role
b have greater freedom in employing practitioners in complementary medicine
c have a greater choice of where they refer patients
d can allocate unused funds as the GPs' own personal income
e have a greater administrative workload

10.17 *Which of the following are the functions of a practice manager*

a drafting the employment contract of the secretary
b ensuring that eligible payments are received from the Health Authority
c ECG recording
d running health promotion clinics
e appointment of receptionists

10.18 *Responsibilities of the health visitor include*

a examination of the mother at home immediately postnatally
b immunization of infants against tetanus, pertussis, diphtheria, and polio
c carrying out the free field distraction hearing test on infants at 7–9 months
d visiting 11 year old children to administer Heaf test and BCG if appropriate
e surveillance of at risk elderly living on their own

10.19 *Compared to the appointment system in general practice, the walk-in system*

a is more efficient for the GPs
b is generally associated with longer waiting time in the waiting room
c requires more time from the ancillary staff
d allows the practice to plan holidays for the doctors and staff more easily
e is currently more commonly used in the UK

10.20 *Which of the following statements is/are true regarding the management of asthma in general practice?*

a a GP with a list of 2000 patients will have about 10 patients with asthma
b every patient with moderately severe asthma should possess a peak flow meter
c patients whose self-monitoring records showed a PEFR of 220 litre/min at night, and yet achieve a PEFR of 550 litre/min when he was seen in the afternoon clinic is likely to be malingering
d oral steroids should be avoided unless the patient is symptomatic whilst on maximal inhaled therapy for at least 72 h
e the patient's inhaler technique should be regularly checked by the practice nurse or the doctor

10.21 *Which of the following activities may constitute part of a medical audit*

a to study whether a new drug is effective in the treatment of diabetes
b to study what proportion of the patients in the practice have their blood pressure recorded
c to study whether patients favour patient-held records or doctor-held records
d to study what proportion of the asthmatic patients in the practice have been admitted to hospital in the last 6 months
e to study the risk of deep vein thrombosis of a new compared with an existing oral contraceptive drug

10.22 *Compared to those from the higher social classes, people of the lower social classes are more likely to*

a smoke
b take part in cervical screening
c be referred to hospital by their GPs for the same illness
d suffer from chronic illness
e be involved in motor vehicle accidents

10.23 *Which of the following statements about motion sickness is/are true?*

a it occurs more frequently in children than in adults

b nausea and vomiting may be prominent symptoms
c it is preferable to occupy the back seats than the front seats for car passengers
d reading a newspaper may alleviate the symptoms
e antihistamines should be taken just before the start of the journey

10.24 *Doctors may divulge information about their patients gained in the course of medical consultation to the relevant other party under which of the following circumstances, without the explicit consent of the patient?*

a the patient has not explicitly stated that the information should be kept confidential to others in the consultation
b a mature 15 year old girl refused to allow her parents to be informed that she is taking oral contraceptives
c a 34 year old bus driver with intractable epilepsy refused to let the Driving and Vehicles Licensing Centre know about his condition, and continues his normal work
d a patient was diagnosed to be suffering from food poisoning, and refused to give consent for his condition was reported to the consultant in communicable disease and control
e a patient suffers from an usual drug reaction to cimetidine, and the reaction was reported to the Department of Health under the Yellow Card scheme

10.25 *Patients with which of the following conditions will not be permitted to drive a family car by the Drivers and Vehicles Licensing centre?*

a a diabetic patient on oral hypoglycaemic agent
b an epileptic patient who only has fits whilst asleep in the last 5 years
c an asymptomatic untreated patient with complete heart block
d a 75 year old patient who is both physically and mentally well
e a patient who makes a good recovery from a myocardial infarct 6 months ago

10.26 *Which of the following must all GPs carry when they are on-call for emergencies?*

a injectable penicillin
b injectable glucagon
c nebulizer
d oral aspirin
e injectable adrenaline

10.27 *In which of the following circumstances should deaths be reported to the coroner?*

a the patient has not been seen by the doctor in the past month
b there is more than one cause of death
c there is no next of kin
d the patient died of suspected suicide
e the patient died instantly of a motor vehicle accident

10.28 *Social workers*

a are employed directly by GPs
b are responsible for allocating home helps
c can only see clients referred to them by GPs
d are closely involved with cases of suspected child abuse
e are involved in the application for compulsory detention and treatment of mentally ill patients

Answers

10.1 a **False** b **False** c **False** d **False** e **True**
There is good evidence that treatment of asymptomatic hypertension would reduce the risk of future ischaemic heart disease and cerebrovascular disease. Hypertension is generally regarded as diastolic blood pressure over 90 mm Hg, or systolic blood pressure over 160 mm Hg. Unless a single blood pressure reading is dangerously high (e.g. above 130 mm Hg, or symptomatic hypertension), treatment should be started only after three readings at different times. Although the elderly are more susceptible to the side-effects of antihypertensive agents, there is now much evidence that treating hypertension in the elderly is beneficial in reducing the risk of future ischaemic heart disease and strokes. General speaking, patients with diastolic blood pressure persistently above 105 mm Hg or a systolic blood pressure persistently above 160 mm Hg should be treated with antihypertensive agents. Patients with a diastolic blood pressure of 90–100 mm Hg should be given general lifestyle advice, and have their blood pressure monitored at least every 6 months. Patients with a diastolic blood pressure persistently above 100 but below 110 mm Hg should be treated if they have other cardiovascular risks. All patients with diastolic blood pressure above 110 mm Hg should all be treated. Patients with diastolic blood pressure above 130 mm Hg should be urgently referred to the hospital for investigation and treatment.

10.2 a **False** b **False** c **False** d **True** e **True**
Just over 30% of patients above the age of 40 who attend the surgery are hypertensive. In general practice, over 95% of these patients have primary hypertension without secondary diseases. The weight, height, body mass index, smoking habits, alcohol intake, and family history of all patients with hypertension should be

recorded, so that the appropriate dietary and lifestyle advice can be given, and the cardiovascular risks assessed. It is especially important to treat those with high personal risk factors. Those with mild hypertension need not have either ECG or chest radiography performed.

10.3 a **True** b **True** c **True** d **False** e **True**
There should be an established protocol for all diabetic patients in the clinic. In addition to the patient's own monitoring records, random glucose, and the patient's perceived problems, it is also important to check glycosylated haemoglobin regularly as an indication of the overall control in the last 8–10 weeks. Cardiovascular examination including blood pressure, peripheral pulses, sensory functions in the feet, and eye examination should also be carried out at least annually.

10.4 a **True** b **True** c **False** d **False** e **True**
Although depression in general practice may present with the classical psychological symptoms of low mood, loss of enjoyment, and hopelessness, it frequently presents with physical symptoms such as chronic tiredness and multiple hypochondriacal symptoms. It may also present with the biological symptoms of depression such as loss of appetite, loss of weight, and insomnia. Alternatively, it may present with alcohol, drug addiction, or marital problems. Hoarse voice for over 3 months should be referred to the ENT to exclude laryngeal carcinoma. Morning headaches exacerbated by cough suggest raised intracranial pressure, possibly due to a intracranial space-occupying lesion.

10.5 a **True** b **True** c **True** d **True** e **False**
Mild to moderate depression may be managed in the general practice in different ways. Listening and sharing the patient's problems is the first important step in establishing a positive therapeutic relationship. Most GPs would treat by prescribing either a tricyclic antidepressant (e.g. amitriptyline) or a 5-HT reuptake inhibitor (e.g. paroxetine). The latter is becoming more popular because it has relatively fewer side-effects, although it is somewhat more expensive. However, there are alternative or complementary treatments such as referral for psychological counselling, referral for cognitive therapy, and referral for social support. A monoamine oxidase inhibitor is an inappropriate first line treatment.

10.6 a **True** b **True** c **True** d **False** e **False**
Insomnia is a common symptom in general practice. Underlying physical disorders (e.g. pain, breathlessness due to asthma or heart failure) and psychological disorders (e.g. depression, anxiety) should first be excluded. The patient should then be reassured, and the physiology of sleep should be explained. Simple advice such as altering the activities just before bedtime should be given. Relaxation techniques (e.g. breathing techniques, relaxation tapes, self-hypnosis, etc.) may be useful. A short-acting benzodiazepine hypnotic may be used in some patients, but the risks of dependency, rebound insomnia on withdrawal, and hangover effect should be carefully considered and explained to the patient. Barbiturates, which were commonly used in the past, should now be avoided owing to the risks of dependency and other side-effects.

10.7 a **False** b **True** c **True** d **True** e **True**
Men who drink more than 28 units per week and women who drink more than 21 units per week are above the recommended safe limits (Department of Health 1996 guidelines). Less than 20% of patients with this level of intake or above are known to their GPs, and the patients often deny the problems. Patients may present in a variety of ways, including fatigue, anorexia, weight loss, recurrent epigastric pain, and physical complications of alcohol such as jaundice and cirrhosis of the liver. They have a higher rate of mental illness such as depression and psychosis, as well as higher incidence of marital problems. They should be encouraged to recognize their problems; support from family, friends, and self-help groups such as Alcoholic Anonymous are valuable.

10.8 a **False** b **False** c **False** d **False** e **False**
Wax is secreted physiologically, and has a protective function. It should be removed by syringing only if it causes symptoms such as hearing loss. Syringing may be carried out by the practice or district nurses, although the GP has to ensure that the nurse is competent and trained to do so. Syringing should not be performed if there is a history of recurrent otitis externa or perforated tympanic membrane. The wax should be softened by olive oil or sodium bicarbonate drops administered twice daily for at least 3 days prior to the procedure. The water must be warmed to body temperature, otherwise the subject will experience severe vertigo. The water jet should be directed upwards and backwards, both to minimize the risk of perforation and to ensure that the wax is removed successfully. The external ear canal should be dried to minimize the risk of otitis externa.

10.9 a **True** b **True** c **False** d **True** e **False**
Indications for receiving influenza immunization routinely include residents of nursing homes or old people's homes, chronic renal failure, chronic respiratory disease (e.g. chronic obstructive airways disease, asthma), chronic heart disease, diabetes, and immunosuppression. There is good evidence from the USA that immunization of everyone over the age of 65 is cost-effective, although the Department of Health has not yet adopted this recommendation.

10.10 a **True** b **True** c **True** d **False** e **True**
In general, all infections which central surveillance is necessary for prevention and control are notifiable. The list is rather long, and includes all bacterial meningitides, meningococcal septicaemia, tuberculosis, measles, mumps, rubella, whooping cough, viral hepatitis, food poisoning, and malaria.

10.11 a **True** b **False** c **False** d **False** e **False**
Most smears are currently taken by practice nurses, who must be thoroughly trained in the technique of smear-taking. Good techniques can significantly reduce the rate of 'inadequate' smears. Women between the age of 20 and 65 are routinely called, although women who have commenced sexual intercourse may be screened from an earlier age. The screening interval currently varies between 3 and 5 years amongst the Health Authorities in the United Kingdom, although there is little evidence that there is any benefits of a 3 yearly interval over a 5 yearly interval. Generally speaking,

women with 'inadequate' smears should be recalled to have the smear repeated. Women who have smears with mild abnormalities should have the smear repeated within 6 months or a year. Women who have smears with more than mild abnormalities should be referred for colonoscopy. Abnormalities of cervical smears (CIN2 or CIN3) do not necessarily imply the presence of invasive carcinoma.

10.12 a **True** b **True** c **True** d **False** e **True**
Side-effects of combined oral contraceptives are relatively rare, and may include nausea, vomiting, mid-cycle bleeding, breast discomfort, and weight gain. Other rarer serious side-effects include arterial thrombosis (e.g. myocardial infarction, cerebral thrombosis), venous thrombosis (e.g. deep vein thrombosis, pulmonary embolism), migraine, and hypertension. Glucose tolerance may be reduced.

10.13 a **True** b **False** c **True** d **False** e **False**
Chickenpox is a common childhood viral illness. The rash characteristically appears in crops, and goes through macular, papular, and vesicular stages before drying to form scabs. There is little to gain from isolating a child from siblings, who have already been exposed to the infection, in any event it may be better to contract the disease in childhood. As the mother is 10 weeks pregnant, there is a risk of contracting chickenpox and congenital varicella syndrome in the fetus if she does not have prior immunity against chickenpox. Hence, the mother should be tested for varicella zoster antibody, and receive a dose of varicella zoster immunoglobulin (VZIG) if it is negative. This may minimize the illness in the mother, but will not prevent congenital varicella syndrome in the fetus. As the child is not immunocomprised, she does not require VZIG.

10.14 a **True** b **False** c **True** d **True** e **True**
Hayfever is due to type I hypersensitivity reaction, usually to pollens. Nasal symptoms (e.g. rhinorrhoea, sneezing) and ocular symptoms (e.g. conjunctivitis) may occur. Appropriate treatments of hayfever include sodium cromoglycate eye drops or nasal drops, steroid nasal drops, and oral antihistamine. If these treatments are ineffective, depot steroid injections may be used, although side-effects may include adrenal suppression and muscle atrophy at the injection site. For severe hayfever, a short course of oral steroids may be used with caution.

10.15 a **True** b **False** c **True** d **True** e **False**
Most GPs are able to carry out injection of tennis elbows, cryocautery of verrucae, and excision of lipomas. Some can carry out sigmoidoscopy, but most cannot carry out colonoscopy. Renal biopsy is a specialist procedure and should only be performed by nephrologists.

10.16 a **True** b **True** c **True** d **False** e **True**
General practice fundholding occurs in the internal market health care system, whereby a practice is allocated a fund for the healthcare expenditure of its patients and the practice staff costs. The practice therefore acts both as a provider of primary health care to its patients, and as a purchaser of secondary health care and community

nursing care. Fundholders have greater choice of where they refer patients, and what they are referred for. They can also employ other health professionals (e.g. dietitians, counsellors, practitioners of complementary medicine) to work in the practice. However, they must allocate the money for the benefit of their patients, and cannot allocate the fund as personal income or for any personal purposes. Fundholders have to keep detailed records of all the referrals they have made and the nature of the referrals and all the prescriptions written, and keep detailed accounts. Hence, they have a greater administrative workload than non-fundholders.

10.17 a **True** b **True** c **False** d **False** e **True**
The practice manager plays an important role in the smooth running of the general practice surgery. The responsibilities include managing the practice ancillary staff (e.g. appointment, issuing of contracts, approving holidays, etc.), managing the finances (e.g. monitoring expenditure and income of the practice, liaison with accountants), ensuring that the practice premises fulfil the legal requirements (e.g. regarding safety), planning stock control of equipment and stationery, and developing and monitoring the strategy of the practice. ECG recording and running health promotion clinics are the responsibility of the district or practice nurses.

10.18 a **False** b **True** c **True** d **False** e **True**
Health visitors are generally qualified nurses or midwives who have undergone further training. Their main statutory roles are in the surveillance of children below the age of 5 years from the time the midwife has left (10 days postnatally), although they are increasingly involved with the elderly. Responsibility of surveillance of children include immunization, developmental assessments (including hearing tests), and surveillance of children at risk of abuse. They are also involved in the surveillance of other individuals, especially the elderly, who are at risk.

10.19 a **False** b **True** c **False** d **False** e **False**
The appointment system allows the practice to plan more efficiently, and the workload to be shared more equally amongst the doctors. The patients are likely to wait for a shorter time in the waiting room. Moreover, it allows special clinics (e.g. antenatal clinics, child surveillance clinics, asthma clinics, etc.) to be more easily organized. On the other hand, patients with non-urgent problems may have to wait for a longer time for their appointments, and more time from the ancillary staff (receptionists) is required. Currently, most general practices in the United Kingdom use the appointment system.

10.20 a **False** b **True** c **False** d **False** e **True**
The prevalence of asthma in the general practice is about 5% in adults, and almost 10% in children. Hence, a GP with a list size of 2000 is likely to have about 100 asthmatic patients. The patients should be managed by the steps approach recommended by the British Thoracic Society. Every patient with moderate or severe asthma should possess a peak flow meter, and record their peak flow regularly. In moderate and severe asthma, there is usually considerable diurnal variation of the severity of the asthma, with peak flow at its lowest in the middle of the night. If the patient shows symptoms

of an acute attack, a course of oral steroids should be prescribed early. It is important to monitor the patient's compliance and technique in using their inhalers.

10.21 a **False** b **True** c **False** d **True** e **False**
Medical audit is a process of comparing our own current medical practice to some agreed standard of performance (e.g. current guidelines, policies, national data). If our current performance falls short of the standard, changes should be implemented, and our practice should be monitored again in future to ensure that the changes have been effective. It is different from research, which has the purpose of answering questions for which no standards exist. Hence, studying whether a new drug is effective, whether patients favour one method of record-keeping over another, or the relative side-effects of a new drug, are examples of research rather than medical audit.

10.22 a **True** b **False** c **False** d **True** e **True**
It has been consistently found over the last 20 years that the lower social classes are at least two times more likely to die from most diseases compared with the higher social classes. The lower social classes are also more likely to suffer from chronic illnesses. There is evidence that this difference is widening. There is little evidence to support the hypothesis that this is due to the sick drifting down the social ladder (social drift hypothesis), but it is generally accepted that being in a high social class promotes health. There are several reasons for this. Firstly, resources available to the higher social classes (e.g. fire guards, smoke alarm) may protect them from illnesses and accidents. Secondly, people of lower social classes are more likely to have a lifestyle which is injurious to health (e.g. smoking, drinking alcohol). Thirdly, those who have the greatest health needs are least likely to obtain health care. Hence, people in lower social classes are less likely to attend health promotion clinics or screening. Moreover, they are less likely to be referred to the hospital by their GPs for the same degree of illness.

10.23 a **True** b **True** c **False** d **False** e **False**
Motion sickness is a common symptom, and it occurs more frequently in children than in adults. Common symptoms include pallor, malaise, nausea, and vomiting. Headaches and sleepiness may also occur. It is caused by mismatch of ocular and vestibular information to the brain. Advice should include good ventilation, looking out of the window, and sitting in the stable part of the vehicle (e.g. in the front seat in a car, and in the middle of a boat or plane). Antihistamine or anticholinergic drugs may be used. They should be taken about 2 h before the journey, as otherwise absorption of the drug may be reduced with the onset of motion sickness.

10.24 a **False** b **False** c **True** d **True** e **True**
Doctors have a duty to keep confidential all information obtained in the course of a medical consultation and not pass it on to third parties, irrespective of whether this was explicitly stated by the patient. However, there are a few exceptions. They include orders from a court of law; statutory duties imposed on doctors (e.g. notification of infectious diseases and abortions); and if the public interests outweigh private interests (e.g. if an epileptic public transport driver refuses to notify the Driver and

Vehicle Licencing Centre (DVLC) and put public safety at risk, or notifying social workers of a case of child abuse). Doctors should respect the rights of confidentiality of a mature 15 year old.

10.25 a **False** b **False** c **True** d **False** e **False**
The regulations for holding a heavy goods vehicle licence or public service licence are much more stringent than for the ordinary driving licence. The DVLC publishes detailed regulations on each condition. In general, diabetic patients are usually granted limited a licence as long as the quality of the control is good. A epileptic patient is usually allowed to drive if the patient had no fits in the last 2 years, or had no fits in the daytime in the past 3 years. A patient who has a myocardial infarct should not drive for at least 2 months. A patient with untreated complete heart block must not drive under any circumstances. Old age alone is not a bar to driving, if there is no significant physical or mental impairment.

10.26 a **True** b **True** c **True** d **True** e **True**
Injectable penicillin is essential in the urgent treatment of suspected meningococcal disease. Injectable glucagon is essential in the treatment of hypoglycaemia, if venous access is difficult. A nebulizer is essential in the initial emergency treatment of an asthmatic attack. It is important for the GP to administer oral aspirin immediately on making a clinical diagnosis of myocardial infarct. Intramuscular adrenaline is important in the treatment of anaphylaxis, and intravenous adrenaline (in appropriate dosage) may be essential in the resuscitation of a patient with cardiac arrest.

10.27 a **True** b **False** c **False** d **True** e **True**
Deaths which should be reported to the coroner include cases where the cause of death is unknown; if the patient has not been seen by the doctor in the last 14 days; suspected suicide, homicide, or deaths under suspicious circumstances; deaths resulting from accidents and injuries; deaths resulting from medical treatments; all cases of poisoning; and if abuse or neglect is suspected.

10.28 a **False** b **True** c **False** d **True** e **True**
Social workers are employed by the Social Services Department of the local authority. They are independent of the health providers and may see clients referred from any source, including self-referrals. They have a wide range of functions, including advising individuals on personal, financial, and welfare issues; allocating resources available from the social services (e.g. meals on wheels, home help); social services to children (e.g. supervising fostering and adoption processes, management and supervision of suspected child abuse cases); and services to the mentally ill (e.g. application for compulsory detention, assessment and treatment orders, follow-up of mentally ill patients). The social services department has recently taken on a purchaser role—to assess the social needs of their clients, and purchase the care from other providers to meet the identified needs.

11 *Problem solving*

Questions

A GP was called out at midnight to visit a 24 year old man with a one day history of increasing shortness of breath and wheezing. He was known to suffer from asthma since childhood and had been maintained on regular salbutamol and steroid inhaler. His usual peak flow had been 550 litre/min. On examination, his pulse was 120 beats/min and his respiratory rate was 50 beats/min. His respiration was very shallow. He had very quiet breath sounds, but no wheeze was detected on auscultation. His peak flow was 120 litre/min.

11.1 It is essential for the GP to elicit the following points in the history and examination

a whether cyanosis was present
b whether the second heart sound was split
c whether the patient was able to speak in words, phrases, or sentences
d family history of asthma
e whether precordial heave was present

11.2 Which of the following is/are recognized appropriate management actions by the GP?

a administer theophylline orally
b administer salbutamol nebulizer and review progress in 4 h time
c arrange admission to hospital immediately
d administer intravenous hydrocortisone
e administer high dose oxygen

11.3 In the event, the patient was immediately transported to the accident and emergency department with no treatment from the GP. Clinical signs were unchanged. After the appropriate drug treatments were given, which of the following investigations must be performed immediately?

a blood gas
b liver function test
c chest radiograph
d calcium level
e spirometry

11.4 ***The patient became increasingly confused and drowsy. In addition to the anti-asthmatic drugs, which of the following are recognized appropriate management actions?***

a prescription of intravenous diazepam
b prescription of oral chlorpromazine
c nursing in a dark room on a medical ward
d lumbar puncture
e immediate transfer to the Intensive Care Unit

A 24 year old woman consulted her GP with a few days' history of bilateral painful red nodules on both shins. On examination, she was mildly pyrexial with temperature 37.5°C and mild cervical lympadenopathy. Examination of the cardiovascular, respiratory system, and the abdomen revealed no abnormalities.

11.5 ***Which of the following points in the history and examination is/are important in clarifying the aetiology of the skin lesions?***

a drug history
b alcohol history
c previous history of jaundice
d symptoms of breathlessness
e symptoms of migraine

11.6 ***A detailed history and examination failed to reveal no further relevant information. However, a chest radiograph showed bilateral hilar lymphadnopathy with no pulmonary shadowing. Which of the following investigations may show abnormalities of associated with the likely diagnosis?***

a calcium level
b magnesium level
c lymph node biopsy
d angiotensin converting enzyme
e renin level

11.7 ***The patient was treated conservatively, and was reviewed by a general physician 6 months after the initial presentation. The skin lesions had resolved, the patient was asymptomatic, and all investigations were normal except that mild bilateral hilar lymphadenopathy persisted on the***

chest radiograph. Which of the following drugs is/are recognized as appropriate for management?

a azathioprine
b erythromycin
c high dose septrin
d prednisolone
e hydroxychloroquine

A GP was called at 2:00 a.m. to see a 12 year old boy with a high fever and a 5 h history of being unwell and vomiting. He had no significant past medical history. He had not been in contact with anyone known to have an infectious disease. He lived with his parents and two brothers, aged 10 and 14. On examination, his temperature was 38.5°C. His pulses were of low volume, and at a rate of 120 beats/min. There was a generalised petechial rash all over his trunk and limbs. He was drowsy, but was orientated in time, place and person. There were no signs of meningism.

11.8 ***Which of the following actions is/are recognized appropriate management by the GP?***

a give an injection of pethidine
b give an injection of chlorpheniramine
c give an injection of benzylpenicillin
d give an injection of metoclopramide
e arrange an appointment with the paediatrician at 9 a.m.

11.9 ***He was seen by the general paediatrician. His physical signs remained unchanged. Appropriate immediate investigations include***

a blood PCR (polymerase chain reaction) test for bacterial antigen
b blood culture
c urinary test for bacterial antigens
d skin scrapings for gram stain and microscopy
e mantoux test

11.10 ***Which of the following are appropriate immediate management by the paediatrician?***

a notify the consultant in communicable disease and control
b withhold antibiotics in the absence of symptoms and signs of meningism
c administer plasma or normal saline via an intravenous infusion
d monitor the level of consciousness closely
e monitor the blood pressure closely

11.11 ***Which of the following are appropriate preventative measures to be taken by either the paediatrician or the public health doctors before the investigative results are available?***

a offer oral benzylpenicillin to his brothers

b offer oral rifampicin to his parents
c offer oral rifampicin to all the pupils in the school
d offer vaccination to all the pupils in the school
e offer vaccination to his brothers

A 30 year old woman was brought to her GP with episodes of restlessness, agitation, intermittent palpitations, and tremor in the last few weeks. There were also episodes of shortness of breath, associated with tingling of the fingers, and the feeling that she was going to die. Most of these episodes appeared occur when she was out of the house. On examination, her thyroid gland was not palpable. There was tremor on her outstretched hands. Her pulse was sinus rhythm at a rate of 90 beats/min. Her reflexes were generally brisk and symmetrical. Examination of her respiratory system reveals no abnormalities. The results of the investigations performed by her GP were as follows:-

plasma thyroxine	75nmol/litre	(70–140 nmol/litre)
TSH	9.0 mU/litre	(0.5–5.7 mU/litre)
calcium (total)	2.50 mmol/litre	(2.12–2.65 mmol/litre)
albumin	40 g/litre	(30–50 g/litre)

11.12 *Which of the following conclusions are true?*

a the investigative results explain most of her presenting symptoms
b the patient is euthymic
c her respiratory symptoms are likely to be due to a chest infection
d her palpitations are likely to be due to supraventricular tachycardia
e the tingling of the fingers is likely to be due to hypomagnesaemia

11.13 *Which of the following treatments is/are appropriate?*

a carbimazole
b thyroxine
c barbiturates
d cognitive behavioural therapy
e anxiety management therapy

A GP was urgently called at 10 p.m. by the mother of a 20 year old man, John. John lived with his mother in a two-bedroomed flat. According to the mother, John has behaved extremely strangely in the last 3 weeks. He had been complaining of enemies 'in the other end of the world' plotting against him, and that their spies had been following him everywhere. In the previous hour, he had armed himself with a kitchen knife and accused his mother of joining these enemies. His mother became so worried that she left the flat quickly and called the GP.

11.14 *Which of the following is/are recognized appropriate management actions by the GP?*

a persuade his mother to go back into the flat to calm John down
b arrange an outpatient appointment the next week with a consultant psychiatrist
c interview John alone in his flat that evening

d sign an application for a compulsory order for admission for assessment in a psychiatric unit based solely on the account given by his mother
e call the police and duty social worker to accompany the doctor to interview John in his flat

In the event, John ran out of the house with a knife, and was disarmed by the police and brought to the local accident and emergency department. He was interviewed by the duty psychiatrist. He was found to be extremely agitated, paranoid, and completely lacking in insight into his illness. He refused to remain in hospital, and had to be restrained by three staff to stop him from leaving.

11.15 *Which of the following are recognized appropriate management by the duty psychiatrist?*

a administer a single dose of intramuscular chlorpromazine against John's will
b detain John whilst awaiting the arrival of the duty social worker to complete the application for compulsory order for admission for assessment
c admit John to the ward without applying for a compulsory order for admission
d ask his mother to sign a consent form for John to be admitted to hospital
e ensure John's agreement to be admitted by threatening to 'section' him if he refuses

John was subsequently admitted to the psychiatric ward. He complained of the 'enemies' putting thoughts into his head, and controlling his actions via electronic equipment.

11.16 *Which of the following is/are likely differential diagnoses?*

a mania
b depression
c schizophrenia
d obsessive compulsive behaviour
e hysteria

A 35 year old man was referred to the ophthalmologist with a 4 day history of sudden and progressive visual loss in the central visual field in his right eye and the feeling that 'everything is darker through the right eye', associated with right periocular pain on moving the eyes. On examination, his visual acuity without glasses were 6/60 in both eyes. He was myopic, but had forgotten to bring his glasses. When the 'swinging flashlight test' (swinging a strong light to shine from one eye to the other every few seconds) was performed, it was found that the right pupil dilated, whilst the left pupil constricted when the light was swung from the fellow eye to it. The conjunctiva was not inflamed, and fundoscopy was normal.

11.17 *Which of the following conclusions is/are true?*

a a left third nerve palsy was present

b a right third nerve palsy was present
c the visual loss in the right eye had been confirmed
d the diagnosis is likely to be iritis in the right eye
e the diagnosis is likely to be central retinal vein thrombosis

11.18 *Which of the following examinations and investigations is/are likely to be abnormal?*

a visual field testing of the right eye
b visual field testing of the left eye
c ishihara colour vision test of the right eye
d intraocular pressure of the right eye
e skull radiograph.

11.19 *Which of the following is/are recognized appropriate management plans for the patient within the next 2 weeks?*

a topical steroid eye drops
b close observation with no active treatment
c referral for neurosurgical opinion
d laser treatment to the peripheral retina
e treatment with prednisolone for a total of 2 weeks

The symptoms settled within 4 weeks with the appropriate management plans. However, he presented 3 years later to his GP with sudden weakness of his left leg. Examination revealed a reduction of the power of the left leg, with brisk right knee and ankle reflexes and up-going right plantar.

11.20 *Which of the following investigations is/are likely to assist in confirming the diagnosis?*

a CT scan
b MRI scan
c visual evoked response
d lumbar spine radiograph
e CSF electrophoresis

A 65 year old Caucasian man presents with a 6 months history of tiredness, malaise and severe weight loss. Physical examination was unremarkable apart from marked weight loss. Investigations reveal:-

Full blood count

Hb	9 g/dl	(13.5–18 g/dl)
MCV	60 fl	(76–96 fl)
MCHC	250 g/litre	(30–360 g/litre)
WBC	8×10^9 /litre	($4.0–11.0 \times 10^9$/litre)
platelet	250×10^9 /litre	($150–400 \times 10^9$/litre)

Urea and electrolytes

sodium	134 mmol/litre	(135–145 mmol/litre)

potassium	3.5 mmol/litre	(3.5–5.0 mmol/litre)
bicarbonate	30 mmol/litre	(24–30 mmol/litre)
urea	7.0 mmol/litre	(2.5–6.7 mmol/litre)

Chest radiograph—normal
Faecal occult blood—positive on three occasions

11.21 Likely causes for the haematological abnormalities include

a folate deficiency
b vitamin B_{12} deficiency
c iron deficiency
d thalassaemia
e haemolytic anaemia

11.22 Further investigations of the man's symptoms should include

a Schilling test
b ferritin level
c sigmoidoscopy
d barium enema
e intravenous pyelogram

A 3 year old boy was brought to see his GP with a 5 day history of generalized bruises all over his trunk and limbs. On examination, he was an active well toddler. There were generalized bruises and petichiae all over his trunk and limbs, and the tip of the spleen was palpable. Investigative results were as follows:

Hb	120 g/litre	(11–15 g/litre)
WBC	8×10^9 /litre	($4.0–11.0 \times 10^9$ /litre)
platelet	12×10^9 /litre	($150–400 \times 10^9$ /litre)

blood film—normal white cell differential and morphology

prothrombin time	12 s	(10–14 s)
APTT	41 s	(35–45 s)

11.23 Probable differential diagnoses include

a haemophilia A
b Von Willebrand disease
c acute leukaemia
d idiopathic thrombocytopenic purpura
e child physical abuse

11.24 Which of the following are recognized appropriate management?

a manage conservatively with frequent haematological monitoring
b perform a bone marrow biopsy

c perform bone marrow irradiation
d advise strict bed rest in hospital
e treat with oral prednisolone

11.25 *The child is at significantly increased risk of which of the following?*

a epistaxis
b rectal bleeding
c haemarthrosis
d bleeding into muscle
e intracranial haemorrhage

The biochemistry results of a 50 year old man were as follows:

calcium	1.96 mmol/litre	(2.12–2.65 mmol/litre)
phosphate	1.75 mmol/litre	(0.8–1.45 mmol/litre)
alkaline phosphatase	200 IU/litre	(30–300 IU/litre)

11.26 *Probable diagnoses include*

a osteomalacia
b Paget's disease
c bone metastases
d hypoparathyroidism
e renal failure

11.27 *Investigations which will further clarify the diagnosis include*

a protein electrophoresis
b parathyroid hormone level
c creatinine level
d calcitonin level
e chest radiograph

A 23 year old man was brought to the accident and emergency department unconscious. Apart from his conscious level, physical examination was unremarkable. The biochemical results were as follows:

Urea and electrolytes

sodium	144 mmol/litre	(135–145 mmol/litre)
potassium	4.8 mmol/litre	(3.5–5.0 mmol/litre)
chloride	100 mmol/litre	(95–105 mmol/litre)
bicarbonate	12 mmol/litre	(24–30 mmol/litre)
urea	6.9 mmol/litre	(2.5–6.7 mmol/litre)

Blood gas

PaO_2	12 kPa	(>10.6 kPa)
$PaCO_2$	2.3 kPa	(4.7–6.0 kPa)
pH	7.34	(7.35–7.45)

11.28 *Which of the following statements are true?*

a there was an element of metabolic acidosis
b there was an element of respiratory acidosis
c the patient was hypoxic
d the anion gap is normal
e the patient was hypoventilating

11.29 *Which of the following investigations must be performed immediately to evaluate the diagnosis?*

a blood glucose
b blood cortisol
c lumbar puncture
d blood salicylate level
e thyroid function test

11.30 *Probable diagnoses include*

a renal tubular acidosis
b acute asthma
c diabetes ketoacidosis
d aspirin overdose
e salmonella gastroenteritis

A house physician was called to set up a continuous aminophylline infusion for a 35 year old man admitted with an acute asthmatic attack. The medical registrar had just assessed the patient, given a loading dose of aminophylline, and asked for a continuous infusion to be given at 500 μg/kg per hour. 10 ml-ampoules of aminophylline at a concentration of 25 mg/ml and 1 litre bags of dextrose saline were available. The patient weighed 75 kg. The house physician decided to mix 1 ampoule of aminophylline with 1 litre of dextrose saline.

11.31 *Which of the following statements is/are true?*

a the patient required 375 mg/h of aminophylline
b each ampoule of aminophylline contains 250 mg of the drug
c each 1010 ml of the mixture prepared by the house physician contains 2500 mg of aminophylline
d each ml of the mixture prepared by the house physician contains about 0.25 mg of aminophylline
e the infusion should be set at about 150 mls/h

A 60 year old woman was brought to the accident and emergency department by her relatives with a 3 day history of fluctuating levels of confusion, which was worse in the evenings. At its worst, she could not concentrate on any task for more than a minute. She also complained of seeing many people moving around the house when there were nobody there. Also, she had slept very poorly in the last few days. Physical examination revealed mild pyrexia, nystagmus, and mild ataxia, but was otherwise unremarkable. Mental state examination revealed that she was restless and agitated. She was disorientated in time and place, but not in person. Her attention span was significant reduced, and she could not register a two-digit number. She described a recent visual hallucinatory experience.

11.32 *Which of the following investigations should be performed immediately?*

a blood glucose
b urea and electrolytes
c full blood count
d red cell transketolase
e urine culture

11.33 *Likely differential diagnoses include*

a alcohol withdrawal
b urinary tract infection
c Wernicke's encephalopathy
d schizophrenia
e dementia

A 25 year old woman attended the accident and emergency department with a 2 day history of central and right iliac fossa pain. Her appetite had been normal until the previous day. There was no history of change of bowel habit. Her last period was about 7 weeks previously, and there was scanty dark vaginal bleeding on the day of admission. On examination, she was mildly pyrexial (37.8°C). Her pulse was 90 beats/min, and her blood pressure was 120/70. The abdomen was not distended. There was tenderness in the right iliac fossa with slight guarding and rebound tenderness.

11.34 *On the basis of these findings, which of the following examination and investigations should be performed immediately?*

a rectal examination
b vaginal examination
c urinary culture
d serum amylase
e abdominal radiograph

11.35 *Probable diagnoses include*

a appendicitis
b diverticulitis
c pelvic inflammatory disease
d ectopic pregnancy
e endometriosis

Her urine was found to be positive for β-HCG.

11.36 *Which of the following is/are appropriate management actions?*

a arrange for dilatation and curettage to be performed

b arrange for appendicetomy to be performed
c no action other than conservative treatment with intravenous fluids
d arrange for ultrasound of the uterus
e arrange for laparoscopy

An 8 year old boy was brought to the accident and emergency department by his mother at 10 p.m. He had been well until an hour previously, when he was suddenly noted to be drowsy and unsteady on his feet. There was no history of prior head injury. He denied headache and there were no other neurological symptoms. He is the only child of a single-parent family, living alone with his mother. His mother had chronic generalized anxiety state. On examination, the child was aprexial. He responded to questioning, but was obviously drowsy. He was clearly ataxic, and finger-nose tests were adversely affected on both sides. There were no signs of neck stiffness, fundi was normal, and there were no other neurological abnormalities. Full blood count was normal with white cell count of 9×10^9/litre, with normal differential.

11.37 *Which of the following is/are recognized appropriate investigations in assessing the cause for his symptoms?*

a EEG
b nerve conduction test
c creatinine kinase
d CAT scan
e urinary drug screen

11.38 *Which of the following is/are recognized appropriate management for the patient before the investigation results are available?*

a intravenous antibiotics
b intravenous acyclovir
c close neurological monitoring
d regular rectal diazepam
e putting the child in an isolation cubicle

In the event, the child was admitted for assessment and investigations. By 6 a.m. the next morning, the child was found to be fully alert and playing happily, with a completely normal gait. A review of the treatment chart revealed that the child had been treated conservatively.

11.39 *Appropriate preventive actions include*

a advising mother to administer rectal diazepam for future pyrexial illness
b advising mother to immunize the child against chickenpox
c advising mother to keep all medicines and drugs safely out of reach of the child
d advising mother to keep her child away from other children of the same age

e notifying all health professionals in the area that the case was a Munchausen by proxy

Jane, a 24 year old woman, was referred by her GP to the gynaecologist for infertility. Jane had been married to John, aged 26, for 3 years, and they had been trying for a baby in the last 18 months. Jane had no significant past medical history. She came off a combined oral contraceptive 12 months ago. Since then, her periods had occurred every 25–31 days. Her GP also enclosed the result of her husband's semen analysis:

volume	3 ml	(>2.75 ml)
sperm count	21×10^6 sperms/ml	(>20×10^6 sperms/ml)
% motile	42%	(>40%)
% normal form	70%	(>60%)

11.40 *Which of the following statements is/are true?*

a it is unnecessary for the gynaecologist to see Jane's husband
b it is important to perform a pelvic examination
c it is important to ask Jane about past history of pelvic infection
d it is almost impossible for Jane to conceive without medical intervention
e it is almost certain that an organic cause for the infertility will be found

11.41 *Which of the following is/are recognized appropriate tests for ovulation?*

a FSH level
b progesterone level at day 21 of cycle
c monitoring follicle development by ultrasound
d oestradiol level at day 7 of cycle
e β-HCG level at day 21 of cycle

The following hormonal results showed:

FSH (luteal phase)	6 U/litre (2–8 U/litre)
LH (luteal phase)	6 U/litre (3–16 U/litre)

11.42 *Which of the following conclusions can be deduced from the results?*

a premature ovarian failure is unlikely
b ovulation is confirmed
c polycystic ovarian syndrome is unlikely
d pituitary microadenoma is unlikely
e an adrenal disorder is likely

11.43 *In addition to the results given above, which of the following is/are also appropriate relevant initial investigations?*

a calcium level
b magnesium level
c skull radiograph

d prolactin level
e thyroid function tests

11.44 *If all appropriate initial investigations are normal, appropriate further investigations include*

a postcoital test
b ovarian biopsy
c dilatation and curettage
d CT scan of the brain
e laparoscopy and dye test

A house physician was called to the ward to review the gentamicin dose of a 45 year old woman who was started on intravenous gentamicin 80 mg three times daily 2 days previously. The results before and after the fourth dose of gentamicin were a follows:

concentration before dose	4.1 mg/litre	(<2 mg/litre)
concentration 30 min after dose	7.2 mg/litre	(5–10 mg/litre)

11.45 *Which of the following is/are recognized appropriate adjustments?*

a continue the same dose
b change to 80 mg twice daily
c change to 60 mg four times daily
d change to 100 mg three times daily
e change to 60 mg three times daily

A house surgeon admitted a 40 year old insulin-dependent diabetic man to a surgical ward electively for an inguinal hernia repair under general anaesthetic for the operating list the next morning. His usual insulin requirements had been 40 U Mixtard in the morning, and 30 U Mixtard in the evening.

11.46 *Which of the following is/are recognized appropriate management by the house surgeon?*

a request for the patient to be placed last on the list
b administer the usual 40 U Mixtard in the morning
c ensure that the patient takes clear fluid only from 6 a.m. on the day of surgery
d set up a 0.9% saline drip on the morning before surgery
e check urea and electrolytes on the morning before surgery

A 50 year old woman complained of hearing problems for the last 6 months. On examination, the Rinne test was positive on the right but negative on the left. The Weber test revealed that the sound was localized to the left ear.

11.47 *The examination findings were compatible with*

a normal hearing in both ears
b conductive deafness in the left ear only
c conductive deafness in the right ear only

d sensorineural deafness in the left ear only
e sensorineural deafness in the right ear only

11.48 *Differential diagnoses include*

a chronic noise exposure
b gentamicin ototoxicity
c wax in the affected ear
d presbyacusis
e perforated eardrum

A 56 year old was referred to the general physician by his GP with an 8 month history of increasing shortness of breath and palpitation. He denied symptoms of orthopnoea. On examination, he had an irregularly irregular pulse of 100 beats/min, and a blood pressure of 140/80. His apex beat was not displaced, but there was a left parasternal heave. His JVP was raised (4 cm above the sternal edge). There was minimal peripheral oedema. On auscultation, there was a loud first heart sound, an opening snap after the second heart sound, and a mid-diastolic murmur maximal at the apex. The lung fields were clear. A smooth 2 cm liver was palpable.

11.49 *Which of the following statements about the patient is/are correct?*

a he was likely to have second degree heart block
b he was at significant risk of systemic embolism
c he had right-sided heart failure
d he did not need to take antibiotics before dental extraction
e he was at significant risk of developing pulmonary hypertension

11.50 *Which of the following investigative results confirm the clinical findings?*

a ECG showed peaked p waves
b R wave of 25 mm in lead V6 and the S wave of 20 mm in V1
c chest radiograph showed mitral valve calcification
d chest radiograph showed dilatation of ascending aorta
e echocardiogram showed left ventricular dilatation

11.51 *Which of the following is/are recognized appropriate management?*

a digoxin
b diuretics
c insert temporary pacing wire
d warfarin
e tricuspid valvotomy

A 20 year old primigravida had an uneventful antenatal period until the week 33 of her pregnancy when she presented in the antenatal clinic with epigastric pain. On examination, she looked well. Her pulse was 90 beats/min, her blood pressure was 140/95, and she had minimal peripheral oedema. Abdominal examination revealed some tenderness in the right hypochondrium. The fundus was 33 cm, the lie was longitudinal, the presentation was cephalic, and the fetal head was free. The fetal heart was heard at a rate of 140 beats/min.

11.52 *Which of the following physical examination may yield relevant information about the cause of her symptoms?*

a rectal examination
b auscultation of lung bases
c tendon reflexes
d ophthalmoscopy
e urine testing

11.53 *Which of the following investigations should be performed?*

a liver function test
b platelet count
c peripheral blood film
d serum amylase
e renal ultrasound

11.54 *Which of the following is/are recognized appropriate immediate management of the patient?*

a prescribe an antacid and review in the antenatal clinic next week
b admit patient to the antenatal ward for observation
c refer the patient to a surgeon to consider cholecystectomy
d isolate the patient
e induce labour

A 15 year old girl consulted her GP with a history of unprotected sexual intercourse 60 h ago. She indicated that she had become sexually active in the past 3 months, and her 20 year old partner usually used a condom. Unfortunately, he ran out of them recently. She requested treatment to prevent pregnancy. However, her GP is a devout Catholic, and did not feel comfortable in prescribing such treatment.

11.55 *Which of the following statements is/are correct?*

a the GP should persuade the girl to discuss the treatment with her parents within the next 2–3 days
b if the parents agreed to the treatment, the GP must prescribe such treatment irrespective of his/her religion and belief
c the girl's partner had committed a criminal offence
d the girl had committed a criminal offence
e the GP should inform the police

In the event, the girl initially agreed to consult her parents. However, she returned an hour later to see another GP in the practice, and stated that she did not want her parents to know about her unprotected sexual intercourse.

11.56 *The GP*

a should inform her parents without the girl' knowledge
b may prescribe the morning-after pill without further enquiries
c may prescribe the morning-after pill only if she was unlikely to have unprotected sexual intercourse again
d may prescribe the morning-after pill only if she appeared mature to the doctor and understood the nature of the morning-after pill treatment
e may prescribe the morning-after pill only if she agreed to leave her partner

11.57 *Which of the following is/are appropriate advice if the GP prescribed the morning-after pill?*

a she should not expect to have a period for another 8 weeks
b the morning-after pill is a single dose treatment
c she must start the treatment as soon as possible
d condoms are not required for the next 2 weeks
e she should take an extra dose should she vomit within 3 h of the treatment

A 17 year old man had presented to his GP with what appeared to be a common cold 3 weeks previously. However, the symptoms gradually changed to fever, yellowish nasal discharge, bilateral facial pain especially on bending forwards, toothache in the upper premolars on both sides, and a cough. On examination, the temperature was 37.5°C, the throat was not inflamed, and there were no cervical lymphadenopathy. The teeth looked healthy to the GP on inspection. The chest was clear.

11.58 *Which of the following actions by the GP is/are appropriate?*

a analgesia with paracetamol
b refer to head and neck surgeon
c order an ultrasound of the maxillary antrum
d refer to the dentist
e order chest physiotherapy

The appropriate treatment was given. However, the patient returned 2 weeks later complaining of painful swelling of the eyelids on the left. On examination, the eyelids on the left were very red and swollen, and completely covered the left eye. However, the conjunctiva was not inflamed. The right eye looked normal. The symptoms of fever and nasal discharge remained unchanged.

11.59 *Which of the following examinations or investigations is/are appropriate?*

a white cell differential count
b skin testing for allergens
c antinuclear antibody
d blood culture
e visual acuity of the left eye

11.60 *Which of the following statements is/are true?*

a the nasal symptoms and the swollen eyelids are unrelated
b oral chlorpheniramine should be prescribed
c the patient should be referred to the ear, nose, and throat surgeon within the next 4 weeks
d the patient should be given intravenous antibiotics
e steroid eye drops should be given

Answers

11.1 a **True** b **False** c **True** d **False** e **False**

The patient was known to have chronic asthma maintained on regular salbutamol and steroid inhalers. The history of increasing shortness of breath and wheezing in the previous day suggests exacerbation of his asthma. The clinical signs of tachycardia, tachypnoea, shallow respiration, silent chest, and markedly reduced peak flow reading (less than 25% of normal) suggest very severe life-threatening asthma. The presence of cyanosis; the ability of the patient to speak in words, phrases, or sentences; the presence of drowsiness or confusion, and the presence of pulsus paradoxus are further indicators of the severity of the asthma. The presence of family history of asthma, the splitting of the second heart sound and the presence of precordial heave would not help in the immediate management.

11.2 a **False** b **False** c **True** d **True** e **True**

In the presence of life-threatening severe asthma attack, the patient should be treated with high dose oxygen, nebulized salbutamol and ipatropium and intravenous hydrocortisone, and immediately admitted to hospital. The GP may also consider giving an initial dose of intravenous aminophylline, although he or she may prefer to leave this until the patient arrives in hospital so that it can be given under ECG monitoring. However, oral theophylline would be inappropriate.

11.3 a **True** b **False** c **True** d **False** e **False**

The most important investigations after the appropriate treatments were initiated are blood gas, chest radiograph, and ECG rhythm monitor. Mechanical ventilation should be considered if PaO_2 level of below 8 kPa, a $PaCO_2$ level of over 6.5 kPa, or a pH of less than 7.3. A chest radiograph should be performed to exclude a pneumothorax, and ECG rhythm should be monitored when aminophylline is being given.

11.4 a **False** b **False** c **False** d **False** e **True**

Confusion and drowsiness are ominous signs, and suggest hypercapnia due to deterioration of his asthma. The patient should be transferred immediately to the Intensive Care Unit and mechanical ventilation should be considered. Prescription of tranquillizers or benzodiazepines is inappropriate, as they reduce the respiratory drive.

11.5 a **True** b **False** c **False** d **True** e **False**
Bilateral painful red nodules on both shins in a 24 year old woman are characteristic of erythema nodosum. This may be idiopathic, but common causes include sarcoidosis and drugs (e.g. sulphonamide, oral contraceptives). Hence drug history and symptoms of breathlessness are important. Rarer causes include streptococcal infection, tuberculosis, Crohn's disease and ulcerative colitis.

11.6 a **True** b **False** c **True** d **True** e **False**
Bilateral hilar lymphadenopathy on the chest radiograph and bilateral erythema nodosum strongly suggest the diagnosis of sarcoidosis. Hypercalcaemia and increased level of angiotensin converting enzyme are associated with increased sarcoid activity. Lymph node biopsy may reveal characteristic sarcoid histology. The positive Kveim test after 4–6 weeks is characteristic of sarcoidosis, although a negative test does not exclude the diagnosis.

11.7 a **False** b **False** c **False** d **False** e **False**
Bilateral hilar lymphadenopathy without pulmonary shadowing almost always resolve spontaneously without treatment. Hence, no treatment was needed, but a chest radiograph should be repeated after a year to ensure resolution of the hilar lympadenopathy. Prednisolone is sometimes used to treat hypercalcaemia, renal disease, lung fibrosis, and uveitis associated with sarcoidosis.

11.8 a **False** b **False** c **True** d **False** e **False**
A history of sudden onset of pyrexia, vomiting, and being unwell, and the physical finding of a generalized petechial rash is characteristic of meningococcal septicaemia. The child should be treated as having meningococcal septicaemia until proven otherwise. An intravenous injection of benzylpenicillin (or a broad spectrum cephalosporin) should be given immediately, and the child should be referred to the paediatrician for admission as a matter of urgency.

11.9 a **True** b **True** c **False** d **True** e **False**
It is important to take appropriate samples to identify the organism responsible for the illness. Blood culture may provide a definitive diagnosis as well as the antibiotic sensitivity of the organism. However, the results may not be available for a few days, and the organisms may not be cultured if antibiotics had been given by the GP before admission. Immediate diagnosis is often possible by gram staining and microscopy of the skin scrapings from the petechial rash. Blood PCR may identify the antigen of the organisms even if antibiotics have been given before admission. An urine specimen is inappropriate for identifying meningococcal antigen. A Mantoux test is inappropriate, as tuberculosis meningitis is usually less acute, and does not give rise to a petechial rash.

11.10 a **True** b **False** c **True** d **True** e **True**
The consultant in communicable disease and control should be notified of a clinical case of meningococcal septicaemia, so that appropriate control measures can be implemented. Meningococcal septicaemia often has a poorer prognosis than meningococcal meningitis. Broad spectrum antibiotics (e.g. cefotaxime) should be

given until the antibiotic sensitivity results are available. Shock and hypotension is often present, and intravenous plasma or normal saline should be given. The child's pulse, blood pressure, and neurological status should be carefully monitored.

11.11 a **False** b **True** c **False** d **False** e **False**
This is an isolated case of meningococcal septicaemia. Prophylactic rifampicin (or ciprofloxacin) should be given to all household and kissing contacts. The head teacher may be advised to send a letter to all parents asking them to be vigilant and seek medical advice early if symptoms occur in their children. However, chemoprophylaxis with rifampicin is not indicated unless there are two or more related cases in the school. Vaccines are only available for groups A and C, but two thirds of meningococcal diseases are currently of group B. Hence, vaccines should be withheld until the organism is identified. If it is proven to be group A or C, vaccines should be offered to household and kissing contacts.

11.12 a **False** b **False** c **False** d **False** e **False**
The presenting features of restlessness, agitation, intermittent palpitations, and tremor suggest a diagnosis of either hyperthyroidism or anxiety state with panic attacks. However, the accompanying symptoms of the feeling that she was going to die suggest an anxiety state. Further, her symptoms of breathlessness associated with tingling of the fingers suggest hyperventilation due to anxiety. However, the investigative results of normal thyroxine but a high TSH levels reveal that she was mildly hypothyroid. Hence, she had two separate disorders—hypothyroidism and an anxiety state.

11.13 a **False** b **True** c **False** d **True** e **True**
Her mild hypothyroidism should be treated with a suitable dose of thyroxine. Her anxiety state may be managed by suitable counselling, anxiety management therapy, or cognitive behavioural therapy. Benzodiazepines may be used in the short term with caution, but barbiturates should not be used.

11.14 a **False** b **False** c **False** d **False** e **True**
According to the account given by his mother, John was clearly psychotic and paranoid. As he was armed with a kitchen knife, it was clearly dangerous for the GP or his mother to approach him alone. This is an obvious emergency which must be dealt with immediately. Legally, the GP must see and assess the mental state of the patient before signing an application for compulsory order for admission. Therefore, the most appropriate action under these circumstances is to interview John in the presence of the duty approved social worker with a view for applying for compulsory order for admission, and with sufficient help from the police so that any violence can be contained.

11.15 a **True** b **True** c **False** d **False** e **False**
John was clearly a danger to himself and others if he was allowed to leave the hospital. Also, it was necessary to administer treatment immediately. The duty psychiatrist can, by common law, administer a single dose of treatment against John's will before

the application for compulsory order for admission under the Mental Health Act is completed. Also, John may be detained against his will whilst awaiting the arrival of the duty social worker to complete the application, as long as the duty social worker had been summoned and that he/she arrives within a reasonable period of time. However, it is illegal to admit John to the ward before the application is completed. Also, his mother had no legal authority to give consent for John's admission, as John is over the age of 18. Obtaining John's agreement to be admitted by duress does not constitute informed consent.

11.16 a **False** b **False** c **True** d **False** e **False**
John had symptoms of thought insertion and passivity feelings. These are Sneider's first-rank symptoms. Hence, the most likely diagnosis is schizophrenia. John's paranoid symptoms are not mood-congruent, and affective disorders are not likely.

11.17 a **False** b **False** c **False** d **False** e **False**
The symptoms of sudden and progressive unilateral visual loss in the central visual field with subjective reduction in brightness, and periocular pain on eye movement, and the signs of afferent pupillary defect in a 35 year old, are characteristic of optic neuritis. The afferent pupillary defect is characteristic of optic nerve lesion. We cannot conclude that there had been deterioration in visual acuity in either eye, as it was measured without glasses. The visual acuity should be remeasured either with a pinhole or with the appropriate corrections.

11.18 a **True** b **False** c **True** d **False** e **False**
Optic neuritis is usually associated with central scotoma in the visual field of the affected eye, and loss of colour discrimination power. It is also associated a subjective reduction in the level of brightness of objects visualized. The intraocular pressure and the skull radiograph would be normal.

11.19 a **False** b **True** c **False** d **False** e **True**
The natural history of optic neuritis is spontaneous recovery within 4 weeks. Hence, many ophthalmologists would manage the condition conservatively. Over 50% with an attack of optic neuritis develop multiple sclerosis later on in life. Treatment with systemic steroids is known to accelerate the rate of recovery of visual loss. Moreover, there is limited evidence that treatment with systemic steroids might reduce the risk of subsequent multiple sclerosis slightly. Hence, other ophthalmologists treat the condition with systemic steroids.

11.20 a **False** b **True** c **True** d **False** e **True**
With subsequent neurological symptoms in the left leg, the most likely diagnosis is multiple sclerosis. Visual evoked response may be delayed in multiple sclerosis. Magnetic resonance imaging of the brain is sensitive to multiple sclerosis plaques, but CT scan is usually normal. CSF electrophoresis may reveal oligoclonal bands.

11.21 a **False** b **False** c **True** d **False** e **False**
The full blood count shows a microcytic hypochromic anaemia (with low MCV and

MCHC indices). The two commonest causes are iron deficiency anaemia and haemoglobinopathies (e.g. thalassaemia, sickle cell disease). As the patient is Caucasian, haemoglobinopathies are unlikely. Both vitamin B_{12} deficiency and folate deficiencies are characteristically associated with macrocytic anaemia. Haemolytic anaemia is characteristically normocytic.

11.22 a **False** b **True** c **True** d **True** e **False**
To confirm that the anaemia is due to iron deficiency, either the ferritin level or the TIBC level should be measured. The Schilling test is a test for vitamin B_{12} absorption. The symptoms of malaise and weight loss, iron deficiency anaemia, and persistently positive faecal occult blood suggest gastrointestinal malignancies as the diagnosis. Hence, sigmoidoscopy, colonoscopy, and barium enema should be performed.

11.23 a **False** b **False** c **True** d **True** e **False**
The haematological investigations showed isolated thrombocytopenia. The most likely diagnosis is idiopathic thrombocytopenic purpura, which is an autoimmune disease. However, a proportion of children with acute leukaemia also presents with this picture with no abnormalities of the white cells in the blood film. Hence, a bone marrow biopsy is sometimes necessary if there are unusual features, or if the platelet level does not recover within a few weeks. Child physical abuse usually causes local rather than generalized bruises, and the platelet count is normal.

11.24 a **True** b **True** c **False** d **False** e **True**
The platelet count is quite low, although the child is asymptomatic. Either conservative management with close haematological monitoring or treatment with oral prednisolone would be appropriate management. As the platelet count is quite low, many paediatricians would perform a bone marrow biopsy. Whether the child is admitted to hospital depends on the social circumstances, but strict bed rest is not indicated.

11.25 a **True** b **True** c **False** d **False** e **True**
Children with low platelets are prone to bleed from the gum, the nose, the gastrointestinal tract, and into the brain. Bleeding into the joints and muscle are more characteristic of disorders of the intrinsic coagulation pathway such as haemophilia A and haemophilia B.

11.26 a **False** b **False** c **False** d **True** e **True**
The calcium level is usually high in bone metastases. In Paget's disease, the calcium and phosphate levels are usually normal, but the alkaline phosphatase level is usually elevated. In osteomalacia, both calcium and phosphate levels are low, but the alkaline phosphatase levels are high. The results given showed a low calcium and a high phosphate level. This may be due to hypoparathyroidism, or chronic renal failure.

11.27 a **False** b **True** c **True** d **False** e **False**
The purpose of further investigations is to distinguish between hypoparathyroidism and chronic renal failure. The latter case is often associated with secondary

hyperparathyroidism. Useful investigations include parathyroid hormone level and renal function tests. Protein electrophoresis is not indicated, as myeloma is associated with a high calcium level.

11.28 a **True** b **False** c **False** d **False** e **False**
The results showed a low bicarbonate level, a low carbon dioxide level, and a near-normal pH. This is a mixed picture of metabolic acidosis and respiratory alkalosis. The respiratory alkalosis may be due to hyperventilation. The patient was not hypoxic as the PaO_2 was normal. The anion gap is measured by $[Na^+] + [K^+] - [Cl^-] - [HCO_3^-]$. In this case, it was 144 + 4.8 – 100 – 12 = 36.8. An anion gap of more than 16 mmol/l is excessive.

11.29 a **True** b **False** c **False** d **True** e **False**
A mixed picture of metabolic acidosis with increased anion gap and respiratory alkalosis is suggestive of aspirin overdose. Other causes of metabolic acidosis include diabetic ketoacidosis, liver failure, shock and uraemia. A urea level of 6.9 mmol/l renders the diagnosis of uraemia unlikely. Immediate investigations should include blood glucose, blood salicylate, and liver function tests.

11.30 a **False** b **False** c **True** d **True** e **False**
Renal tubular acidosis causes loss of acid and a biochemical picture of metabolic acidosis with normal anion gap. Acute asthma is usually associated with hypoxia. Salmonella gastroenteritis may cause metabolic acidosis with normal anion gap.

11.31 a **False** b **True** c **False** d **True** e **True**
The patient requires (500 µg × 75 = 37.5 mg) of aminophylline per hour. Each ampoule of aminophylline contains (25 mg × 10 = 250 mg). As 1 ampoule of aminoophylline was mixed with each litre bag of dextrose saline, each 1010 ml of the mixture contains 250 mg of aminophylline. Each ml of the mixture prepared contains about (250 mg/1010 = 0.25 mg) of aminophylline. Hence, the infusion should be set at 37.5/0.25 = 150 ml/h.

11.32 a **True** b **True** c **True** d **True** e **True**
The presentation is that of acute delirium, characterized by fluctuating course of disturbances of consciousness, attention, cognition, and the sleep-wake cycle. There are many causes for delirium, such as hypoxia; cerebrovascular accident; electrolyte and metabolic disturbances such as hypercalcaemia, hyponatraemia, hypoglycaemia, liver failure; alcohol and substance withdrawal, and infections (e.g. pneumonia, meningitis, encephalitis). However, the presence of nystagmus and ataxia should raise the suspicion of Wernicke's encephalopathy. Immediate investigations should include full blood count, infection screen, urea and electrolytes, liver function tests, blood and glucose. Red cell transketolase should also be performed in this case to exclude Wernicke's encephalopathy.

11.33 a **True** b **True** c **True** d **False** e **False**
See answers to question 11.32. The recent and acute onset of symptoms made dementia unlikely.

11.34 a **True** b **True** c **True** d **False** e **False**
Acute appendicitis should be considered in the presence of right iliac fossa tiredness with guarding and rebound tenderness. However, her delayed period and abdominal pain preceding vaginal bleeding should strongly raise the suspicion of ectopic tubal pregnancy. Rectal examination and vaginal examination should be performed to evaluate these possibilities. Another diagnosis to consider is urinary tract infection. Pancreatitis is unlikely, and abdominal radiograph is not indicated.

11.35 a **True** b **False** c **False** d **True** e **False**
See answer to question 11.34 above. Whilst pelvic inflammatory disease and diverticulitis are possible diagnoses, they are very unlikely. Endometriosis may cause dyspareunia, but seldom causes acute abdominal pain.

11.36 a **False** b **False** c **False** d **True** e **False**
The fact that her urine was positive for β-hCG strongly raised the suspicion of ectopic pregnancy. However, another possibility is intrauterine pregnancy. Hence, a pelvic ultrasound, if available, should be performed. However, if this is not available, it is appropriate to arrange for laparoscopy when both ectopic pregnancy and appendicitis may be either confirmed or excluded.

11.37 a **False** b **False** c **False** d **True** e **True**
The child presented with an extremely acute history of drowsiness and ataxia. There was no symptoms and signs of meningitis. EEG, nerve conduction test, and creatinine kinase are all inappropriate investigations. The main differential diagnoses were accidental or non-accidental overdose and acute encephalitis. An unlikely diagnosis is intracranial thrombosis or bleeding. CAT scan and urinary drug screen should be performed initially. MRI scan and lumbar puncture might be indicated later.

11.38 a **False** b **False** c **True** d **False** e **False**
As the child was apyrexial with a normal white cell count and differential, bacterial meningitis or herpes encephalitis were very unlikely diagnoses. The child should have frequent neurological observations.

11.39 a **False** b **False** c **True** d **False** e **False**
The child recovered fully in less than 12 h with no treatment. The most likely diagnosis was benzodiazepine overdose from taking his mother's medication. The most likely cause was accidental, and the mother should be advised to keep all medicines safely locked up out of reach of the child. Although non-accidental poisoning was a remote possibility if frequent episodes occurred, there was little evidence in the history to suggest that this was the case.

11.40 a **False** b **True** c **True** d **False** e **False**
It is extremely important to see the couple together to explore the technique, frequency and timing of sexual intercourse. It is important to enquire about a past history of pelvic infection, as this is an important cause of loss of tubal patency. A pelvic examination may reveals pathologies such as fibroids and fixed retroverted uterus.

About 90% of couples who have regular intercourse conceive within a year. However, a significant proportion of the 10% who do not ultimately conceive without medical intervention. Important major causes for infertility are reduction of sufficient healthy sperms for the male partner, annovulation, tubal blockage, hostile mucus, and psychological causes. However, no causes are found in over a quarter of all cases.

11.41 a **False** b **True** c **True** d **False** e **False**
There are several appropriate tests for ovulation. Crude observations include basal temperature rise during mid-cycle and monitoring of the stretchiness of cervical mucus. More reliable tests include a progesterone level of over 30 nmol/l at day 21 of cycle, detecting LH surge with suitable kit, and monitoring follicle development by ultrasound.

11.42 a **True** b **False** c **True** d **False** e **False**
In premature ovarian failure, the FSH level is characteristically high due to lack of feedback inhibition from oestrogen. In polycystic ovarian syndrome, the LH to FSH level is characteristically high. No conclusions can be drawn regarding ovulation from the results. Most pituitary microadenoma secretes prolactin.

11.43 a **False** b **False** c **False** d **True** e **True**
Hyperprolactinaemia is a common cause for annovulation and infertility. Hypothyroidism may also cause infertility. Skull radiograph is not indicated unless the prolactin level is raised.

11.44 a **True** b **False** c **False** d **False** e **True**
Laparoscopy and dye test is useful to detect endometriosis and to confirm the patency of the fallopian tubes. A post-coital test is useful to exclude cervical mucus hostility. CT scan of the brain is not indicated unless prolactin level is elevated.

11.45 a **False** b **True** c **False** d **False** e **False**
The results shows that the trough concentration was high, but the peak concentration was just above the therapeutic level. The high trough concentration is potentially nephrotoxic and ototoxic. To reduce the trough concentration, the frequency of administration must be reduced. To maintain the same peak concentration, the individual dosage may remain the same.

11.46 a **False** b **False** c **False** d **False** e **True**
Diabetic patients admitted for routine surgery should be placed first on the list if possible, to reduce the uncertainty about the time of surgery. Patients must be kept nil by mouth for at least 6 h prior to the administration of general anaesthetics. Otherwise, the patient may risk aspiration of the stomach contents during induction of anaesthetic. The urea and electrolytes should be checked on the day of surgery, and an intravenous infusion of dextrose or dextrose saline should be given. Different anaesthetists may have their own favourite insulin regime. In general, the morning dose of subcutaneous insulin should be omitted, and a sliding scale of intravenous insulin according to the blood glucose level should be given.

11.47 a **False** b **True** c **False** d **False** e **False**
A Rinne test is positive when the air conduction is better than bone conduction, and may occur in normal ears and in sensorineural deafness. A negative Rinne test indicates conductive deafness. Weber's test is localized to the affected ear in conductive deafness, and to the contralateral ear in sensorineural deafness. The sound appears central if both ears are normal.

11.48 a **False** b **False** c **True** d **False** e **True**
Chronic noise exposure, gentamicin ototoxicity and presbyacusis are causes of sensorineural deafness; wax and perforated ear drum are causes of conductive deafness.

11.49 a **False** b **True** c **True** d **False** e **True**
The clinical symptoms and signs were characteristic of pure mitral stenosis causing atrial fibrillation and right-sided heart failure. As the patient was in atrial fibrillation, he was at significant risk of systemic embolism. He was also at significant risk of pulmonary hypertension. All patients with valvular disorders with a high pressure gradient (including mitral stenosis) should take antibiotics before dental extraction to prevent bacterial endocarditis.

11.50 a **False** b **False** c **True** d **False** e **False**
The ECG was expected to show atrial fibrillation with no p waves. An R wave of 25 mm in lead V6 and 20 mm in S wave of V1 is indicative of left ventricular hypertrophy. Mitral valve calcification is sometimes present on CXR in chronic mitral stenosis. Dilatation of ascending aorta occurs in aortic stenosis.

11.51 a **True** b **True** c **False** d **True** e **False**
Recognized appropriate treatments include digoxin and diuretics to control symptoms; and anticoagulation to minimize the risk of systemic embolus. If this is ineffective, mitral valvotomy or balloon valvoplasy may be needed.

11.52 a **False** b **False** c **True** d **True** e **True**
Epigastric pain, right hypochondrial tenderness, and a raised blood pressure during pregnancy should immediately raise the suspicion of symptomatic pre-eclampsia. In pre-eclampsia, the tendon reflexes are characteristically brisk, and haemorrhages may be seen in the optic fundus. Urine testing shows heavy proteinuria. Note that oedema is not a necessary criteria for the diagnosis of pre-eclampsia.

11.53 a **True** b **True** c **True** d **False** e **False**
Symptomatic pre-eclampsia is often associated with the HELLP syndrome (haemolysis, elevated liver enzyme, and low platelet count). Hence, liver function tests, platelet count and peripheral blood film should be performed. Clotting screen should also be performed. Levels of urea and electrolytes and urate should be measured. Serum should be saved so that cross-match may be performed with the minimum of delay should need arise. Ultrasound of the fetus may be performed to determine the well-being and growth of the fetus.

11.54 a **False** b **True** c **False** d **False** e **False**
Symptomatic pre-eclampsia is a potentially serious condition, and the patient should be immediately admitted to the antenatal ward for bed rest and close observation of her symptoms, blood pressure, proteinuria, urine output, and urate level. Antihypertensives should be considered if the blood pressure remains elevated. Induction of labour might be considered if the pre-eclampsia becomes uncontrolled, and the prematurity of the fetus must be taken into account in reaching this decision.

11.55 a **False** b **False** c **True** d **False** e **False**
The usual postcoital contraceptive treatment for a young girl is the morning-after pill unless the patient presents more than 72 h after unprotected sexual intercourse, or there are specific contraindications to morning-after pill treatment. If the prescription of the morning-after pill is against the GP's religion and belief, he or she has no duty to prescribe the treatment but does have a duty to ensure that the girl has access to the service of another doctor. Sexual intercourse with a girl under the age of 16 is a criminal offence for the male partner, but not for the girl. However, the GP is not justified in breaching confidentiality by informing the police.

11.56 a **False** b **False** c **False** d **True** e **False**
According to the House of Lord judgement in the Gillick case in 1986, the doctor should persuade a girl under the age of 16 to consult her parents and obtain their consent for the medical treatment. However, if she refuses, the doctor may treat if it appears to the doctor that the girl is sufficiently mature and that she understands the general nature of the treatment and the implications for the treatment.

11.57 a **False** b **False** c **True** d **False** e **True**
The morning-after pill treatment consist of two tablets followed by another two tablets exactly 12 h later. The first dose should be taken within 72 h of the unprotected intercourse. If vomiting occurs within 3 h of a dose, an extra dose should be taken. The next period may be earlier or later than expected. However, if she does not have a period within 5 weeks, pregnancy should be excluded. It is important to warn the patient that she would need to use barrier contraceptives until her next period.

11.58 a **True** b **False** c **False** d **False** e **False**
A history of purulent nasal discharge following a common cold, facial pain especially on bending forwards, and toothache in the upper teeth are characteristic of acute sinusitis. The patient should be treated with analgesia, oral antibiotics (e.g. doxycycline or amoxycillin). Ephedrine nasal drop may be considered. Toothache is likely to be due to referred pain from the maxillary antrum, and does not require the attention of a dentist.

11.59 a **True** b **False** c **False** d **True** e **True**
Severely swollen and red left eyelids following an episode of sinusitis are extremely suggestive of left orbital cellulitis due to spread of infection from the sinuses. This is potentially a very serious condition, and may cause meningitis, brain abscess,

cavernous sinus thrombosis, and blindness from occlusion of the central retinal artery. White cell differential count and blood culture should be performed. Visual acuity should be carefully monitored.

11.60 a **False** b **False** c **False** d **True** e **False**
The correct management is urgent referral to the ENT surgeon, intravenous antibiotics, and close monitoring of the visual acuity. The ENT surgeon should liaise closely with the ophthalmologist. If the condition fails to respond to antibiotics, or the visual acuity deteriorates, the infected sinuses and/or the orbit need to be drained surgically.

Index